Ten Years of Images from Circulation

JOURNAL OF THE AMERICAN HEART ASSOCIATION

Ten Years of Images from Circulation

JOURNAL OF THE AMERICAN HEART ASSOCIATION

Hugh A. McAllister, Jr., MD
Clinical Professor of Pathology (retired),
The University of Texas Medical School in Houston
and Baylor College of Medicine
Chief, Department of Pathology (retired),
Texas Heart Institute and St. Luke's Episcopal Hospital

James T. Willerson, MD
President: The University of Texas Health
Science Center in Houston
President-Elect and Medical Director: Texas Heart Institute
Alkek-Williams Distinguished Professor of Medicine:
The University of Texas Medical School in Houston

American Heart Association®
Learn and Live℠

Acquisitions Editor: Frances R. DeStefano
Managing Editor: Nicole Dernoski
Project Manager: Jennifer Harper
Manufacturing Coordinator: Kathleen Brown
Marketing Manager: Angela Panetta
Design Coordinator: Risa Clow
Production Services: International Typesetting and Composition
Printer: Walsworth Publishing Company

Printed in the USA

Library of Congress Cataloging-in-Publication Data

Ten years of images from Circulation / [edited by] Hugh A. McAllister Jr., James T. Willerson.
p. ; cm.
Presents images previously published in Circulation from 1993 to 2005.
ISBN-13: 978-0-7817-6706-4
ISBN-10: 0-7817-6706-7
1. Cardiovascular system—Diseases—Atlases. I. McAllister, Hugh A. II. Willerson, James T., 1939- III. Circulation.
[DNLM: 1. Cardiovascular Diseases—diagnosis—Atlases. 2. Cardiovascular Diseases—diagnosis—Collected Works. 3. Diagnostic Imaging—Atlases. 4. Diagnostic Imaging—Collected Works. WG 17 T289 2007]
RC669.9.T46 2007
616.1'00222—dc22

2006031129

Care has been taken to confirm the accuracy of the information presented and to describe generally accepted practices. However, the authors, editors, and publisher are not responsible for errors or omissions or for any consequences from application of the information in this book and make no warranty, expressed or implied, with respect to the currency, completeness, or accuracy of the contents of the publication. Application of this information in a particular situation remains the professional responsibility of the practitioner. Statements, opinions, and results of studies published in *Circulation* are those of the authors and do not reflect the policy or position of the American Heart Association, and the American Heart Association provides no warranty as to their accuracy or reliability.

The authors, editors, and publisher have exerted every effort to ensure that drug selection and dosages set forth in this text are in accordance with current recommendations and practice at the time of publication. However, in view of ongoing research, changes in government regulations, and the constant flow of information relating to drug therapy and drug reactions, the reader is urged to check the package insert for each drug for any change in indications and dosages and for added warnings and precautions. This is particularly important when the recommended agent is a new or infrequently employed drug.

Some drugs and medical devices presented in this publication have Food and Drug Administration (FDA) clearance for limited use in restricted research settings. It is the responsibility of the healthcare provider to ascertain the FDA status of each drug or device planned for use in their clinical practice.

To purchase additional copies of this book, call our customer service department at **(800) 638-3030** or fax orders to **(301) 223-2320.** International customers should call **(301) 223-2300.**

Visit Lippincott Williams & Wilkins on the Internet at LWW.com. Lippincott Williams & Wilkins customer service representatives are available from 8:30 AM to 6 PM, EST.

10 9 8 7 6 5 4 3 2 1

Preface

In this book we present interesting and relatively unusual images of the cardiovascular system that should be of interest to all who care for patients with cardiovascular disease. These images were published in *Circulation* from 1993 to 2005, and after 1998, many were published in the electronic version of the journal. We believe that it is useful, however, to have them in one book where they might be available for review by students and practitioners of cardiovascular medicine toward the goal of always improving patient care.

HUGH A. MCALLISTER, JR., MD
JAMES T. WILLERSON, MD

Contents

Section II
Coronary Arteries

Chapters

Section III
Intracardiac Masses

Chapters

Section IV
Endocardium and Valves

Chapters

Section V
Pericardium and Myocardium

Chapters

Section VI
Congenital Heart Disease

Chapters

Ten Years of Images from

Circulation

JOURNAL OF THE AMERICAN HEART ASSOCIATION

Section I

Pulmonary Arteries, Aorta, Peripheral Vessels

1

Multilocualted Myxoid Cyst of the Popliteal Artery

Norman M. Rich, MD; Hugh A. McAllister, Jr, MD

From the Department of Surgery, Uniformed Services University of the Health Sciences, Bethesda, Md, and the Department of Pathology, St Luke's Episcopal Hospital, Houston, Tex.

(*Circulation*. 1993;88:1334–1335.)

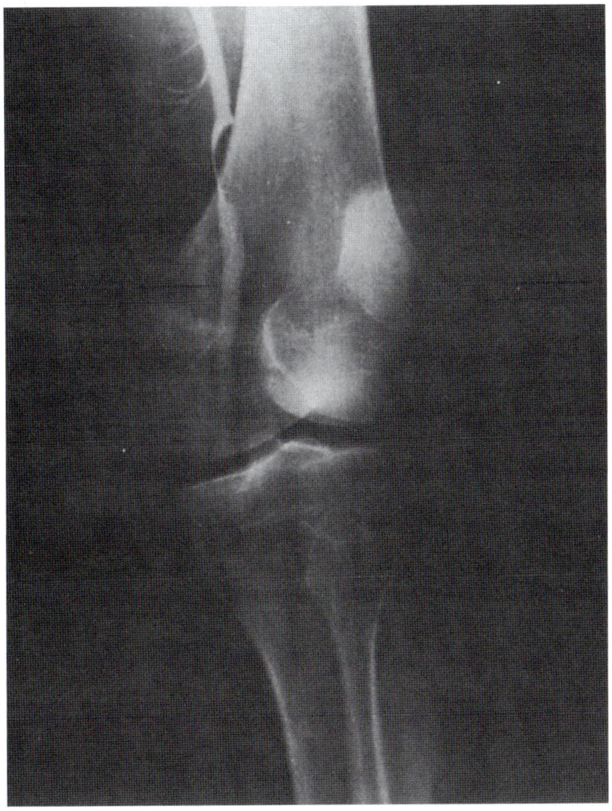

Figure 1. Popliteal arteriogram from a 22-year-old man with claudication. Note the smooth curvature of the defect. Although these cysts have been described in the external iliac, ulnar, and radial arteries, they are much more common in the popliteal artery.

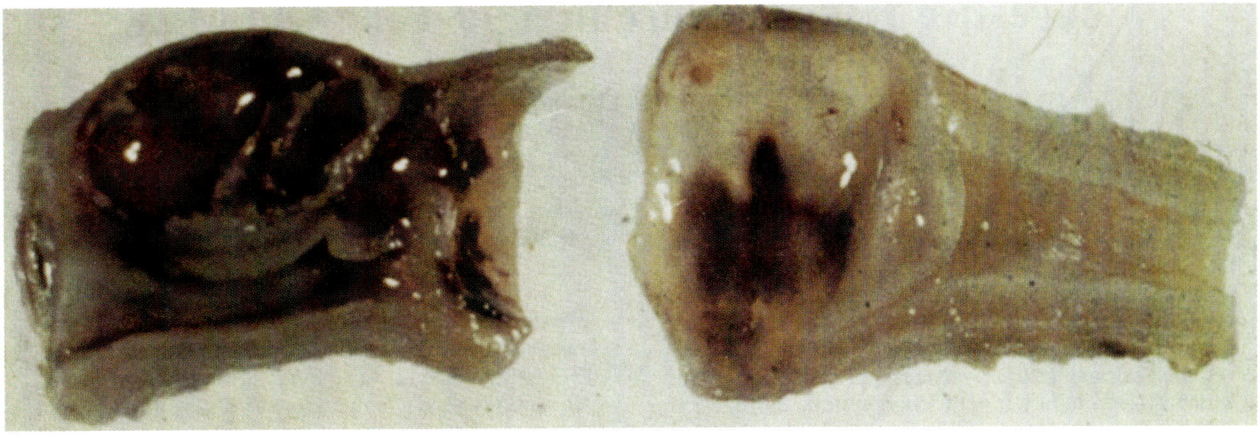

Figure 2. Resected popliteal artery containing a multiloculated cyst between the media and adventitia (left). Progressive enlargement of the multiloculated cyst encroaches upon the arterial lumen, eventually producing thrombosis. The length of the involved arterial segment varies from 2 to 8 cm.

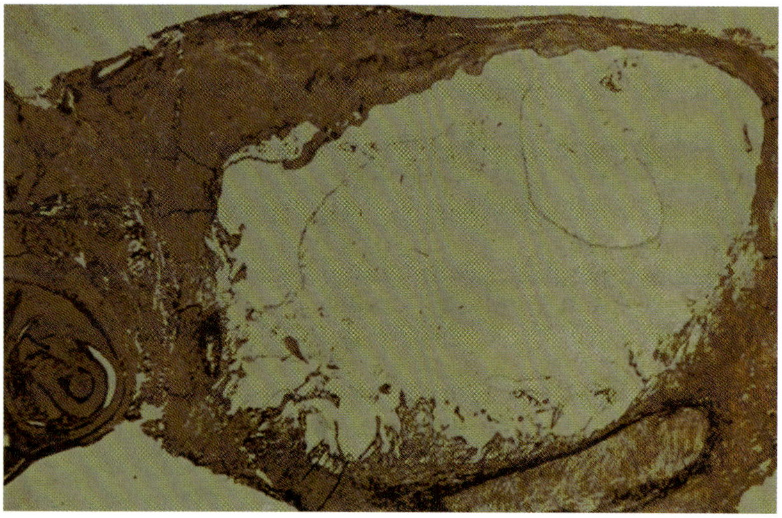

Figure 3. Photomicrograph of a section of the popliteal artery cyst illustrated in Figures 1 and 2. These cysts contain acid mucopolysaccharide and are identical in microscopic appearance to the myxoid cysts of tendon sheaths (*ganglion*).

2 Membranous Obstruction of the Inferior Vena Cava Treated by Percutaneous Balloon Angioplasty

Tsung O. Cheng, MD; Xue-liang Yang, MD; Chuan-rong Chen, MD

From The George Washington University, Washington, DC (T.O.C.), 150th PLA Hospital, Luoyang, China (X.Y.), and Guangdong Cardiovascular Institute, Guangzhou, China (T.O.C., C.C.).

(*Circulation*. 1994;89:896–897.)

A 30-year-old Chinese man (case 5), who underwent surgical sympathectomy 12 years earlier for Budd-Chiari syndrome, developed recurrence of progressive ascites, dyspnea, leg edema, and esophageal varices over the past 5 years. Angiography revealed incomplete membranous obstruction of the inferior vena cava just below the right atrium (Fig. lA). The obstruction was successfully relieved by percutaneous transluminal angioplasty (Fig. lB). The patient remained asymptomatic for a follow-up period of 3.5 years.

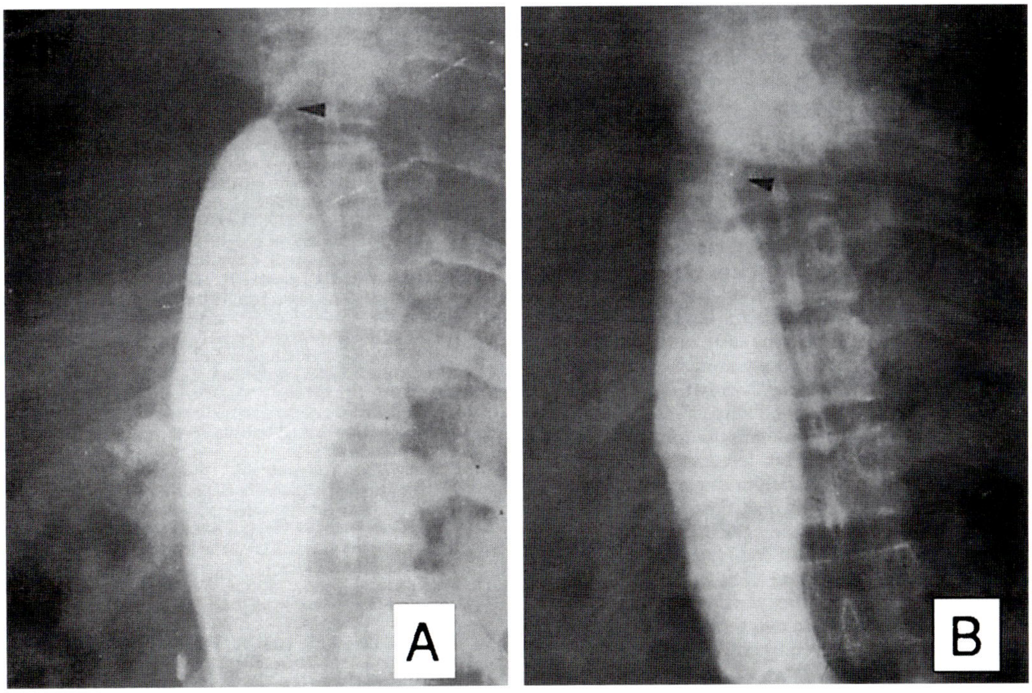

Figure 1. Inferior vena cavogram (case 5) shows a membranous obstruction of the inferior vena cava (MOVC) 1 cm below the right atrium (arrowhead in **A**) with caval dilatation below the obstruction and ample collaterals. After percutaneous transluminal angioplasty (PTA), the caval diameter at the site of MOVC increases from 2 to 20 mm (arrowhead in **B**); the caval diameter below the MOVC decreases from 48 to 40 mm; the collaterals have completely disappeared; and the right atrium, which is barely visualized before PTA, is now well opacified.

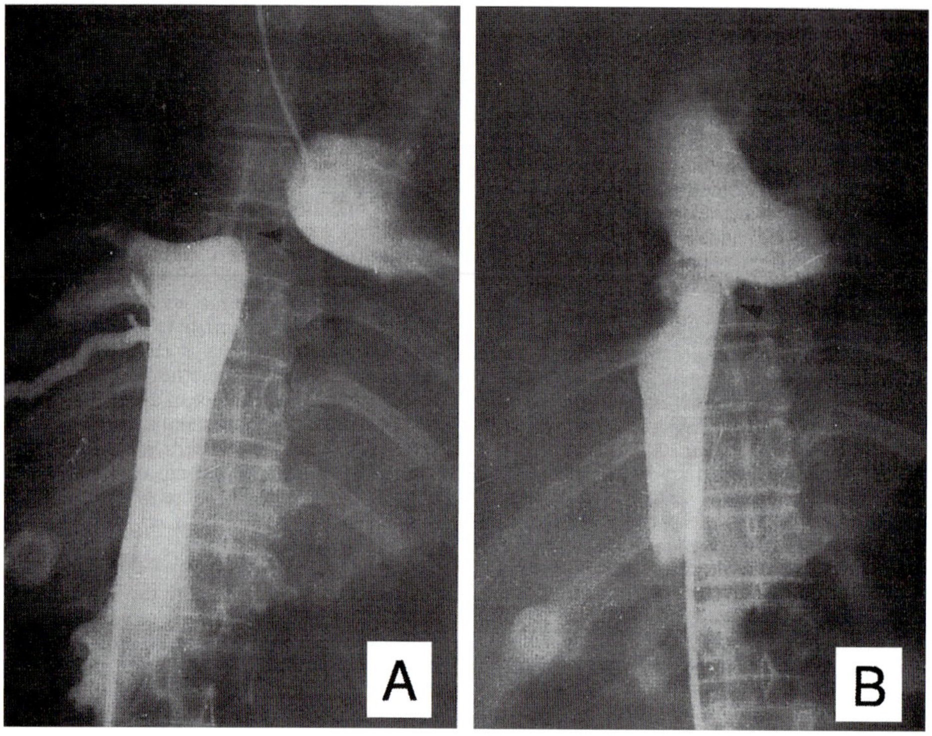

Figure 2. Inferior vena cavogram in case 9 shows complete membranous obstruction of the inferior vena cava (MOVC) just below the level of the diaphragm (arrowhead in **A**) with profuse collaterals below the MOVC; the right heart is opacified by simultaneous right atrial angiography through a National Institutes of Health catheter introduced through the superior vena cava. After successful PTA **(B),** the caval diameter below the MOVC decreases from 29 to 21 mm; the collaterals have disappeared; and the right heart can now be visualized readily after contrast injection into the inferior vena cava.

A 32-year-old Chinese woman (case 9), with almost identical symptoms as the previous patient, was shown on angiography to have complete membranous obstruction of the inferior vena cava just below the level of the diaphragm (Fig. 2A). The obstruction was successfully relieved by percutaneous transluminal angioplasty (Fig. 2B). The patient remained asymptomatic for a follow-up period of 2.5 years.

These two patients were among the 30 patients with membranous obstruction of the inferior vena cava whom we have successfully treated by percutaneous transluminal angioplasty with the Inoue balloon catheter. With the exception of one patient (case 8), who died from massive pulmonary embolism occurring immediately after percutaneous transluminal angioplasty, there were no complications. Long-term results with a follow-up period of as long as 5 years have been very satisfactory.

3

Erosion of Lumbar Vertebral Bodies due to Abdominal Aortic Aneurysm

Kyuhyun Wang, MD; Morrison Hodges, MD

From the Division of Cardiology, Hennepin County Medical Center, University of Minnesota, Minneapolis, Minn.

(*Circulation*. 1994;89:1317.)

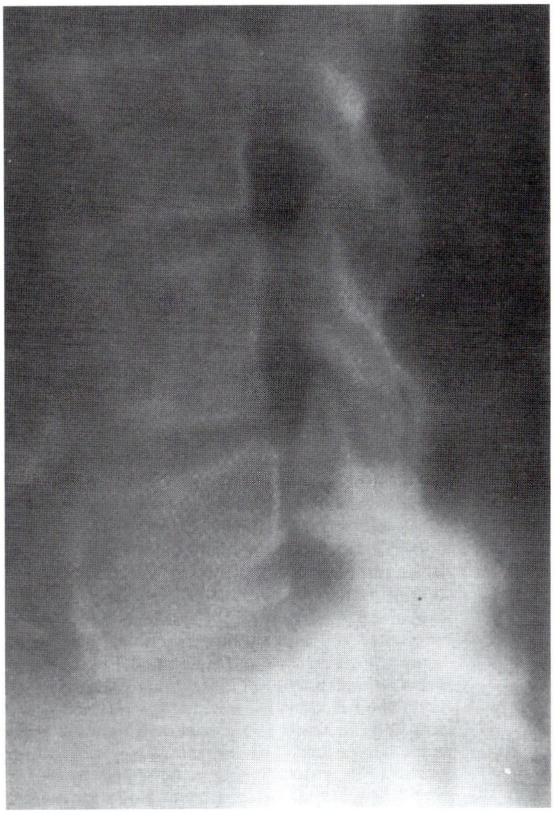

Figure 1. Radiograph shows erosion of lumbar vertebral bodies simulating osteolytic lesions such as from malignancy. It involves three consecutive lumbar vertebral bodies and has a curvature corresponding to the abdominal aortic aneurysm that this patient proved to have. This is a result of the aneurysm's pounding on the vertebral bodies 70 to 80 times per minute for many years, just like the rib notchings secondary to tortuous intercostal arteries in patients with coarctation of the aorta. Back pain in a patient with a proven abdominal aortic aneurysm should raise suspicions of either an expanding or leaking aneurysm, but on rare occasions it may be due to erosion of the spine, as in this case.

4

Metallic Mercury Embolism

Herbert L. Fred, MD; David Marcus, MD

From the Department of Internal Medicine, the University of Texas Health Science Center at Houston, and the Department of Radiology, Baptist Hospital, Pensacola, Fla.

(*Circulation*. 1995;91:3020–3021.)

Venous embolization of metallic mercury is rare. It results from the accidental or deliberate injection of mercury into a peripheral vein. In most cases, the clinical manifestations, if any, are mild and of short duration; supportive care suffices; and prognosis is good.

Findings on chest radiograph are striking and should immediately suggest the diagnosis. One or both lungs invariably contain multiple, tiny, dense spherules diffusely distributed or confined primarily to dependent areas. These spherules sometimes appear as beaded chains filling pulmonary arterioles, giving an *angiogram effect*. Occasionally, mercury can be seen in the heart, especially in the right ventricle where it tends to pool.

Because mercury can pass through the pulmonary capillary bed or around it via shunts, mercury emboli may be visible in radiographs of the head, neck, abdomen, or pelvis. The presence of metallic densities in these sites or in the heart, coupled with the aforementioned pulmonary abnormalities, differentiates mercury embolism from all other diagnostic considerations, particularly aspiration of mercury. We present here three cases that illustrate different degrees of metallic mercury embolism.

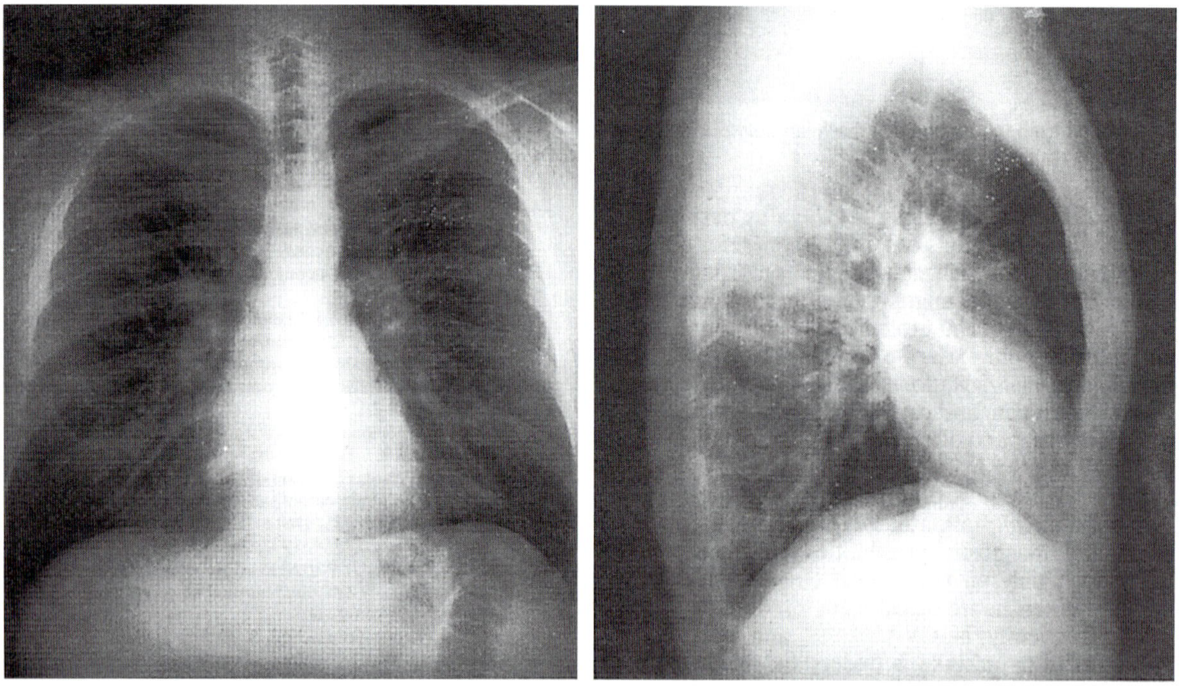

Figure 1. Case 1: Chest radiographs showing multiple metallic densities in both lungs, especially the left. Nine months earlier, this patient had attempted suicide by injecting himself with mercury intravenously.

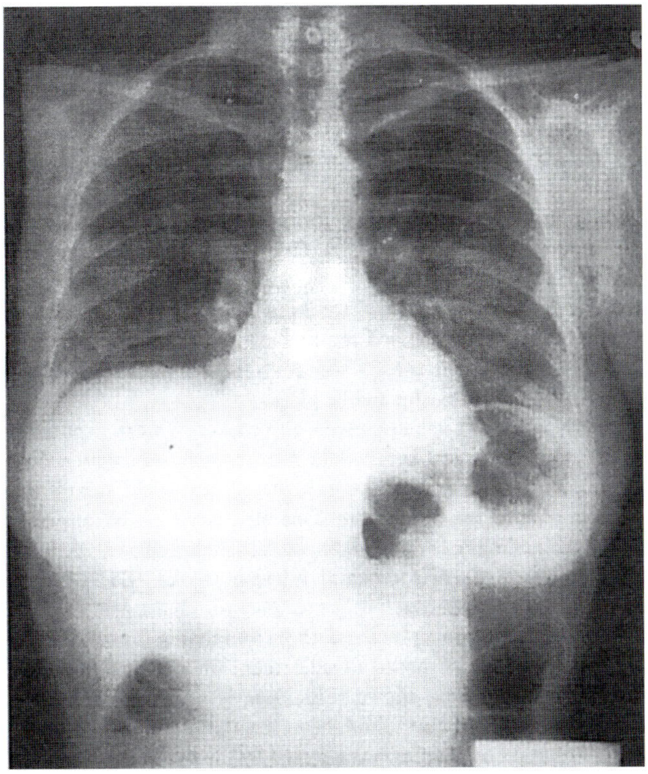

Figure 2. Case 2: Chest radiograph showing tiny metallic densities in the lungs. Similar densities were evident in the liver, pelvis, and brain. Mercury had accidentally entered this patient's vein during blood sampling with a mercury-sealed syringe.

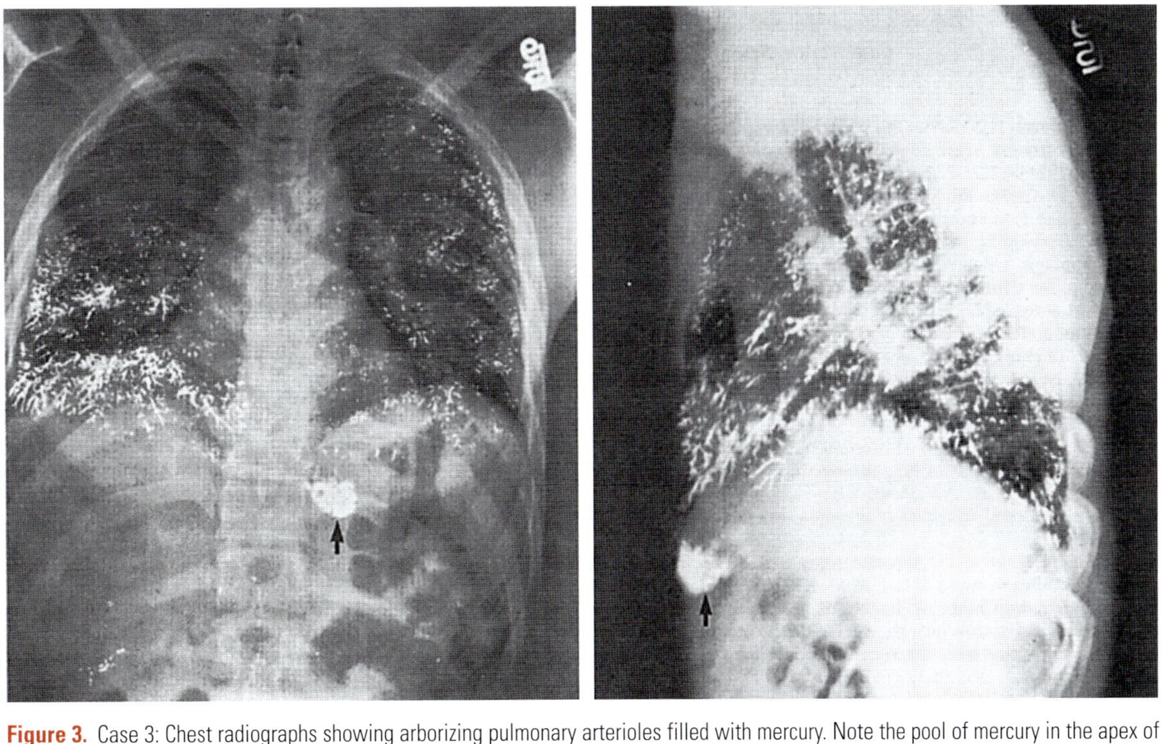

Figure 3. Case 3: Chest radiographs showing arborizing pulmonary arterioles filled with mercury. Note the pool of mercury in the apex of the right ventricle (arrows) and the metallic densities in the upper abdomen and paravertebral plexus. This patient, a schizophrenic, had injected mercury into the forearm.

5

Intra-Aortic Thrombus Producing Embolic Arterial Vascular Disease

P. Lozano, MD; E. Al Mousa, MD; C.F. Wei, MD; F.T. Thandroyen, MD

From The University of Texas Medical School at Houston and Lyndon B. Johnson Hospital, Division of Cardiology, Houston, Tex.

(*Circulation*. 1996;93:1471.)

A 45-year-old man presented with acute onset of claudication of the lower limbs and abdominal pain. Echocardiography of the heart was normal. Intra-aortic thrombi were considered to be the source of emboli producing arterial vascular occlusion, splenic infarction, and renal infarction.

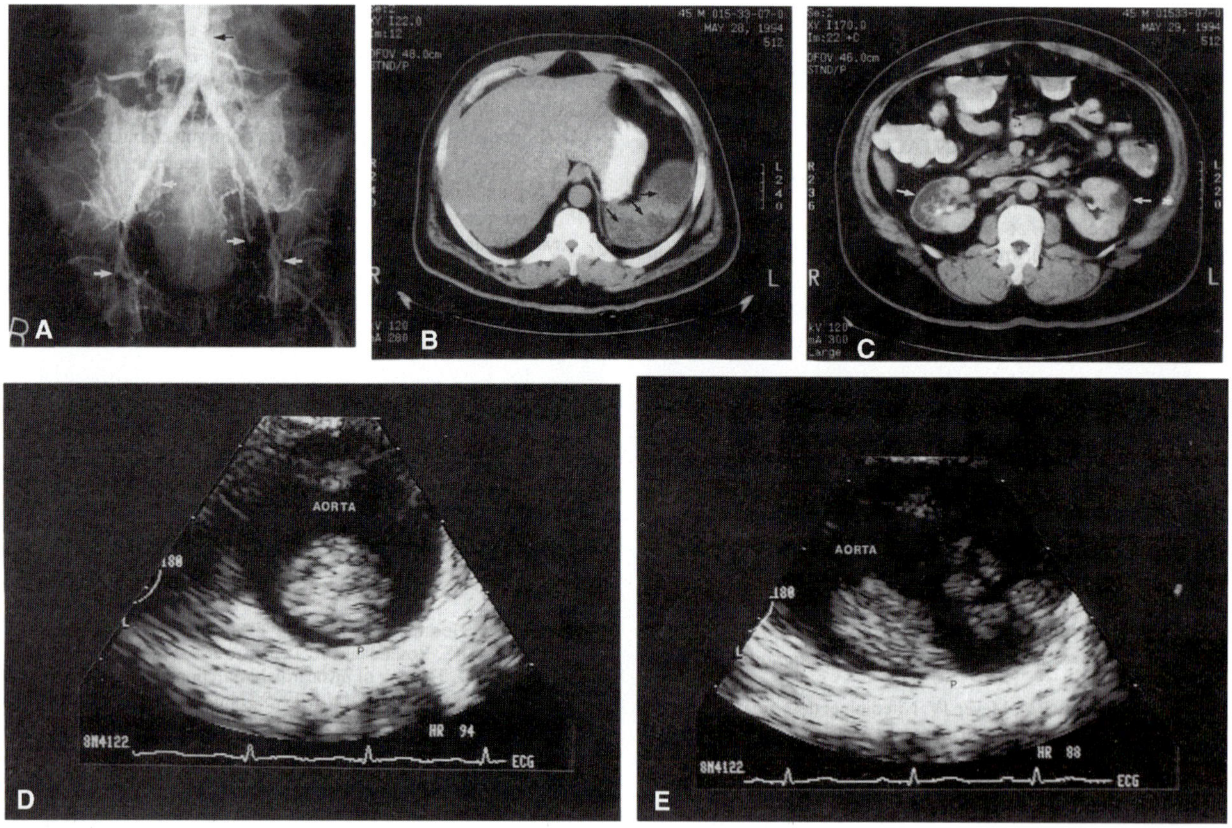

Figure 1. A, Abdominal aortogram showing occlusion (white arrows) of external and internal iliac arteries with extensive collateral circulation. In addition, a filling defect (black arrow) is visualized proximal to the bifurcation of the abdominal aorta. The filling defect most likely represents an intra-aortic thrombus. **B** and **C,** Contrast-enhanced abdominal computerized tomographic scans show multiple large hypodense areas in the spleen (B) in keeping with multiple splenic infarcts. In addition, there are multiple hypodense areas in the kidneys (C) in keeping with multiple renal infarcts. D and E, Transesophageal two-dimensional echocardiographic images of the descending thoracic aorta are shown in two planes. **D,** Short-axis image at 0° illustrates a large intra-aortic mass (≈12 mm) attached to a plaque (P) on the wall. **E,** Long-axis plane at 111°C illustrates the above-mentioned intra-aortic mass arising from the plaque (P) on the wall. In addition, a second multilobulated mass arising from the wall of the aorta is seen. The intra-aortic masses are in keeping with intra-aortic thrombi.

6

Percutaneous Balloon Angioplasty with Adjunctive Stent Placement in the Mesenteric Vessels in a Patient with Takayasu Arteritis

Erol Ozdil, MD; Zvonimir Krajcer, MD; Paolo Angelini, MD

From the Department of Adult Cardiology, Texas Heart Institute at St Luke's Episcopal Hospital, Houston, Tex.

(*Circulation*. 1996;93:1940–1941.)

A 49-year-old woman from Italy with a history of Takayasu arteritis presented with worsening hypertension and symptoms consistent with mesenteric ischemia. The patient had previously undergone aortobifemoral bypass for Leriche syndrome and peripheral angioplasty of the right subclavian artery. At the present hospital admission, peripheral angiography revealed multiple arterial stenoses: 90% stenosis in the left renal artery, 80% in the right renal artery, 90% in the celiac trunk (Fig. lA), and 99% in the superior mesenteric artery (Fig. 2A and 2B). Pressure gradients were 130 mm Hg across the celiac ostium, 145 mm Hg across the superior mesenteric ostium, 135 mm Hg across the right renal artery, and 45 mm Hg across the left renal artery. The patient underwent percutaneous balloon angioplasty, with excellent results in the renal arteries. The mesenteric vessels, however, did not respond adequately to angioplasty because of persistent elastic recoil, despite prolonged inflation of the balloon.

Therefore, an 8 × 40 mm balloon was used to place a Palmaz P204 (Johnson & Johnson) intraluminal stent in the ostium of the superior mesenteric artery (Fig. 2C and 2D). Similarly, an 8 × 30 mm balloon was used to place a Palmaz P154 stent in the ostium of the celiac trunk (Fig. 1B). No residual stenosis or pressure gradient was noted after stent placement. The patient tolerated the procedure well

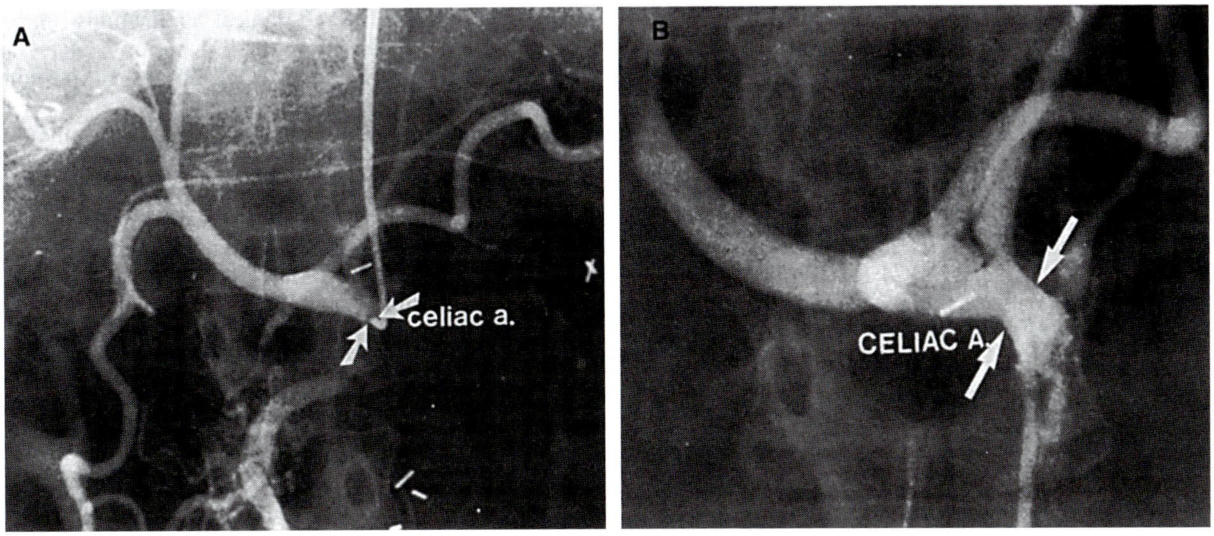

Figure 1. Selective injection in the anteroposterior view **(A)** demonstrating a critical lesion in the ostium of the celiac artery. Anteroposterior view **(B)** demonstrates successful percutaneous transluminal angioplasty and adjunctive placement of a Palmaz stent in the ostium of the celiac artery.

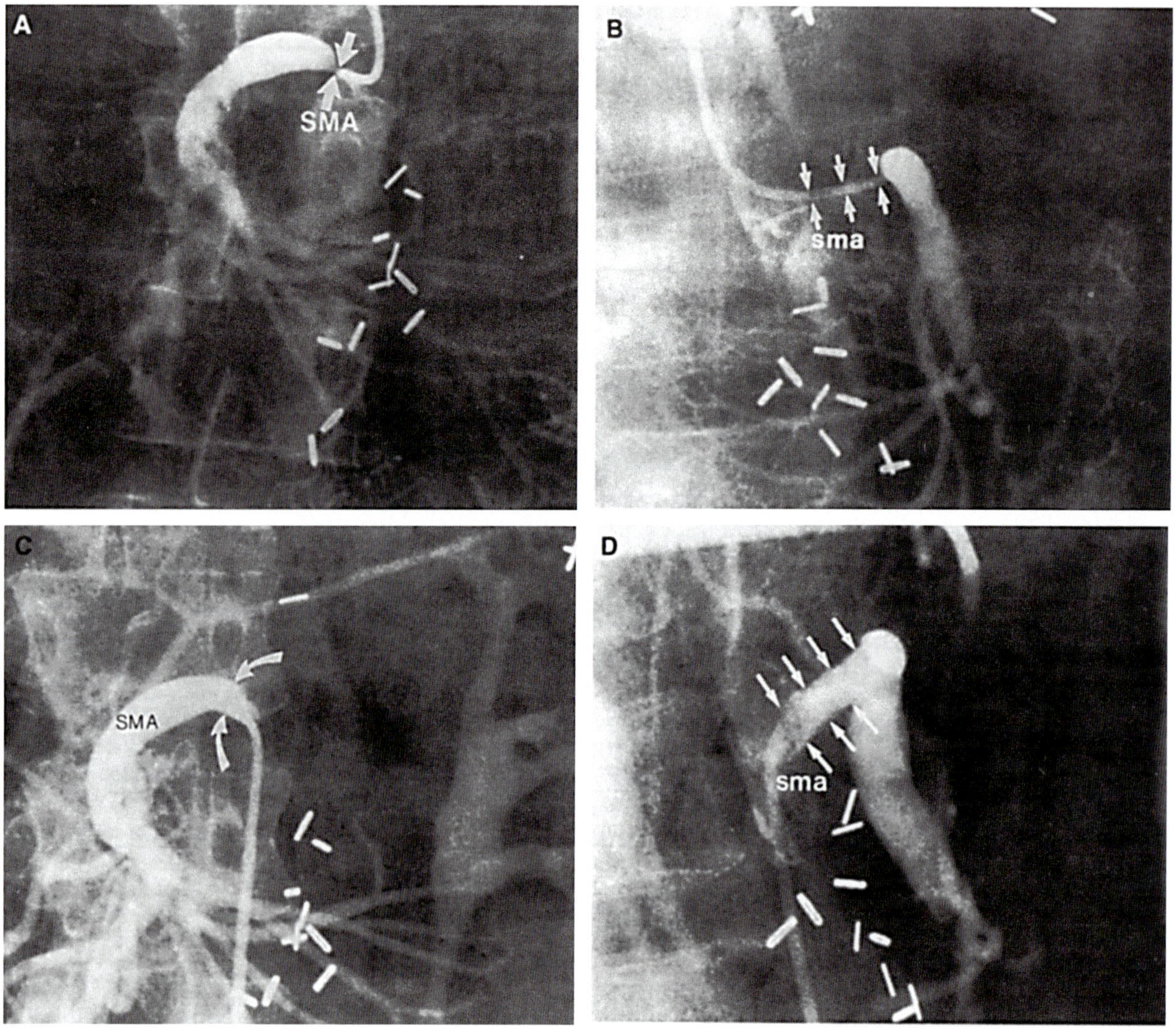

Figure 2. Selective injection in the anteroposterior view **(A)** and lateral view **(B)** demonstrating a critical lesion in the ostium of the superior mesenteric artery (sma). Anteroposterior view **(C)** and lateral view **(D)** demonstrate successful percutaneous transluminal angioplasty and adjunctive placement of a Palmaz stent in the ostium of the superior mesenteric artery; no residual lesion is visible.

and was discharged. At 8-month follow-up, the patient reported no abdominal pain and had no hypertension on medical therapy. Dense fibrotic lesions are often present during the late occlusive phase of Takayasu arteritis. High inflation pressures may be required to dilate these lesions, which are associated with significant elastic recoil, especially in the ostial locations. Stents may be beneficial in treating lesions in which persistent elastic recoil prevents adequate results with balloon angioplasty.

7

Mycotic Aneurysm of the Descending Thoracic Aorta

Donald Oxorn, MD, CM, FRCPC; Stuart Bell, MB, BS, FRCPC
From the Sunnybrook Health Science Centre, University of Toronto, Ontario, Canada.

(*Circulation*. 1997;95:1972–1973.)

A 58-year-old man presented to hospital with atypical chest pain, chills, and fever. Although blood cultures grew *Staphylococcus aureus,* no primary source of infection was evident. Transesophageal echocardiography revealed false aneurysm formation in the lower thoracic aorta 38 cm from the incisors (Fig. 1A). The false aneurysm contained spontaneous echo contrast indicative of low flow. Extravasated blood surrounded the aorta. Angiography (Fig. 1B, arrow), contrast-enhanced computed tomography (CT) (Fig. 1C, arrow), and three-dimensional reconstructed CT (Fig. 1D, arrow) confirmed the presence of an aneurysm arising from the posteromedial aspect of the aorta at the level of the 10th thoracic vertebra. The patient was treated with intravenous cloxacillin and taken to the operating room, where a leaking mycotic aneurysm was resected and a synthetic graft interposed. Intraoperative cultures of the aneurysm grew *Staphylococcus aureus*. The patient made an uneventful recovery and was left with no long-term sequelae.

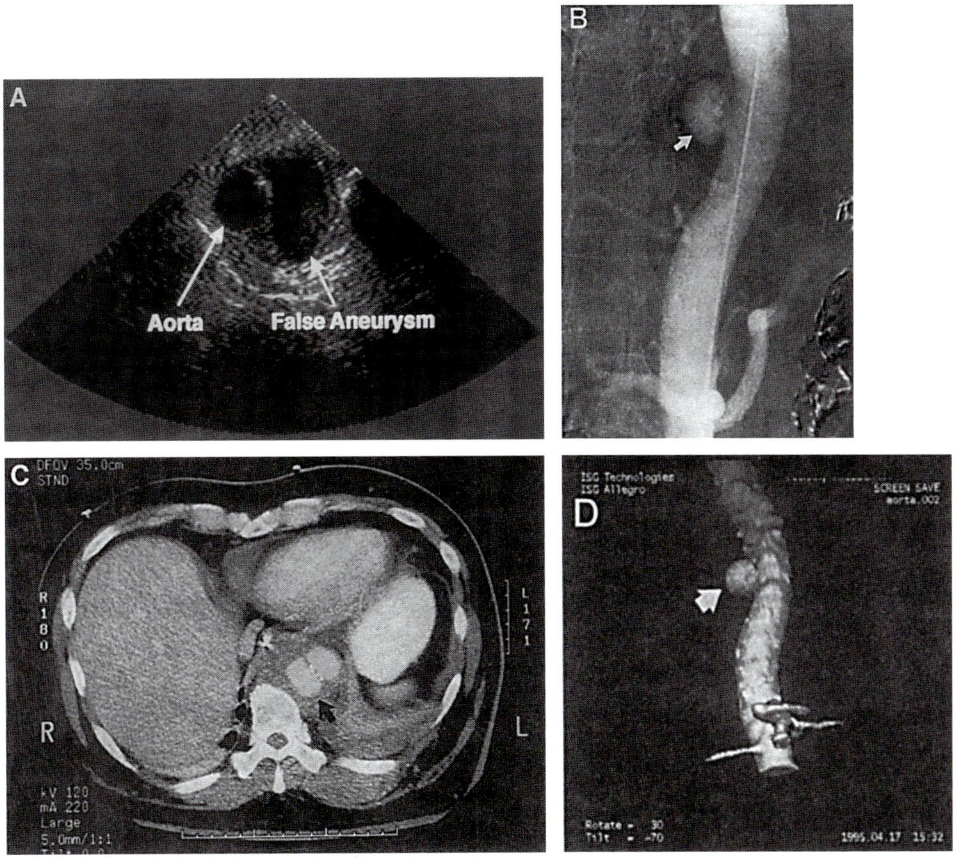

Figure 1.

8 Cholesterol Embolization: Unrecognized Complication of Thrombolysis

G. Pettelot, MD; J. Bracco, MD; D. Barrillon, MD; M. Baudouy, MD; P. Morand, MD
From the Departments of Cardiology and Nephrology, Hôpital Pasteur, Nice, France.

(*Circulation*. 1998;97:1522.)

A 62-year-old man was admitted to the hospital because of myocardial infarction. Treatment with 100 mg of recombinant tissue plasminogen activator was given intravenously for 90 minutes. On the second day, he presented with abdominal and lower limb pain. Physical examination showed a toe and leg livedo reticularis (Fig. 1). The biological evolution showed a progressive increase of creatinine, from 127 to 350 μmol/L until day 20.

A skin biopsy performed on the livedo confirmed the diagnosis of cholesterol embolization exhibiting cholesterol crystals in the intima of small arteries and in the lumen of the capillaries (Fig. 2). The patient did not have any arterial catheterization. Fibrinolysis, by destroying the platelet-fibrin thrombus of the atheromatous ulcerated plaques, allowed the liberation of the cholesterol crystals in the arterial circulation.

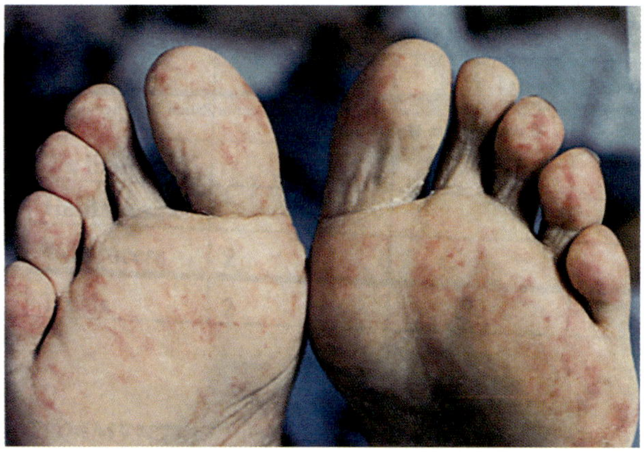

Figure 1. Toe livedo reticularis.

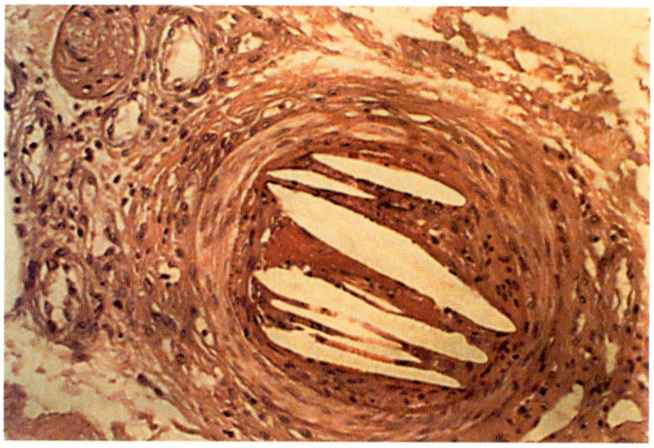

Figure 2. Biconvex, needle-shaped clefts surrounded by fibrin deposition in lumen of an arteriole. Clefts represent site where cholesterol crystals were lodged before they were dissolved for preparation of biopsy.

9

Successful Transcatheter Retrieval of an Air Gun Pellet and Adherent Thrombus from a Pulmonary Artery Branch

Joselyn C.R. Lee, MD; Raymond H. Dominici, MD; Fred A. Crawford, Jr, MD; Wolfgang A.K. Radtke, MD

From the South Carolina Children's Heart Center, Medical University of South Carolina, Charleston, and Clarendon Memorial Hospital (R.H.D.), Manning, SC.

(*Circulation*. 1998;97:1755–1756.)

With his toy gun, a 9-year-old boy inflicted a high-velocity pellet gun shot to his own right thigh, with entry in the upper anterolateral aspect. The initial radiograph in the local emergency room showed the gun pellet in his left posterior pelvic region. He was asymptomatic except for pain in the right groin and thigh. The patient was placed on intravenous fluids and antibiotics and was admitted for observation. A repeat radiograph of his pelvis after 17 hours did not show the pellet. A subsequent chest radiograph located the pellet in the right lower medial lung field. The pellet had presumably migrated through the bloodstream into a right lower-lobe branch of the pulmonary artery. His examination remained normal except for pain when he moved his right thigh. The patient was referred for further treatment and was taken to the pediatric cardiac catheterization laboratory the same day, where he underwent successful transcatheter retrieval of the pellet with a 5F Teflon four-wire basket through a check-flow III blue Mullins 8F sheath via a 12F sidearm sheath in the left femoral vein.

A right pulmonary arteriogram (Fig. 1A) by hand injection through the Mullins sheath showed the 4.5-mm-diameter pellet lodged in a right lower lobe pulmonary artery branch, resulting in decreased flow distal to the pellet. A small radiolucent thrombus was seen adjacent to the pellet. The wire basket was manipulated into the same branch and alongside the pellet (Fig. 1B). The basket was rotated around the pellet, and Figure 1C shows the pellet in the wire basket at the distal tip of the catheter and sheath being removed from the patient. Figure 2 shows the gun pellet with adherent thrombus after removal from the patient inside the wire basket (Fig. 2A) and released from the basket (Fig. 2B).

There were no complications. Fluoroscopy time was 20:05 minutes. The patient was observed for 1.5 days after the procedure to rule out perforation of pelvic or abdominal organs and then was discharged home in good condition.

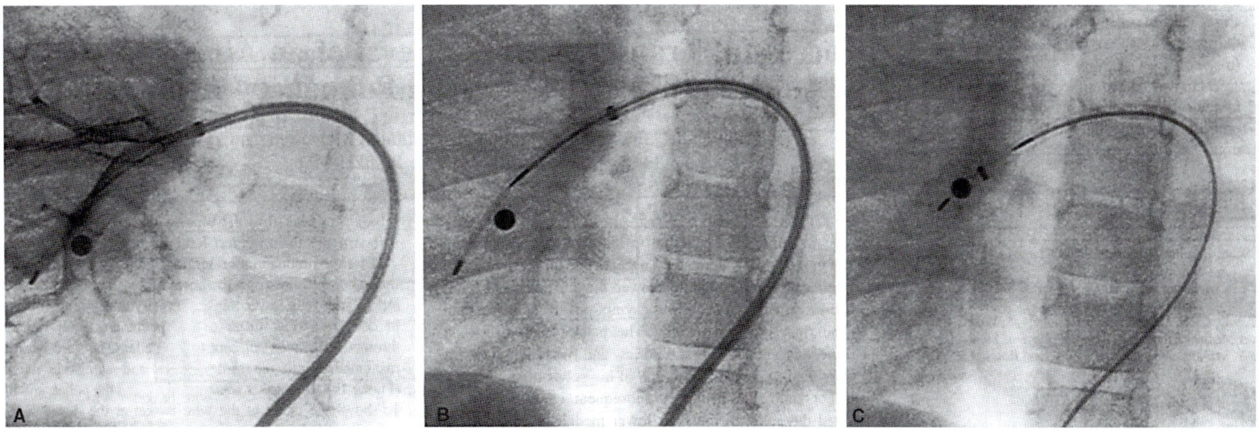

Figure 1.

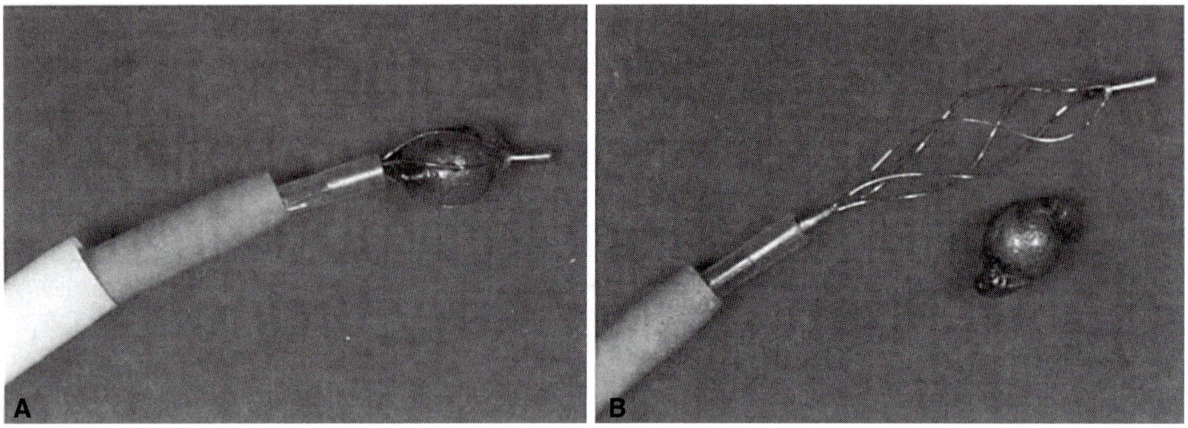

Figure 2.

10

Unusual Manifestation of Subaortic Membrane

Wen-Shiann Wu, MD; Jeng-Kai Teng, MD, PhD; Liang-Miin Tsai, MD; Wei-Chuan Tsai, MD; Lin-Jen Lin, MD; Yi-Heng Li, MD; Jyh-Hong Chen, MD, PhD; Yu-Jen Yang, MD

From the Division of Cardiology, Cardiac Surgery (Y.-J.Y.), National Cheng Kung University Medical College and Hospital, and Chi-Mei Foundation Hospital (W.-S.W.), Tainan, Taiwan.

(*Circulation.* 1998;97:605–606.)

A 52-year-old man complained of dyspnea on exertion for 1 month. On auscultation, a grade 3/6 to-and-fro murmur was heard at the left lower sternal border and was well-transmitted to the apex. Figure 1 is the transesophageal echocardiographic image of this patient at that time. Figures 2 and 3 were produced by cardiac catheterization. There was no significant pressure gradient among aorta, subaortic chamber, and left ventricle.

The patient underwent open-heart surgery several days later. Surgery revealed a 1 × 2 cm defect at the right coronary sinus of Valsalva and a huge subaortic membrane (10 × 20 cm) adhering to the right coronary cusp and interventricular septum (Fig. 4). There was an orifice in the subaortic membrane for communicating with the left ventricle.

The aortic valve was replaced, and the subaortic membrane was successfully excised. The postoperative course was smooth, and the patient was discharged.

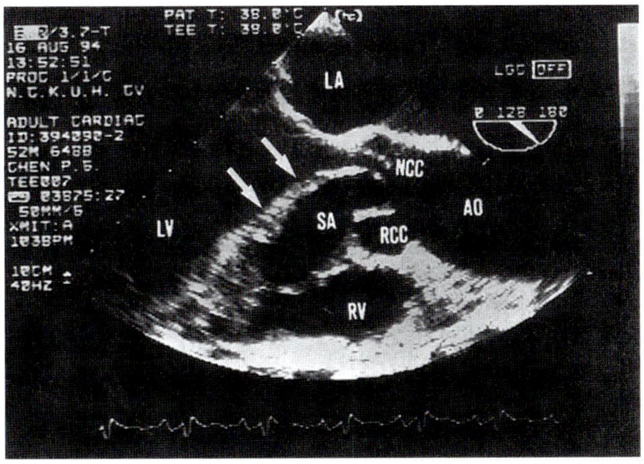

Figure 1. Transesophageal echocardiography demonstrated a calcified aortic valve and a serpentine, elongated subaortic membrane adhering to right coronary cusp and interventricular septum. AO indicates aorta; LA, left atrium; LV, left ventricle; NCC, noncoronary cusp; RCC, right coronary cusp; Arrows, subaortic membrane; SA, subaortic chamber; and RV, right ventricle.

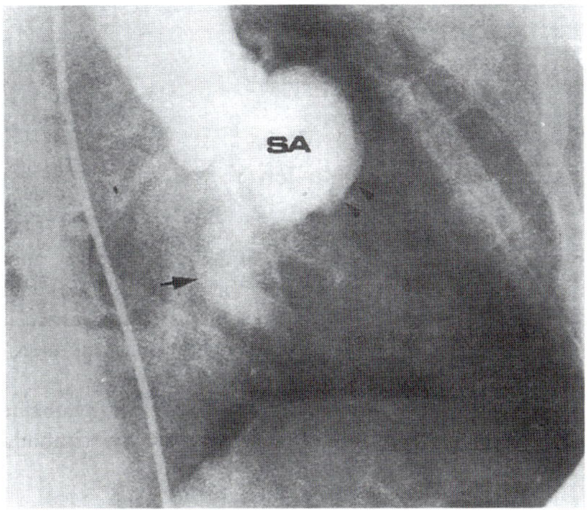

Figure 2. Aortogram with right anterior oblique projection showed an eccentric regurgitant jet (arrow) from the aorta toward left ventricle, and an abnormal subaortic chamber (SA) was also simultaneously visualized. Two arrowheads outline subaortic membrane.

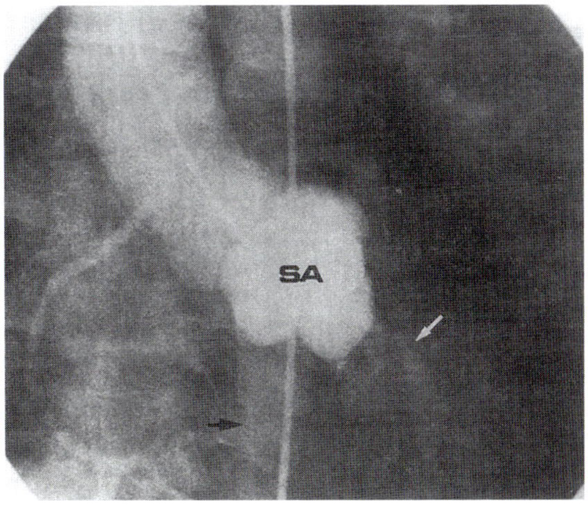

Figure 3. Atypical subaortic membrane with chamber (SA) was demonstrated in left anterior oblique projection with cranial beam angulation. Side hole of catheter was placed at subaortic chamber, and contrast medium was injected. Jet (white arrow) formed by regurgitation of contrast medium through narrow orifice in membrane into left ventricle was found. Another jet (black arrow) was aortic regurgitation.

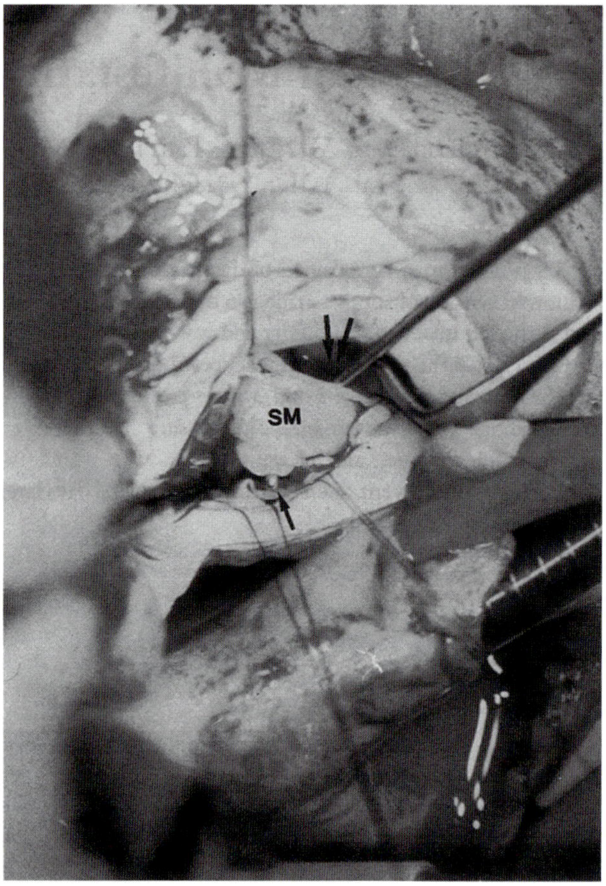

Figure 4. At surgery, tricuspid valve was displaced and subaortic membrane (SM) was exposed. Probe was placed from defect of right coronary sinus of Valsalva (double arrow) to another defect in subaortic membrane (single arrow).

11

Ultrasonographic Images of Takayasu Arteritis

Yoshihisa Matsumura, MD; Keisuke Morimoto, MD; Mitsuko Ishikawa, MT; Hiroaki Kitaoka, MD; Yoshinori L. Doi, MD, PhD

From the Department of Medicine and Geriatrics and the Clinical Laboratory Department (M.I.), Kochi Medical School, Japan.

(*Circulation*. 1998;98:1585–1586.)

A 41-year-old woman was first admitted in August 1992 because of a persistent fever of 102.2°F and chest pain. Her sedimentation rate was 91 mm in the first hour, and C-reactive protein was 9.0 mg/dL. Angiography at that time showed occlusion of the left upper pulmonary artery (Fig. 1A) and normal bilateral common carotid and vertebral arteries (Fig. 1B). A diagnosis of Takayasu arteritis in the acute stage was made. Her condition improved rapidly after the initiation of prednisolone 30 mg/d.

In March 1996, the patient developed bilateral neck tenderness associated with elevated γ-globulin and leukocytosis. Diffuse circumferential thickening of the intima-media complex was found in bilateral proximal common carotid arteries by B-mode ultrasonographic study, resulting in long segmental narrowing of the lumen (2.6 mm in luminal diameter) (Figs. 1C and 1D) that was also shown by angiography (Fig. 1E). She was once again put on prednisolone 30 mg/d, and her bilateral neck tenderness gradually resolved. Reduction in thickness of the intima-media complex was noted after steroid therapy for 2 months (3.2 mm in luminal diameter) (Fig. 1F).

This ultrasonographic demonstration of the inflammatory process of the intima-media complex is consistent with the pathological observation of inflammatory changes seen mainly in the media associated with secondary intimal thickening and may be useful in the diagnosis of Takayasu arteritis.

(Figures follow on next page.)

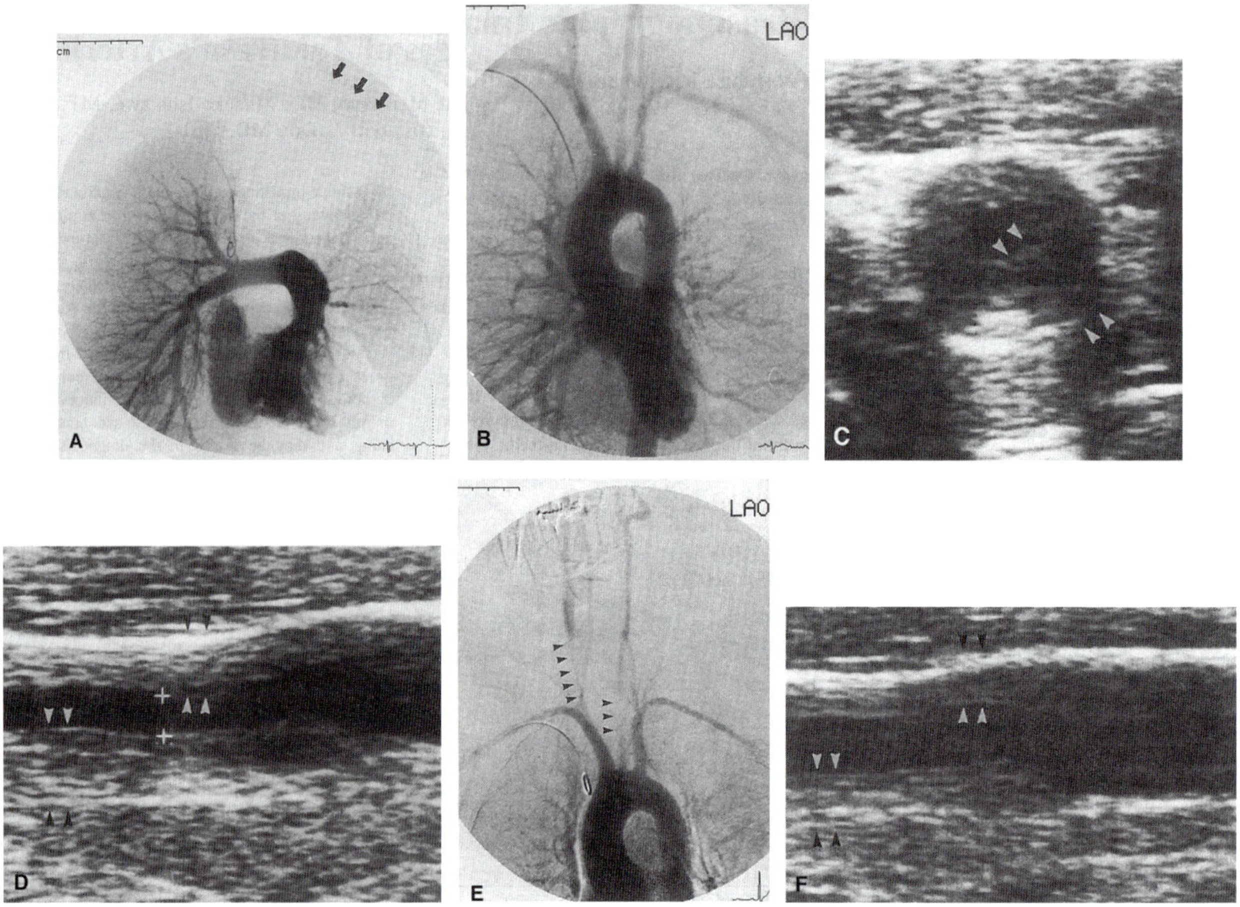

Figure 1.

12 Inflammatory Abdominal Aortic Aneurysm

Yuzuru Sakakibara, MD; Mikia Doy, MD

From the Department of Surgery, Institute of Clinical Medicine, University of Tsukuba (Y.S.), and the Department of Pathology, Tsukuba Medical Center Hospital (M.D.), Tsukuba Science City, Ibaraki, Japan.

(*Circulation*. 1998;98:1823.)

A 73-year-old woman who had been losing weight progressively (–6 kg) over a period of 6 months came to our hospital after experiencing growing abdominal pain for 2 weeks. A computed tomography (CT) of the abdomen revealed a 6-cm infrarenal abdominal aortic aneurysm surrounded by a contrast-enhancing mantel (Fig. 1). Her C-reactive protein value was 4.3 mg/dL. Other laboratory tests revealed no specific findings. The aneurysm was treated with a prosthetic Y-graft through a transperitoneal approach. The characteristic white glistening perianeurysmal fibrosis and severe thickening were noted on the aortic and iliac arterial walls during operation (Fig. 2). Her postoperative course was uneventful. Histopathological examination of the iliac arterial wall was performed, and the dominant finding was an inflammatory reaction with an infiltration of lymphocytes and plasma cells in thickened, collagen-rich tissue (Fig. 3). Plasmacytosis may play a causal role in so-called inflammatory abdominal aortic aneurysm.

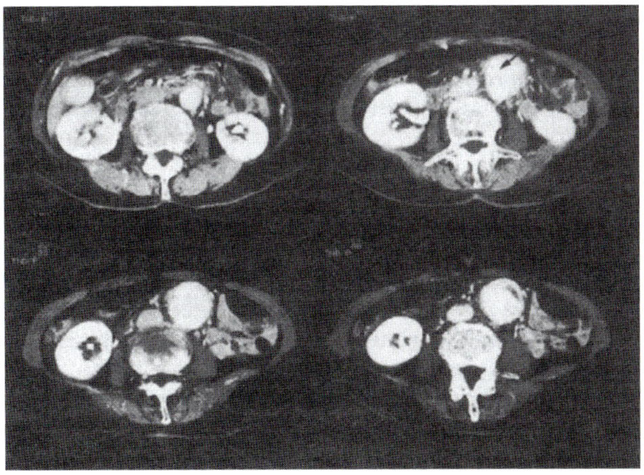

Figure 1. CT of abdomen.

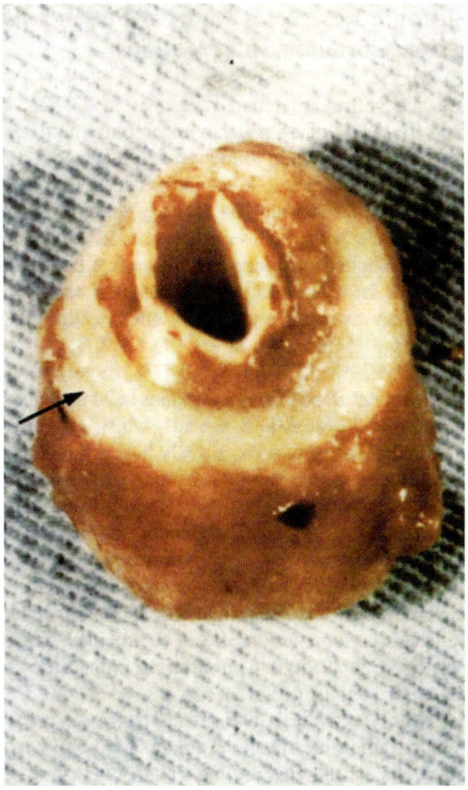

Figure 2. Periarterial thickening of common iliac artery.

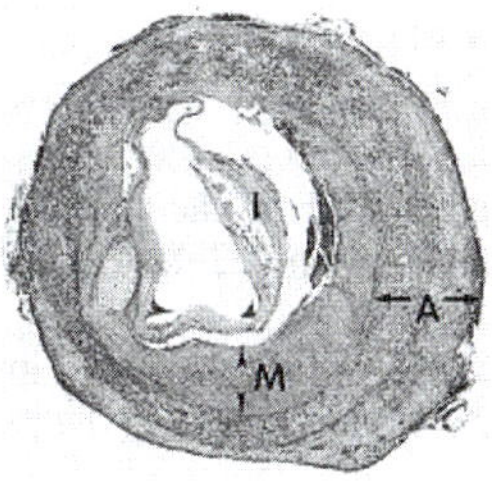

Figure 3. Histopathological findings of aneurysmal wall. M indicates media; A, adventitia.

13

Spiral Computed Tomography Images of Acute Massive Pulmonary Embolism before and after Thrombolysis

Kevin C. Chang, MD, PhD; Nitinkumar Bhatt, MD; William F. Graettinger, MD; Lee B. Darrah, MD

From the Department of Medicine and Radiology (L.B.D.), VA Medical Center, University of Nevada School of Medicine, Reno.

(*Circulation*. 1998;98:2501–2502.)

A 73-year-old man was admitted to the intensive care unit because of sudden onset of dyspnea followed by syncope. On admission, the arterial blood gas (ABG) showed pH 7.45, $PaCO_2$ 25.2 mm Hg, PaO_2 53 mm Hg, bicarbonate 17.6 mEq/L, and SaO_2 89.5% with the patient breathing 2 L/min O_2 via nasal cannula. One year earlier, he had been diagnosed as having a pulmonary embolism, for which he received Coumadin for 6 months. The diagnosis of recurrent pulmonary embolism was made, and the patient was empirically anticoagulated with intravenous heparin. Several hours after anticoagulation was started, the patient became hypotensive, and his respiratory condition deteriorated. A repeat ABG showed pH 7.49, $PaCO_2$ 21.3 mm Hg, PaO_2 44 mm Hg, bicarbonate 16.4 mEq/L, and SaO_2 84.6% with the patient on 100% oxygen through a nonrebreathing mask. A spiral computed tomography (CT) scan of the thorax showed large intramural thrombi in both right and left pulmonary arteries (Figs. 1A and 1B). Because of the hemodynamic and respiratory significance of the emboli, the patient was given intravenous alteplase for thrombolysis.

Approximately 4 hours after thrombolysis, the patient's respiratory condition improved dramatically, with an SpO_2 of 95% on room air. Follow-up spiral CT on the third day after thrombolysis showed resolution of intramural thrombi (Figs. 1C and 1D).

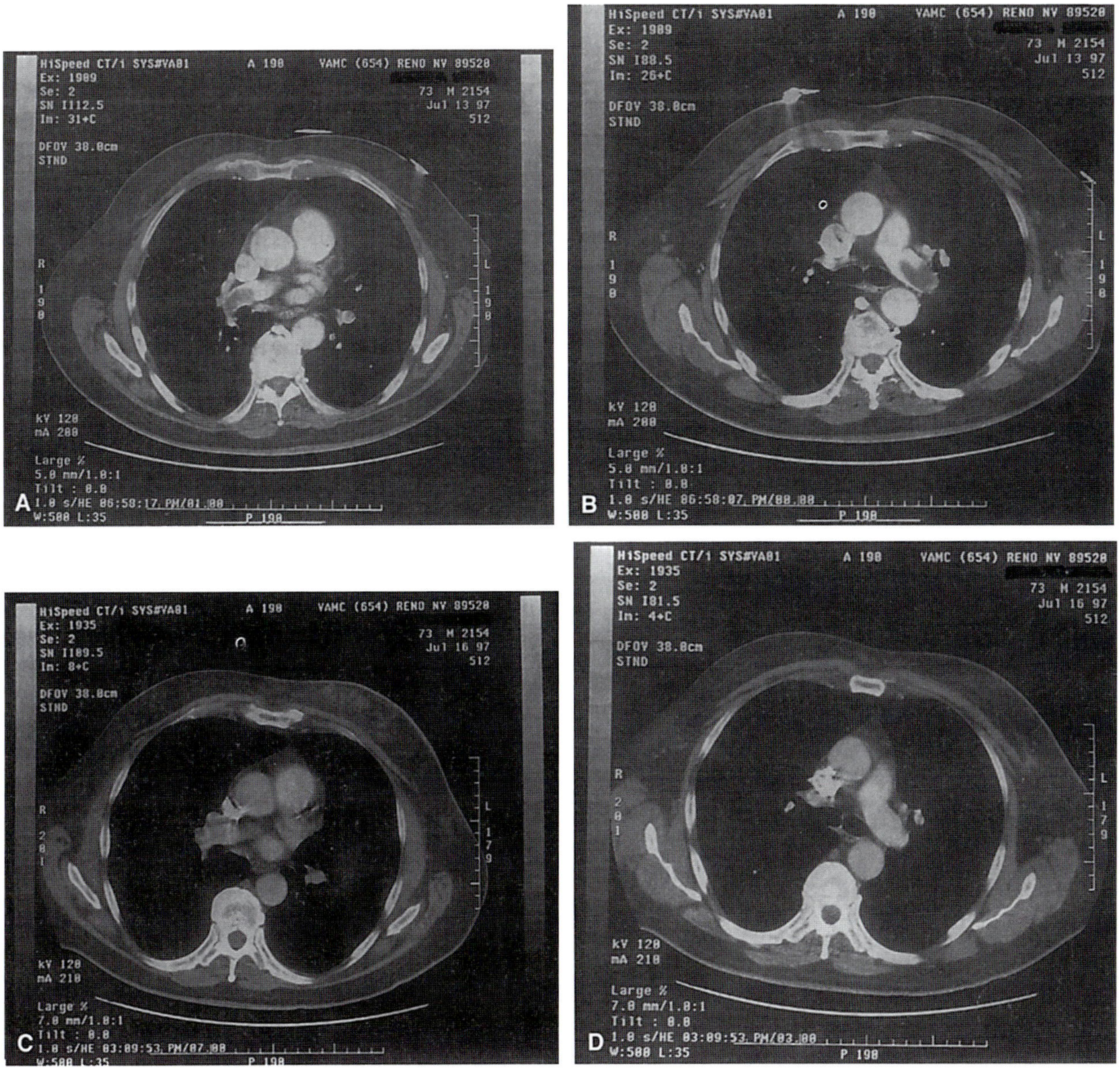

Figure 1.

14 Three-Dimensional Contrast-Enhanced Magnetic Resonance Angiography in a Patient with Chronic Thromboembolic Pulmonary Hypertension before and after Thromboendarterectomy

Karl-Friedrich Kreitner, MD; Eckhard Mayer, MD; Thomas Voigtlaender, MD; Manfred Thelen, MD; Helmut Oelert, MD

From the Departments of Radiology (K.-F.K., M.T.), Cardiothoracic and Vascular Surgery (E.M., H.O.), and Internal Medicine (T.V.), Division of Cardiology, University Hospital, Johannes Gutenberg-University Mainz, Germany.

(*Circulation*. 1999;99:1101.)

The patient was a 69-year-old man with progressive dyspnea during the previous 5 years and no history of thromboembolic events. By means of spiral computed tomography (CT) scanning and multiplanar digital subtraction angiography of the pulmonary arteries, chronic thromboembolic pulmonary hypertension was diagnosed. Mean pulmonary artery pressure and pulmonary vascular resistance were elevated to 46 mm Hg and 890 dyne s cm^{-5}, respectively. The patient underwent successful pulmonary thromboendarterectomy, whereby mean pulmonary artery pressure and pulmonary vascular resistance could be substantially reduced to 20 mm Hg and 237 dyne s cm^{-5}, respectively. Three-dimensional (3-D) contrast-enhanced magnetic resonance (MR) angiography of the pulmonary vasculature clearly depicted the thromboembolic lobar and segmental artery occlusions and stenoses in both lungs as well as the marked postoperative improvement of pulmonary perfusion (Figs. 1A and 1B).

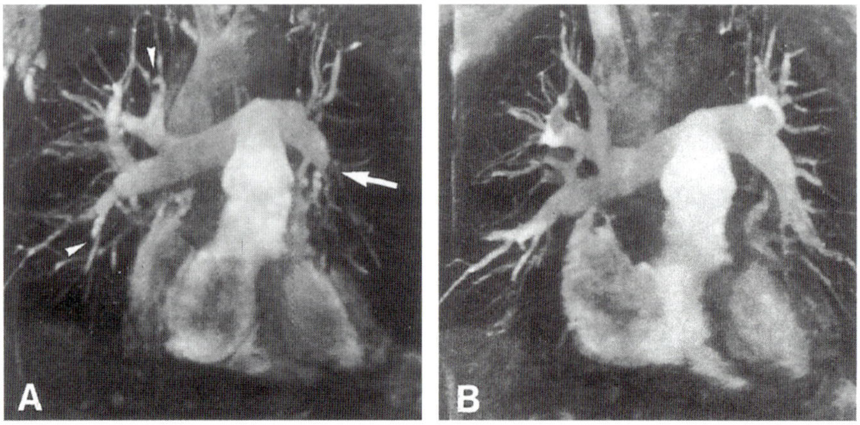

Figure 1. (3-D) contrast-enhanced MR angiography of pulmonary vasculature. **A,** reoperative and B, postoperative "maximum-intensity projection" reconstructions of (3-D) data sets that were acquired in 25 seconds during suspended respiration. Before surgery, there is marked occlusion of several segmental arteries due to thromboembolic material in left lower lobe artery, extending into segmental arteries (arrow) as well as in peripheral segmental arteries of right lung (arrowhead) (A). After surgery **(B),** a nearly complete normalization of arterial vasculature of left lung and improvement of right lung perfusion were demonstrated.

15

Twenty-First-Century Imaging for a Nineteenth-Century Disease

Didier de Canniere, MD, PhD; Thierry Simonart, MD; Jean-Luc Jansens, MD; Dominique Parent, MD, PhD

From the Departments of Cardiac Surgery (D.d.C., J.-L.J.) and Dermatology (T.S., D.P.), Erasmus University Hospital, Brussels, Belgium.

(*Circulation*. 1999;100:884–885.)

Syphilis has become an extremely unusual cause of ascending aortic aneurysms, with barely 41 reported cases since the era of penicillin. The surgical strategy depends on two determinants: the need to replace the aortic valve, if it is involved, and the existence of a collar of normal aortic tissue upstream to the brachiocephalic trunk, enabling the surgeon to clamp the aorta and insert the prosthesis graft without circulatory arrest and reimplantation of the cephalic trunks.

Imaging is thus of paramount importance to decide prospectively between four very different procedures: a Bentall operation, an arch repair in circulatory arrest, a combination of the two, or a simple ascending aortic replacement. We report the case of a 54-year-old White man in whom a routine chest radiograph revealed an aortic aneurysm that proved to be of syphilitic origin (Venereal Disease Research Laboratories [VDRL]+ at 1:4; fluorescent *Treponema* Absorption [FTA]+ at 1:400; *Treponema pallidum* hemagglutination assay [TPHA]+ at 1:400; human immunodeficiency virus [HIV]−). In this case, only a tridimensional CT scan reconstruction of the ascending aorta (and neither angiography [Fig. 1] nor nuclear magnetic resonance [NMR] [Fig. 2]) enabled us to answer the above-mentioned questions by showing the landmarks with the adjacent structures. A successful operation in circulatory arrest followed by a 2-week course of intravenous penicillin led to complete recovery.

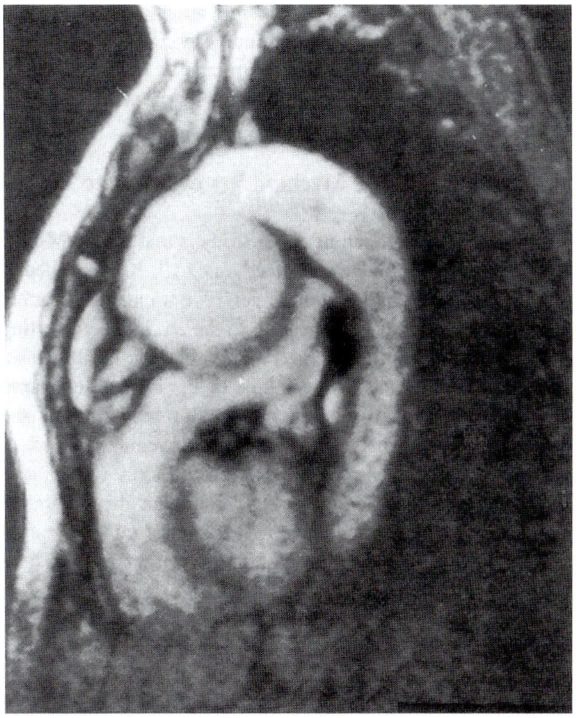

Figure 1. Anglo NMR showing aneurysm compressing pulmonary artery but not precise landmarks of aortic valve, brachiocephalic trunk, or carotid artery.

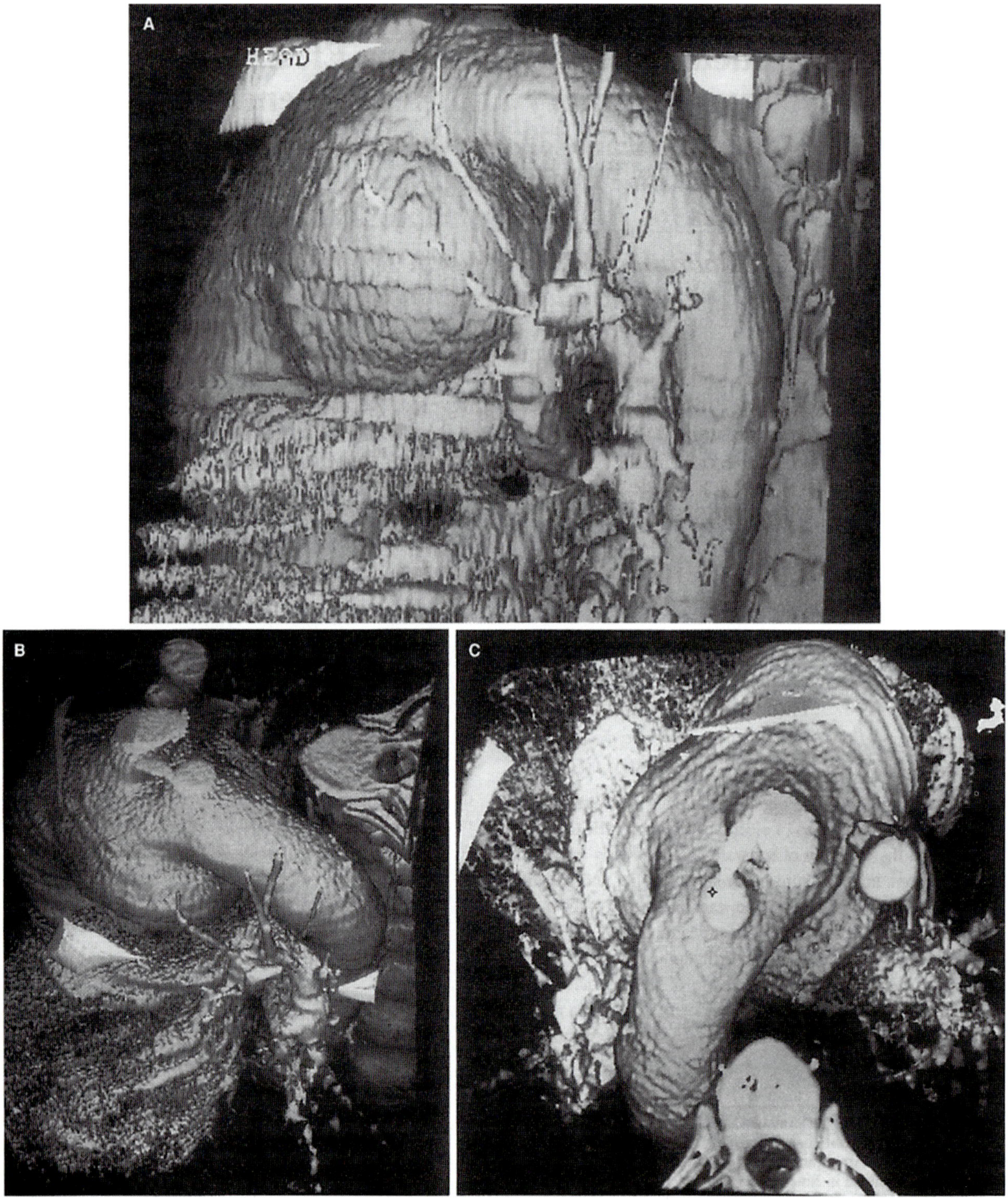

Figure 2. Tridimensional reconstructions of thoracic aorta and adjacent structures. Involvement of brachiocephalic trunk in aneurysmal bag is clearly highlighted. **A,** Left profile. **B,** Left profile +30° rotation. **C,** View from above.

16 Cerebral Arterial Embolism from a Protruding Atheroma of the Aortic Arch after a Nonpenetrating Chest Trauma

Roberto Corti, MD; Mario Alerci, MD; Carlo Tosi, MD; Paolo Tutta, MD; Thomas Hany, MD; Augusto Gallina, MD

From the Divisions of Vascular Medicine and Cardiology (R.C., P.T., A.G.) and Radiology (M.A.), Ospedale San Giovanni, Bellinzona; the Division of Neurology (C.T.), Ospedale Civico, Lugano; and the MRI Center, Department of Radiology (T.H.), University Hospital, Zurich, Switzerland.

(*Circulation*. 1999;100:1009–1010.)

A 60-year-old bricklayer was referred to our hospital because of acute bilateral blindness, vertigo, and bifrontal headache occurring within 10 seconds after a violent shock to the right shoulder while he was trying to open a closed door. On physical examination, the patient presented with bilateral tubular vision and strabismus with diplopia consistent with the clinical diagnosis of a *top of the basilar* syndrome. This syndrome is generally associated with an acute transitory embolic occlusion at the bifurcation of the basilar artery with consequent possible ischemia in the mesencephalic and occipital region. Extensive investigations to detect possible embolic causes (duplex-ultrasound; magnetic resonance angiography of the carotid, vertebral, and basilar arteries; transthoracic echocardiography) were negative.

Transesophageal echocardiography, however, showed multiple atheromatous plaques of the aortic arch with mobile peduncles (Fig. 1, arrows). Spiral computed tomography (CT) confirmed the presence of atherosclerotic plaques of the aortic arch, one located opposite the left subclavian artery (Fig. 2).

Virtual endoluminal reconstruction by magnetic resonance angiography shows the roof of the aortic arch with the origin of the left subclavian artery and left common carotid artery and their relationship with the plaques (Fig. 3).

The causal link between the pedunculated mobile plaques and the cerebral embolism cannot be definitively proved. Nevertheless, the temporal relationship between the shock to this overweight patient and the neurological sequelae in the area supplied by the basilar artery strongly suggest that the nonpenetrating chest trauma may have caused embolization of the large protruding atheroma lying just opposite the left subclavian artery.

This unique case confirms the importance of the thoracic aorta as a possible source of arterial embolism and the crucial role of transesophageal echocardiography as well as the complementary role of new diagnostic techniques, such as magnetic resonance and spiral CT, for the diagnosis of this condition.

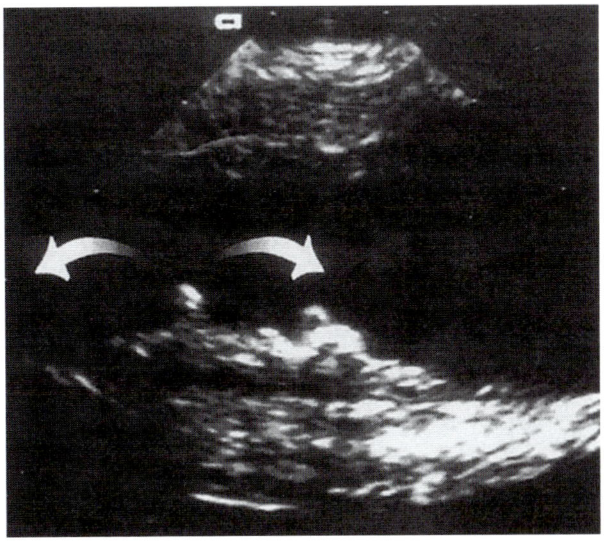

Figure 1. Transesophageal echocardiography shows details of a large calcified plaque (22 × 18 mm) of aortic arch with a mobile peduncle (4 × 2 mm) on top of plaque. Curved arrows on both sides of the mobile peduncle indicate movement of the peduncle into the aortic lumen.

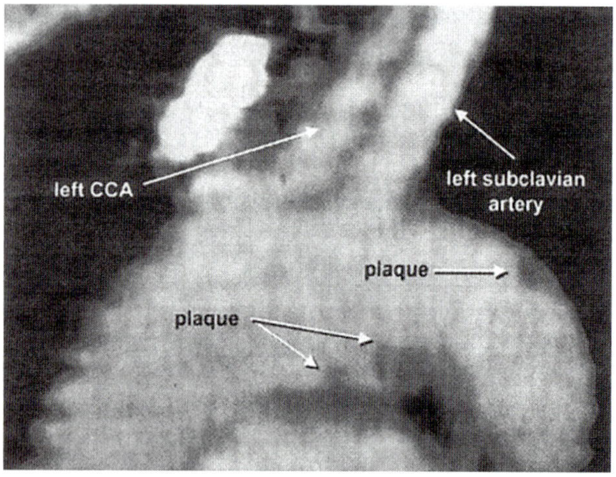

Figure 2. Spiral CT of aortic arch shows presence of multiple atherosclerotic plaques, one of them located just opposite left subclavian artery. CCA indicates common carotid artery.

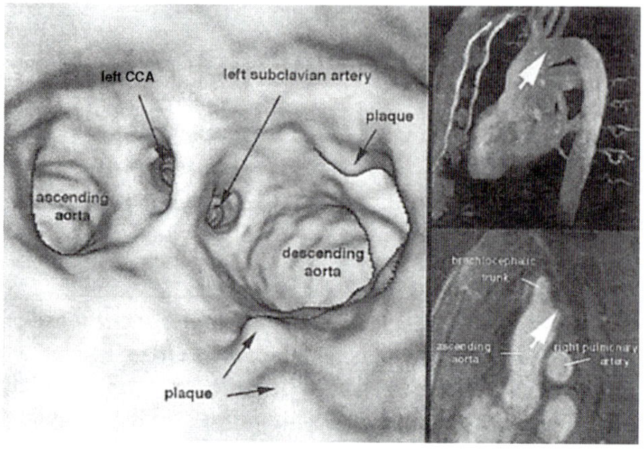

Figure 3. Virtual endoluminal reconstruction by magnetic resonance angiography of aortic arch shows presence of plaques and their relationship to origin of left subclavian artery and left common carotid artery (CCA). White arrows indicate perspective of virtual endoluminal reconstruction.

17

Exclusion of an Aneurysmal Segment of the Thoracic Aorta with Covered Stents

R.H. Stables, MA, MRCP; R. Mohiaddin, FRCR, FESC; J. Panting, BSc, MRCP; DJ. Pennell, FRCP, FESC; J. Pepper, BChir, FRCS; U. Sigwart, MD, FRCP

From the Royal Brompton Hospital, London SW3 6NP, UK.

(*Circulation*. 2000;101:1888–1889.)

The patient was an 80-year-old woman who presented to her local hospital with left-sided chest pain. A computed tomography (CT) scan of the thorax demonstrated an aneurysm of the middle third of the thoracic aorta with a diameter of 9.5 cm. The patient presented a significant operative risk, with marked comorbidity, including chronic venous ulceration and poor respiratory function secondary to lifelong smoking. Initial surgical opinion maintained that the risks of operative intervention were too high to justify the performance of surgical repair. She was referred to a cardiothoracic surgeon at this institution for a second opinion,

Three-dimensional contrast-enhanced magnetic resonance (MR) angiography performed at the Royal Brompton Hospital (Fig. 1A, Pre-stenting) confirmed the existence of a saccular aneurysm of the descending thoracic aorta. The aneurysm began shortly after the origin of the left subclavian artery and measured 9.2 cm in diameter and 12 cm in length. Mural thrombus was noted along the left and posterior walls of the diseased segment. The paucity of contrast in the image presented was related to an acute angulation at the distal end of the aneurysmal portion.

The aneurysm was excluded with a covered stent. Under general anesthesia, the right femoral artery was exposed and cannulated with an angiographic catheter. Contrast images of the arch and descending aorta were acquired, and patency of the femoral and iliac system was confirmed.

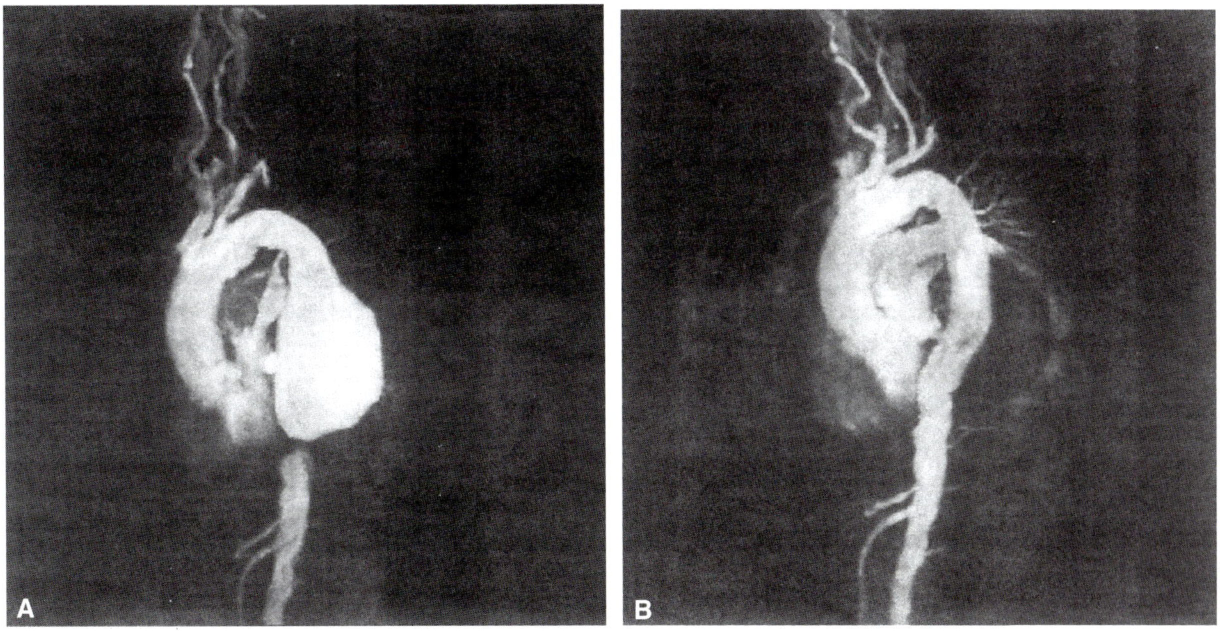

Figure 1. A, Pre-stenting. **B,** Post-stenting

A 31 × 150-mm stent device with a GoreTex coating (WL Gore Thoracic Excluder Endoprosthesis PB-31-15-00) was inserted via a 22F introducer and deployed. Contrast angiography after deployment revealed that the lower portion of the aneurysmal segment had not been excluded, and an additional shorter device (31 × 70 mm) was deployed.

Postimplantation dilation was performed with a perfusion balloon system (WL Gore PD-26-31-10). The femoral arteriotomy was closed with a vein patch, and the patient made an uncomplicated recovery.

A follow-up MR angiogram performed 3 days after stent implantation (Fig. 1B, Post-stenting) showed the stent to be patent along its length and 32 mm in diameter. The aortic lumen outside the stent graft was largely thrombosed. An area of signal enhancement around the distal third of the stented portion was compatible with a small leak at the junction of the two stent devices. A further follow-up scan performed 1 month after the procedure demonstrated that this communication with the false lumen had closed.

18

Magnetic Resonance Imaging and Asymptomatic Aortic Dissection

Stephen G. Worthley, MB BS, FRACP; Gerard Helft, MD, PhD; Zahi A. Fayad, PhD; Valentin Fuster, MD, PhD; Azfar G. Zaman, MB ChB, MRCP, MD; Meir Shinnar, MD, PhD; Juan J. Badimon, PhD

From the Zena and Michael A. Wiener Cardiovascular Institute (S.G.W., G.H., Z.A.F., V.F., A.G.Z., M.S., J.J.B.) and the Department of Radiology (Z.A.F., M.S.), Mount Sinai Medical Center, New York, NY.

(*Circulation*. 2000;101:2771.)

Aortic dissection is a well-known complication of Marfan syndrome. Aortic dissection in patients with Marfan syndrome is associated with aortic root dilatation. As imaging techniques have improved, it has become clear that some patients with Marfan syndrome, in the absence of symptoms, may have evidence of a prior aortic dissection. A 47-year-old White man with documented Marfan syndrome and no prior symptomatology referable to aortic dissection had elective high-resolution magnetic resonance imaging (MRI) of the aorta for an unrelated research project. Importantly, he had no known risk factors for atherosclerotic disease. The magnetic resonance (MR) images showed that his aortic root was not dilated, with a diameter of 36 mm (Fig. lA). His ascending aorta was not dilated, with normal wall thickness and no evidence of an intimal flap (Fig. lB). However, a small defect was evident in the wall of the descending thoracic aorta that was more readily appreciated on magnified views of the region (Fig. 2). Proton density-weighted (Fig. 2A) and T2-weighted (Fig. 2B) images clearly showed a very small but distinct defect within the aortic wall, consistent with a false lumen. Review of the complete series of MR images confirmed a small, limited type B dissection, beginning just beyond the origin of the left subclavian artery and extending distally into the descending thoracic aorta for ≈5 cm. No communicating channels were identified between the two lumens.

With improvements in vascular imaging techniques that permit high-resolution noninvasive analysis of the arterial wall, we may find more asymptomatic, previously undetected aortic dissections in patients with Marfan syndrome. Generally, it has been assumed that this occurs in association with aortic root dilatation; in this case, however, the dimensions of the aortic root were within normal limits. The natural history of this phenomenon in patients with Marfan disease is unclear.

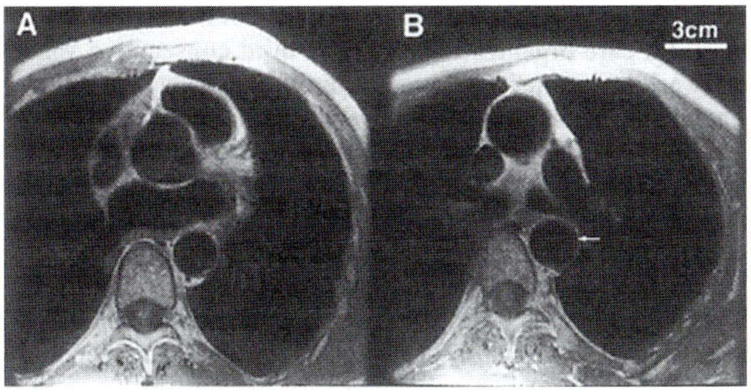

Figure 1. Axial proton density-weighted MR images obtained with cardiac-gated double inversion recovery fast spin-echo sequence at different levels through thorax. Small aortic dissection can be seen in descending thoracic aorta in **B** (arrow). Note normal appearance of aortic root **(A)**.

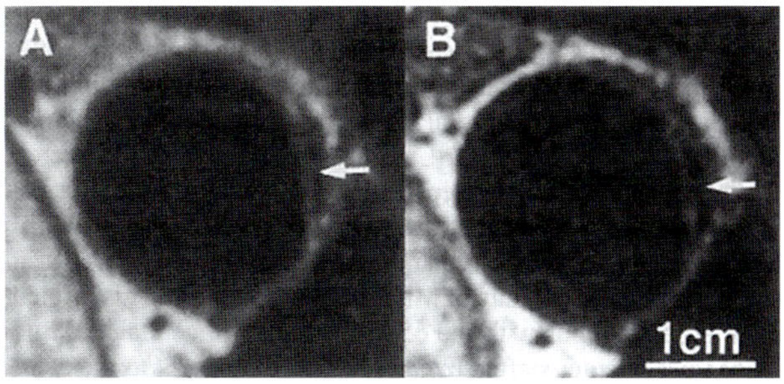

Figure 2. Magnified axial MR images of descending thoracic aorta at same site as Figure 1B, demonstrating small aortic dissection (arrow). False lumen is clearly seen with both proton density-weighted **(A)** and T2-weighted **(B)** images.

19

Penetrating Stab Injury of the Thoracic Aorta

Beat Kipfer, MD; Thierry P. Carrel, MD

From the Clinic for Cardiovascular Surgery, University Hospital, Bern, Switzerland.

(*Circulation*. 2000;102:1068.)

A 36-year-old male psychiatric nurse was stabbed in the back with a knife by a patient suffering from acute psychosis. After initial treatment in an outside hospital, he was transferred in stable cardiopulmonary condition to our department because a lung injury was suspected (Fig. 1). Computed tomography performed while the knife was still in place showed that the blade had penetrated the proximal part of the descending aorta. A periaortic hematoma had developed, but no injury of the lung parenchyma was demonstrated (Fig. 2).

The patient was transferred immediately to the operating room, and an exploratory thoracotomy was performed using left-heart bypass through femoral cannulation as an adjunct. After cross-clamping the aorta, a longitudinal arteriotomy was performed in the anterior part of the vessel wall, and the tip of the blade, which had injured two-thirds of the circumference, was exposed (Fig. 3).

After removal of the knife, the posterior wall was closed from inside using a running polypropylene suture. The aortotomy was closed in a similar fashion, and the patient was weaned from cardiopulmonary bypass without problems. Postoperative recovery was uneventful, and the patient was discharged 5 days after the surgery.

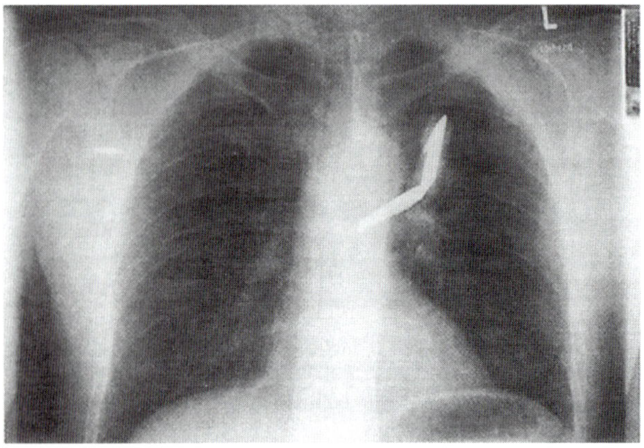

Figure 1. Conventional x-ray demonstrating knife in place in left hemithorax.

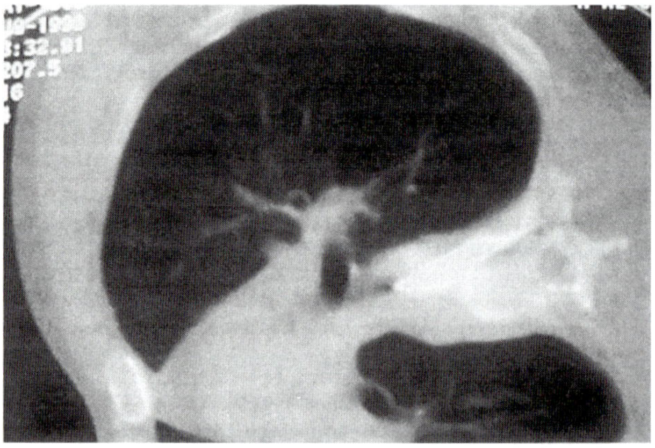

Figure 2. Penetration of tip of the blade into the descending aorta, without lung injury.

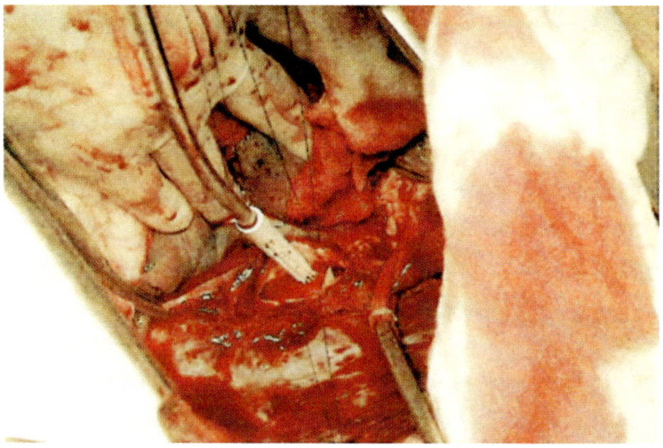

Figure 3. Opened aorta with tip of the blade inside the vessel.

20 Granulomatous Aortitis Presenting as an Acute Myocardial Infarction in Crohn Disease

Michael H. Goldman, MD; Bechara Akl, MD; Shayryar Mafi, MD; Lucia Pastore, MD
From Fairfax Medical Center, Fairfax, Va.

(*Circulation*. 2000;102:3023–3024.)

A 33-year-old man was admitted emergently with evidence of an acute inferior apical myocardial infarction. He had no previous cardiac history but did have a 20-year history of symptomatic Crohn disease. His subsequent coronary angiography revealed a long filling defect in the apical portion of the left anterior descending coronary artery, consistent with intraluminal thrombus (Fig. 1). Left ventriculography demonstrated inferior apical akinesia. Visualization of the ascending aorta during ventriculography unexpectedly revealed a filling defect above the aortic valve. Aortography was performed, and it confirmed the presence of an apparently pedunculated mass (≈4 cm) above the valve, with no evidence of aortic insufficiency (Fig. 2A).

A transesophageal echocardiogram demonstrated a mobile, pedunculated mass attached to the ascending aorta, which was suggestive of an intimal flap and/or possible thrombus. No clear dissection was demonstrated (Fig. 2B). Magnetic resonance imaging (MRI) (Fig. 2C) and computed tomography (CT) scans (Fig. 2D) demonstrated a "linear defect" consistent with a limited dissection.

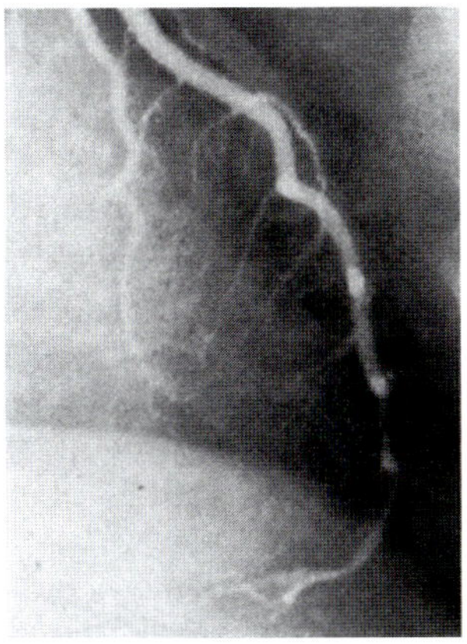

Figure 1. Coronary angiography in right anterior oblique projection reveals a filling defect in apical portion of left anterior descending coronary artery, consistent with a coronary embolus.

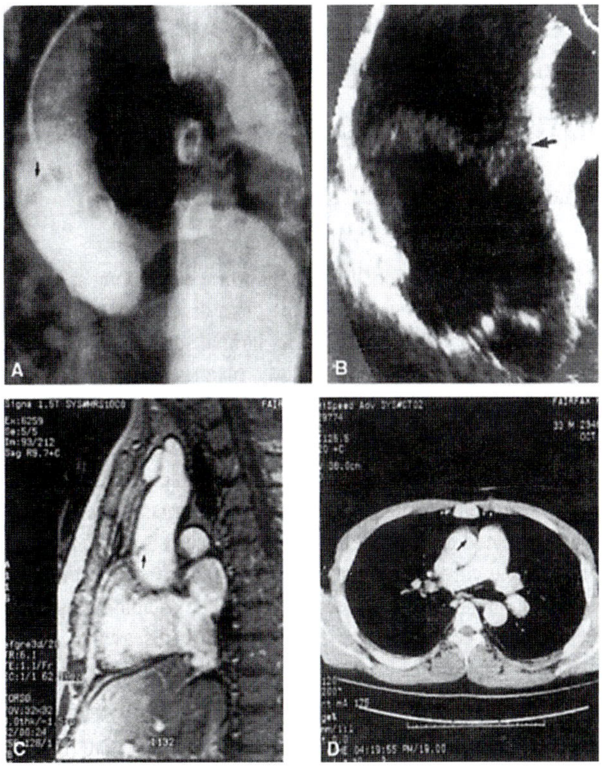

Figure 2. A, Aortography in left anterior oblique projection reveals a filling defect (arrow) in aorta above aortic valve. **B,** Transesophageal echocardiography reveals a mobile mass (arrow) attached to anterior surface of aorta. **C,** MRI reveals small linear defect (arrow). **D,** CT scan reveals faint linear defect (arrow).

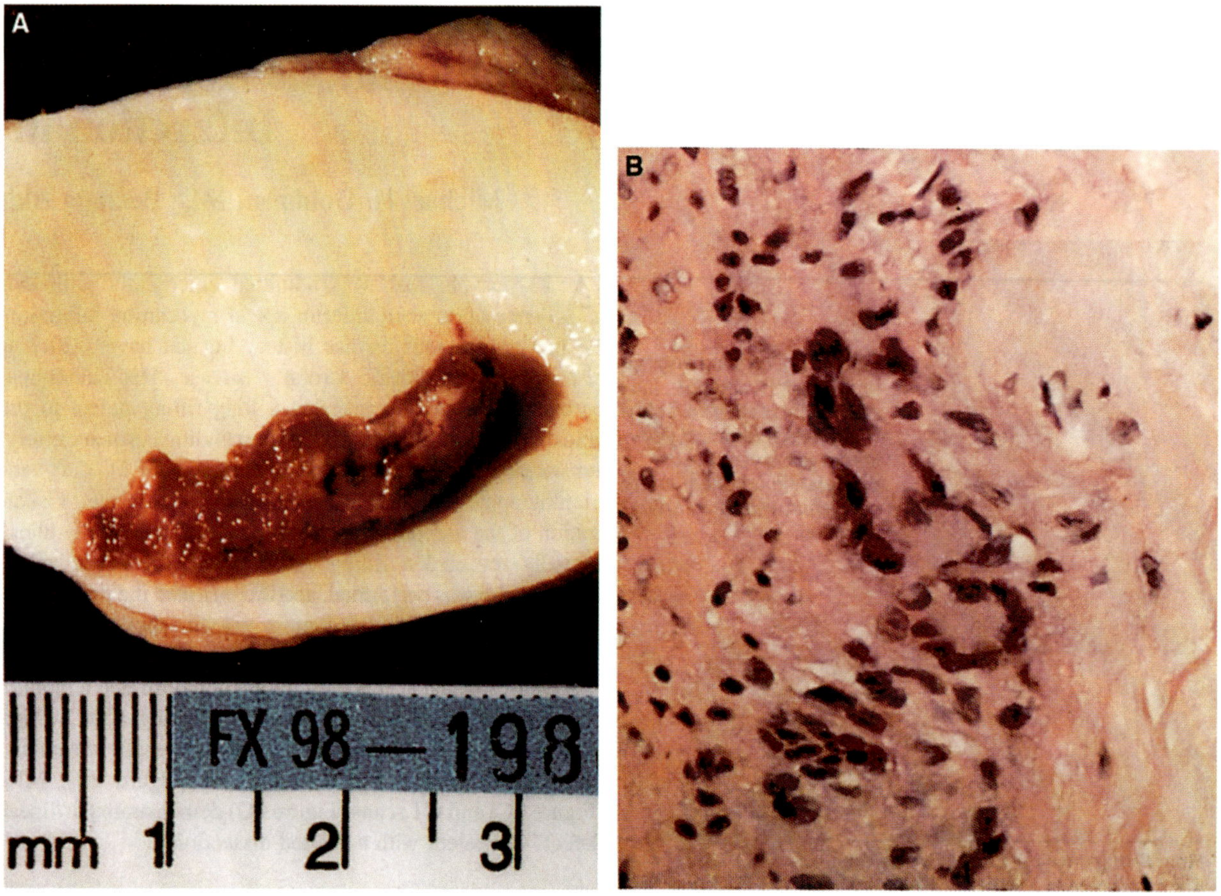

Figure 3. A, Resected portion of aorta with an adherent, pedunculated, sterile fibrin thrombus. **B,** Giant cell granulomas of inner media aorta with focal necrosis (hematoxylin and eosin; magnification, 40×).

At surgical exploration, the outer surface of the aorta appeared normal, without evidence of hematoma, dissection, or enlargement. The aorta was transected. Its intimal surface was smooth, with occasional scattered fibrofatty plaques. Adherent to the aorta was a pedunculated and friable sterile fibrin thrombus measuring $2.5 \times 0.6 \times 0.5$ cm (Fig. 3A). A short segment interposition graft was placed. Microscopic examination of the aorta revealed circumferential granulomatous aortitis with multinucleated giant cells, multifocal necrosis of the media, and perivascular chronic inflammation of the adventitia (Fig. 3B).

These findings were consistent with the granulomatous aortitis seen in giant cell arteritis and Takayasu disease.

The patient was subsequently continued on prednisone and methotrexate, as well as aspirin and Plavix (clopidogrel). During his hospitalization, blood cultures were negative. A full rheumatological evaluation (including HLA-B27 typing) was normal. There was no hematological evidence of hypercoagulability. One year later, he remains asymptomatic on prednisone and methotrexate.

Abnormalities of the ascending aorta in Crohn disease are almost always associated with ankylosing spondylitis and often a positive HLA-B27 phenotype. There have been 5 reports of aortic insufficiency in the absence of ankylosing spondylitis and HLA positivity. There have been no previous reports of Crohn disease-associated aortitis without aortic dilatation or valvular insufficiency.

21 Three-Dimensional Visualization of Pulmonary Thromboemboli in Chronic Thromboembolic Pulmonary Hypertension with Multiple Detector-Row Spiral Computed Tomography

Dominik Fleischmann, MD; Christine Scholten, MD; Walter Klepetko, MD; Irene M. Lang, MD

From the Department of Radiology (D.F.), the Department of Internal Medicine II, Division of Cardiology (C.S., I.M.L.), and the Department of Surgery, Division of Cardiothoracic Surgery (W.K.), University of Vienna, Austria.

(*Circulation.* 2001;103:2993.)

A 36-year-old man experienced new-onset dyspnea on exertion. His previous medical history was unremarkable except for a motorcycle accident 16 years ago with multiple fractures of his right leg requiring surgery. Echocardiography showed severe right heart enlargement with impaired right ventricular function in the absence of intracardiac shunts or valvular heart disease. Venous duplex scanning demonstrated old organized thrombus in the right popliteal and femoral veins. Hemodynamic evaluation at rest disclosed pulmonary hypertension with a pulmonary vascular resistance of 600 dynes s cm^{-5}. Selective digital subtraction angiography showed irregular contours of the central pulmonary arteries, filling defects, and pruning of smaller, subsegmental arteries (Fig. 1A). Contrast medium-enhanced multiple detector-row (or multi slice) spiral computed tomography (CT) with three-dimensional (3-D) rendering clearly demonstrated the organized thromboembolic masses, thus confirming the diagnosis of chronic thromboembolic pulmonary hypertension (Fig. 1B). The patient underwent a successful bilateral pulmonary thromboendarterectomy, yielding 25 g of whitish-reddish, partly organized thromboembolus (Fig. 1C), with subsequent normalization of pulmonary hemodynamics and exercise capacity.

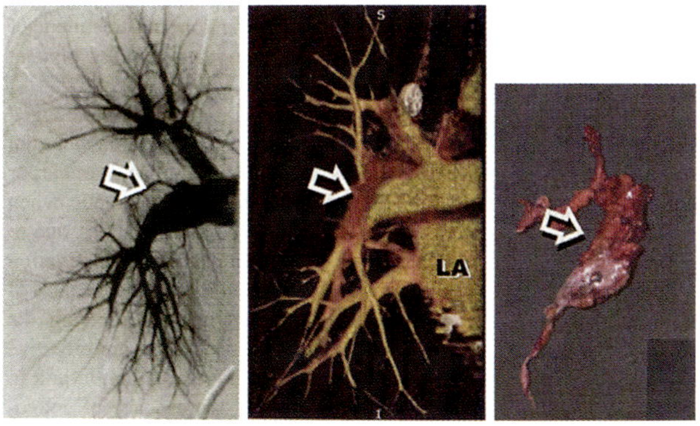

A B C

Figure 1. A, Selective digital subtraction angiography of the right pulmonary artery. The angiogram shows wall irregularities and filling defects (arrow) at the right lower lobe artery. Note that the thrombus itself is not visualized with digital subtraction angiography. Thus, the true size of the pulmonary artery is underestimated. **B,** CT angiography with 3-D volume-rendered image with a cut plane through the right pulmonary artery. Contrast material-filled vessels (arteries and veins) are shown in yellow; thrombus is displayed in red. Note the extensive, wall-adherent thrombotic masses (arrow) within the right pulmonary artery. The white elliptical structure medial to the upper lobe artery represents the azygos vein. LA indicates left atrium. **C,** Surgical thromboendarterectomy specimen from the right pulmonary artery. Thrombus was harvested from the pulmonary artery as far distal as the subsegmental branches. The specimen represents endothelialized thrombus (arrow) with portions of fibroblast-rich organized thrombus parenchyma.

22 Maffucci Syndrome

M. Jermann, MD; K. Eid, MD; T. Pfammatter, MD; R. Stahel, MD
From the Departments of Oncology, Traumatology, and Radiology, University Hospital, Zurich, Switzerland.

(*Circulation*. 2001;104:1693.)

A 30-year-old woman presented with painful hemangiomas (Figs. 1A and 1B) and enchondromas (Fig. 1C) in her arms, predominantly in the left hand. The hemangiomas had existed since childhood. They were slowly increasing in size, especially the girth of the left thumb. Multiple resections of enchondromas and transarterial carpal embolizations of the hemangiomas with polyvinyl alcohol particles had been performed during the previous 9 years. At the age of 22, the small finger of the left hand was removed. At the age of 25, a pathological fracture of the left humerus occurred due to an enchondroma.

A contour reduction and partial excision of the most important nodules was performed. Serum levels of vascular endothelial growth factor and basic fibroblast growth factor were elevated twofold and sevenfold, respectively. The patient is in good clinical health and works part-time as a secretary.

Maffucci syndrome is a rare nonhereditary mesodermal dysplasia. It consists of multiple hemangiomas of the soft tissue and multiple enchondromas, which are most often found in the phalanges and long bones. The bone and vascular lesions exist at birth or occur during childhood and may be progressive. The syndrome can be associated with benign or malignant tumors (goiter, parathyroid adenoma, pituitary adenoma, hemangioendothelioma, adrenal tumor, ovarian tumor, chondrosarcoma, breast cancer, astrocytoma).

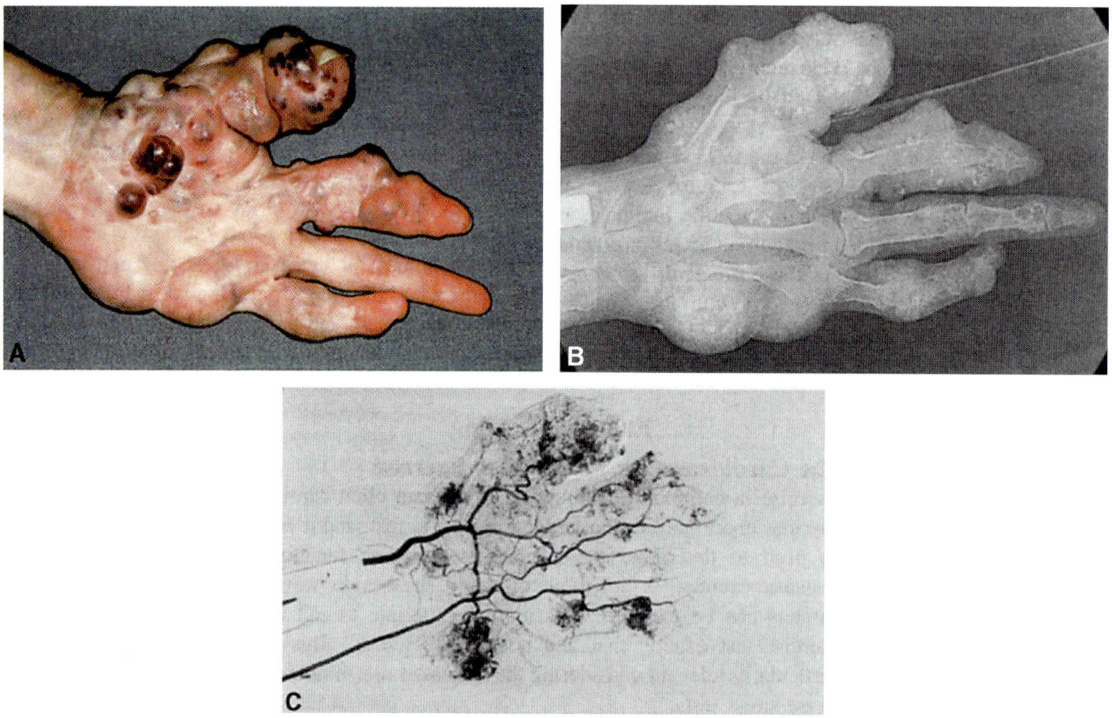

Figure 1. A, Left hand of patient showing extensive hemangiomas. The fifth finger had to be removed 8 years previously. **B,** Radiograph of the left hand showing multiple calcifications within the hemangiomas (e.g., first finger, base of fifth finger) and multiple enchondromas (e.g., metacarpophalangeal joint of the fourth finger, proximal and distal interphalangeal joints of second through fourth fingers). **C,** Arterial angiograph of the left hand showing multiple hemangiomas.

23

Clubbing due to Peripheral Hypervascularization: Recognition by Contrast-Enhanced Three-Dimensional Magnetic Resonance Angiography

Frank Wiesmann, MD; Meinrad Beer, MD; Ulrich Krause, MD; Thomas Pabst, PhD; Werner Kenn, MD; Dietbert Hahn, MD; Georg Ertl, MD

From the Medizinische Universitätsklinik (F.W., G.E.) and the Institut für Röntgendiagnostik, Universität Würzburg (M.B., U.K., T.P., W.K., D.H.), Würzburg, Germany.

(*Circulation*. 2001;104:2503.)

A 23-year-old medical student presented with slowly progressive swelling of the terminal digits that had a duration of 3 years (Fig. 1). There was no family history of clubbing or cyanosis. The patient had no signs of cyanosis or a history of cardiac, pulmonary, or inflammatory bowel disease. His physical activity, including field sports and regular workouts, was unlimited. On examination, he had normal cardiac, lung, and abdominal findings. Furthermore, lung function tests, electrocardiography, Doppler echocardiography, and chest x-ray revealed normal results. Laboratory tests, including vasculitis-associated antibodies and thyroid function, also produced normal results.

Contrast-enhanced three-dimensional (3D) magnetic resonance (MR) angiography of the left hand showed no evidence of arterial stenosis, arteriovenous shunting, or vasculitis. However, there was marked hypervascularization in the terminal digits (Fig. 2), reflecting a potential source of clubbing.

This example demonstrates the potential of MR angiography for diagnostic visualization of vascular abnormalities, without performing invasive arterial catheterization or applying ionized radiation.

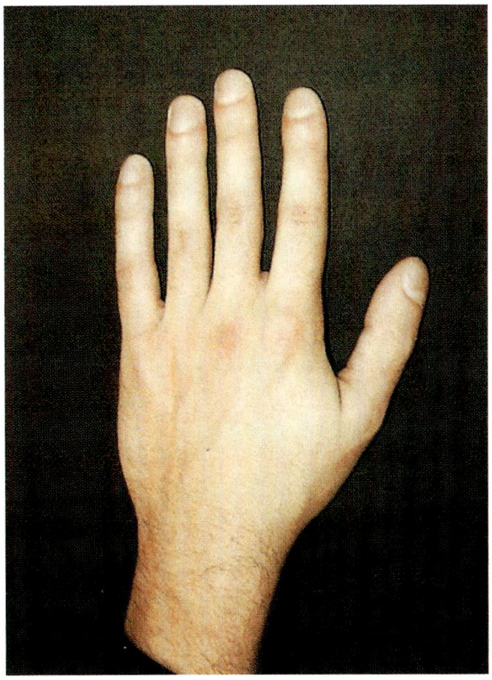

Figure 1. Photograph of the patient's left hand showing clubbing.

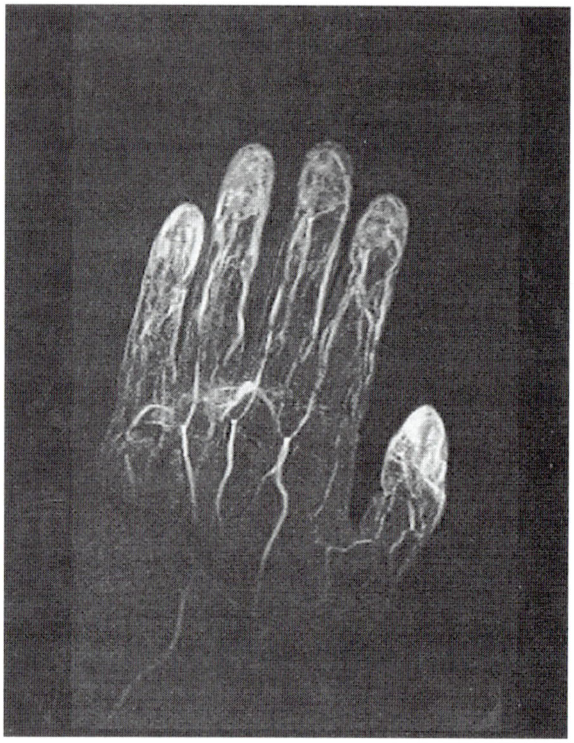

Figure 2. Maximum intensity projection reconstruction of a 3-D contrast-enhanced MR angiogram of the patient's left hand. Note the peripheral hypervascularization in the terminal digits, particularly of the first, fourth, and fifth fingers. There is no evidence of vasculitis or arterial stenosis or occlusion.

24 Fulminant *Clostridium septicum* Aortitis

Marco A. Zenati, MD; Gianluca Bonanomi, MD; Dean Kostov, BS; Robert Lee, MD

From the Divisions of Cardiothoracic Surgery and Pathology, University of Pittsburgh Medical Center, Pittsburgh, Pa.

(*Circulation*. 2002;105:1871.)

An 87-year-old man was admitted to our cardiothoracic surgical service complaining of epigastric and interscapular pain of 3 days' duration. His temperature was 101°F; white blood cell count, 19,100/mm^3; and hemoglobin, 11.3 gm/dL. An ECG and serial cardiac enzyme measurements were negative for myocardial ischemia. An echocardiogram demonstrated normal left ventricular function, mild aortic stenosis, and mild biatrial enlargement. Mediastinal enlargement on chest film prompted a computed tomography (CT) scan of the chest and abdomen. A gas collection dissecting the outer layer of the aortic wall was identified from the level of the left subclavian artery all the way down to the intra-abdominal aorta (≈2 cm) above the celiac axis (Fig. 1). Small bilateral pleural effusions were noted, but no ascites or free air was identified, and the structures within the upper abdomen were unremarkable. Blood cultures were drawn and empirical broad-spectrum antibiotics started. A barium swallow and upper gastrointestinal endoscopy ruled out any infection or perforation of the esophagus. On day three after admission, the patient complained of increased upper abdominal pain not relieved by morphine. A repeat CT scan showed a dramatic increase in the gas collection dissecting within the wall. The large amount of gas surrounding the descending thoracic aorta was associated with left periaortic fluid and soft tissue density. Four days after admission, blood cultures drawn on admission grew anaerobic gram-positive rods, speciated to be *Clostridium septicum,* and therapy with clindamycin and ofloxacin was immediately started. The patient further developed diffuse abdominal tenderness and the onset of renal failure with a creatinine level rising from 1.1 to 1.8 mg/dL. He and his family refused any invasive procedures, and he died on the sixth hospital day.

Autopsy showed severe calcified atherosclerosis of the thoracic and abdominal aorta, with aneurysmal dilation and extensive aortic dissection extending proximally from the right innominate artery and distally to the renal arteries. Aortic rupture at the level of the carina on the right side had resulted in a right hemothorax. The entire length of the dissection was notable for acute inflammatory exudates associated with gram-positive bacilli (Fig. 2). In addition, a 6-cm moderately differentiated adenocarcinoma of the cecum, invading the subserosal fat and involving one omental lymph node was present, a finding consistent with the reported 85% incidence of *Clostridium septicum* infections associated with gastrointestinal or hematologic malignancy.

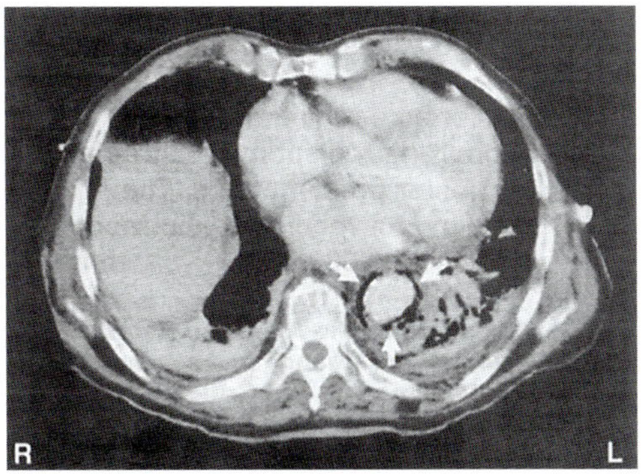

Figure 1. CT demonstrating extensive dissection of the descending thoracic aorta (arrows) due to gas collection from *Clostridium septicum* infection associated with a left periaortic inflammatory reaction. R indicates right; L, left.

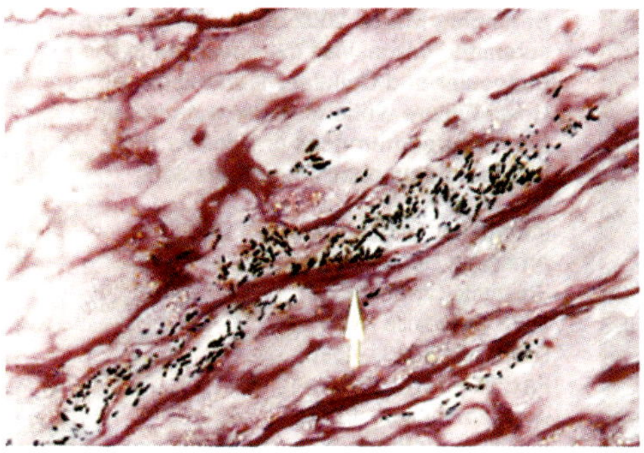

Figure 2. Photomicrograph (magnification ×60) of a section of the descending thoracic aorta showing dissection of the external layer of the vessel wall and infiltration of acute inflammatory exudates associated with clusters of Gram-stained *Clostridia* (arrow).

25

Deep Vein Thrombosis Demonstrated by Magnetic Resonance Direct Thrombus Imaging

J. Kelly, MRCP; BJ. Hunt, MD; A. Moody, MD

From the Department of Haematology, St Thomas' Hospital, London (J.K., B.J.H.), and Department of Academic Radiology QMC, Nottingham (A.M.), UK.

(*Circulation.* 2003;107:2165.)

DOI: 10.1161/01.CIR.0000063426.21085.8C

Magnetic resonance direct thrombus imaging (MRDTI) is a new application of magnetic resonance technology that capitalizes on the fact that thrombus is associated with a substantial reduction in T1 (spin-lattice relaxation time). A T1-weighted magnetization-prepared three-dimensional gradient echo sequence is used with a selective water-excitation radiofrequency pulse to abolish fat signal. The effective inversion time is chosen to null the blood signal, so that thrombus shows up as a high signal on Tl-weighted images against a background of suppressed blood and fat without requiring intravenous contrast. The technique is highly accurate for deep vein thrombosis (DVT) (Fig. 1) and pulmonary embolism (PE) and can be performed using a standard scanner with a lower limb acquisition time of only 7 minutes.

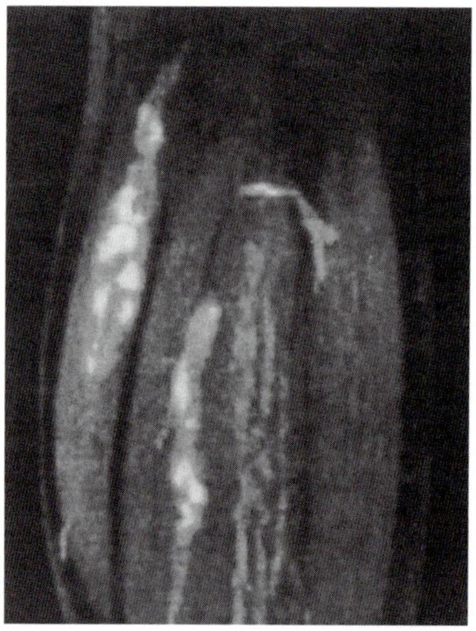

Figure 1. Coronal section of calf showing extensive below-knee DVT.

MRDTI has two major advantages over conventional imaging modalities. Firstly, direct visualization of thrombus not only overcomes many of the pitfalls of alternative techniques that have either identified thrombus as a filling defect or in terms of surrogate markers, but it also provides additional information about thrombus characteristics. Secondly, simultaneous imaging of the legs and chest allows a comprehensive assessment of thrombus load, minimizing the importance of overlooked subsegmental PE (where the prognosis is that of the source), and potentially facilitating a more titrated approach to treatment.

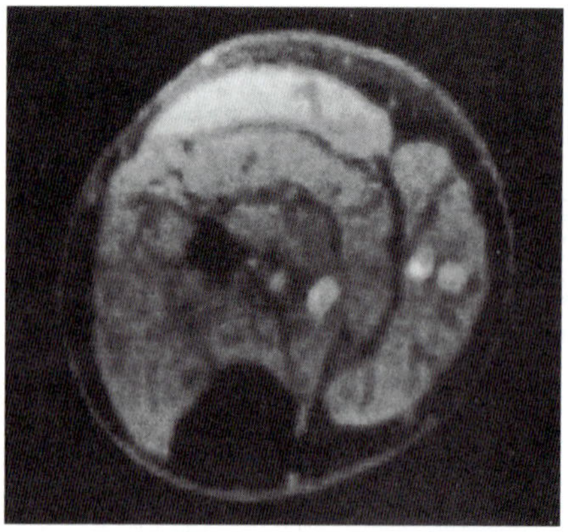

Figure 2. Axial view from the same patient showing the target sign.

The high T1 signal is thought to be due to formation of methemoglobin within red cells in thrombus, which has strong paramagnetic properties. Initially, this occurs subjacent to the endothelium before propagating centripetally so that recent thrombus viewed axially exhibits a characteristic target appearance (Fig. 2).

26 Huge Calcified Pulmonary Arterial Aneurysm

Wen-Shiann Wu, MD

From the Division of Cardiology, Chi-Mei Foundation Hospital, Tainan, Taiwan.

(*Circulation*. 2003;107:2280–2281.)

DOI: 10.1161/01.CIR.0000063924.01337.0C

A 71-year-old woman presented with dyspnea on exertion for one year. On auscultation, a grade 3/6 systolic murmur was heard at the upper sternal border. Chest radiographs (Figs. 1A and 1B) revealed a huge calcified lesion in the left lung field (arrows).

Chest computerized tomographic scan image (Fig. 2) showed a huge saccular aneurysm (5 × 6 × 12 cm) of the main pulmonary trunk with calcified wall (arrow). The patient's condition is stable after 1.5 years of medical therapy.

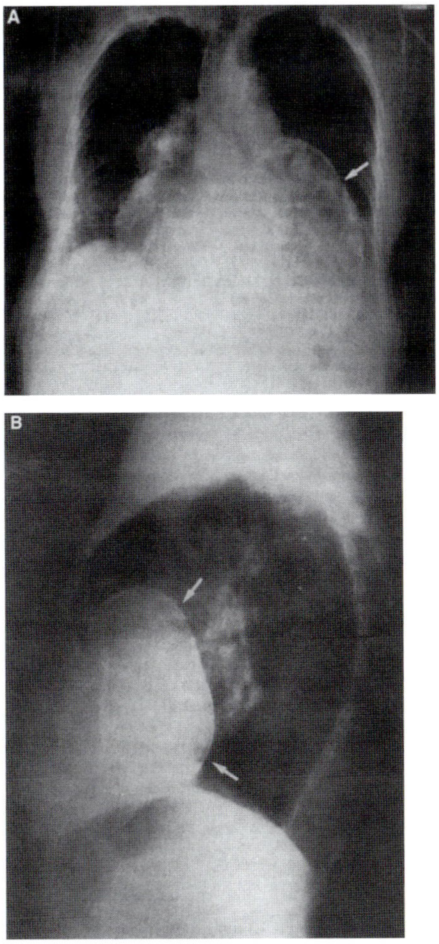

Figure 1. Chest radiographs (posteroanterior **(A)** and lateral **(B)** views) showing a huge calcified lesion in the left lung field (arrows).

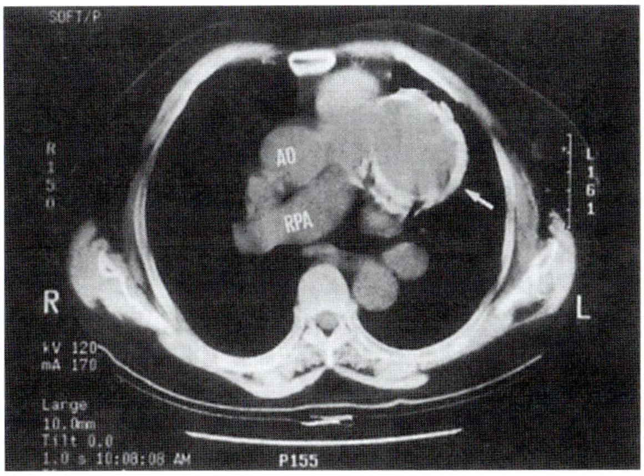

Figure 2. Chest computerized tomographic scan image showing a huge calcified lesion (arrow) originating from the pulmonary artery. RPA indicates right pulmonary artery; AO, aorta.

27 Detection of Carotid Atherosclerotic Plaque Ulceration, Calcification, and Thrombosis by Multicontrast Weighted Magnetic Resonance Imaging

Baocheng Chu, MD, PhD; Marina S. Ferguson, MT; Hunter Underhill, MD; Norihide Takaya, MD, PhD; Jianming Cai, MD, PhD; Michel Kliot, MD; Chun Yuan, PhD; Thomas S. Hatsukami, MD

From the Departments of Radiology (B.C., M.S.F., H.U., N.T., J.C., C.Y.) and Surgery (M.K., T.S.H.), University of Washington, Seattle, and VA Puget Sound Health Care System (T.S.H.), Seattle, Wash.

(*Circulation*. 2005;112:e3–e4.)

A 62-year-old man presented to the emergency department with a chief complaint of severe headache and decreased vision in his left eye. Initial physical examination demonstrated a new-onset left homonymous hemianopsia, which warranted a stroke workup. The patient's head computed tomography (CT) was significant for a 2.3 × 3.7 cm acute hemorrhage in the right posterior parietal and occipital lobes. Conventional angiography was performed and interpreted as >90% stenosis of both internal carotid arteries without ulceration. The remainder of the workup, including echocardiogram, was negative. An ensuing carotid magnetic resonance examination with a phased-array carotid coil and high-resolution (0.3 × 0.3 mm pixel size) multicontrast weighted sequences confirmed the stenosis and demonstrated ulceration and calcification in both carotids and mural thrombus formation in the left carotid (Figs. 1 and 2). After completely recovering from the stroke, the patient underwent staged bilateral carotid endarterectomies. Histological examination of the specimens confirmed the magnetic resonance imaging (MRI) findings of bilateral ulceration and left mural thrombus formation (Fig. 3).

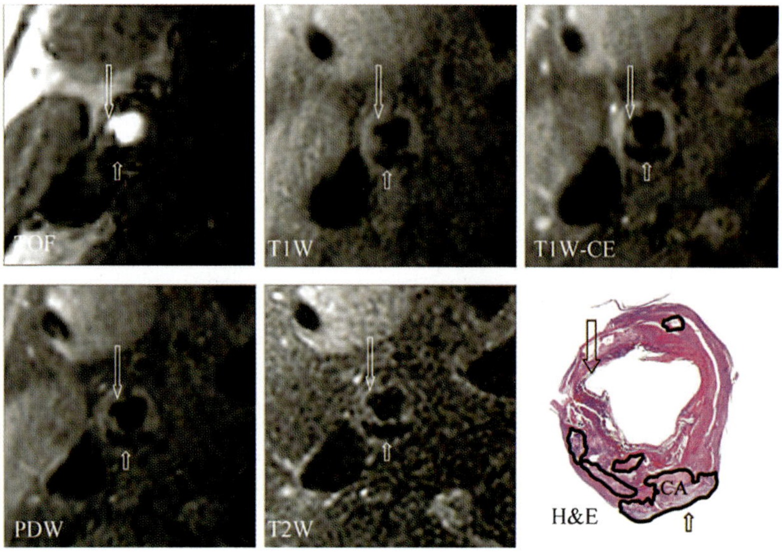

Figure 1. 3-D time-of-flight (TOF) image shows a surface ulcer (long arrow) in the distal right common carotid artery. Black-blood, fast-spin echo, T1-weighted (T1W), postcontrast-enhanced T1W (T1W-CE), proton density weighted (PDW), and T2-weighted (T2W) images confirm surface discontinuity. The hypointense areas on all four weightings correspond to calcifications (short arrows).

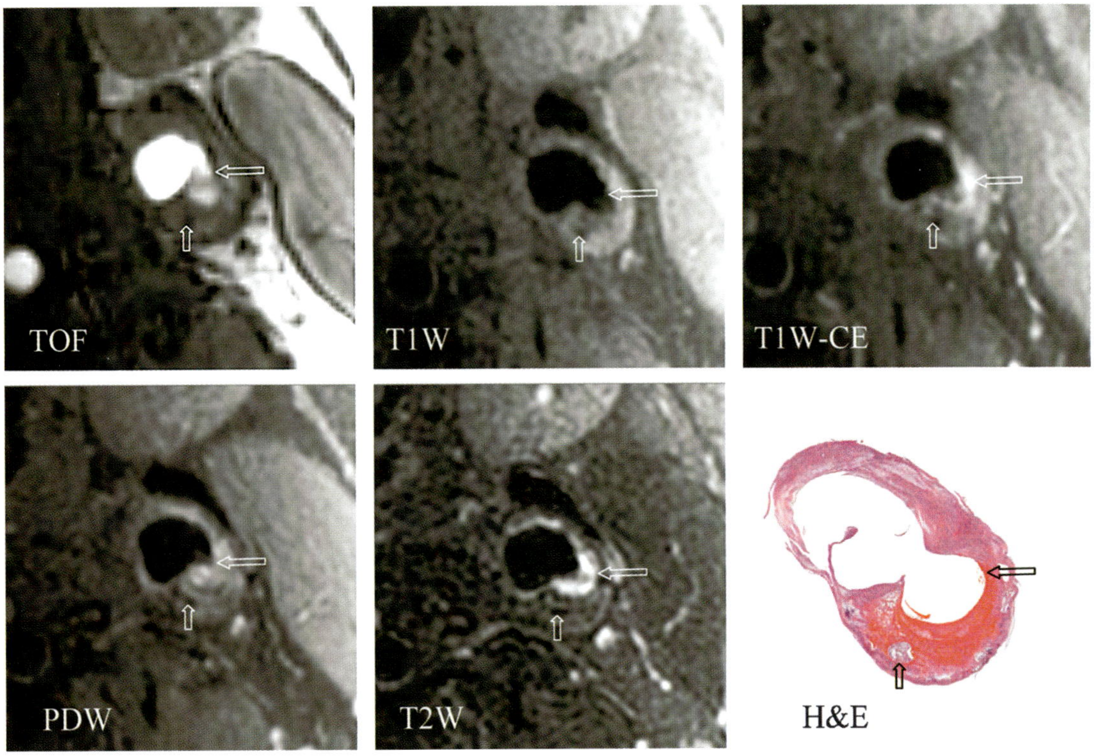

Figure 2. All weightings of the left carotid artery show a distinct ulcer (long arrows) and a small calcification (short arrows). The striking hyperintensity on the ulcer surface in the T2W image indicates the presence of a mural thrombus. Focal contrast enhancement on T1W-CE indicates vasculature at the base of the thrombus.

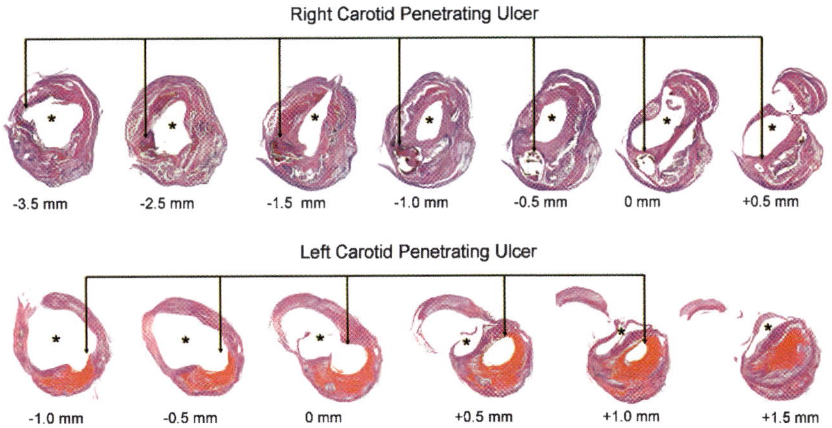

Figure 3. Hematoxylin and eosin (H&E) stain of right and left carotid endarterectomy specimens. The right plaque contained extensive calcifications and fibrosis. A well-defined penetrating ulcer extends 4 mm from the lumen surface through a fibrotic matrix. A penetrating ulcer with mural thrombus formation is seen in the left carotid endarterectomy specimen. Asterisks are placed in the lumen of the common and the internal arteries of both carotids. Location indicators are millimeter distance to the bifurcation. + indicates locations in the internal carotid artery; –, locations in the common carotid artery.

28

Transient Occlusion of the Middle Cerebral Artery by Macroembolism during Carotid Stenting for Traumatic Dissection of the Common Carotid Artery

Eisuke Furui, MD; Yoshikazu Okamoto, MD; Shinya Kida, MD; Junkoh Yamashita, MD; Osamu Matsui, MD; Masahito Yamada, MD

From the Department of Neurology & Neurobiology of Aging (E.F., M.Y.), Department of Neurosurgery (Y.O., S.K., J.Y.), and Department of Radiology (O.M.), Kanazawa University Graduate School of Medical Science, Kanazawa, Japan.

(*Circulation*. 2005;112:e33–e34.)

DOI: 10.1161.CIRCULATIONAHA.104.417698.

Carotid stenting has been used more frequently not only for atherosclerotic carotid stenosis but also for dissection of the carotid artery. Transcranial Doppler ultrasound (TCD) has been reported to be able to detect circulating cerebral microembolic signals in patients with ischemic stroke. TCD can provide useful online information about hemodynamic change and cerebral embolism during carotid endarterectomy. We present our findings during carotid stenting in a patient to illustrate an obstruction of the middle cerebral artery (MCA) main trunk by a macroembolus resulting in ischemic stroke. A 27-year-old man with traumatic dissection of the left common carotid artery with the intimal flap underwent carotid stenting without the use of a distal protection device. We used a TCD machine (Multi-Dop X4, DWL) with two 2-MHz probes mounted on a head frame to insonate the bilateral MCA through the transtemporal window. The dissection was stented with a self-expanding, 8 × 27 mm Wallstent. An 8 × 40 mm balloon was introduced to dilate the stent further, but was removed later without inflation because of the mismatch between the length of the balloon and that of the stent. During this manipulation, we detected three embolic signals from the left MCA having unique chirping sounds. Thereafter, the left MCA mean velocity suddenly decreased from 68 to 16 cm/s (Fig. 1). The patient developed aphasia and right hemiparesis. Within 5 minutes of this episode, the MCA velocity returned to the previous value with no additional embolic signals. The cerebral angiogram obtained after the normalization of the MCA velocity showed left MCA branch occlusion (Fig. 2). A microcatheter system was advanced and located near the occluded artery. Although intra-arterial infusion of 300,000 U urokinase was administered, recanalization was not obtained. Diffusion-weighted images performed 3 days later revealed a fresh cortical infarct in the left MCA territory (Fig. 3). One month later, the patient had almost completely recovered from aphasia and right hemiparesis.

This case demonstrates an obstruction of the MCA main trunk by a macroembolus probably being dislodged from the carotid dissection, followed by spontaneous recanalization and distal embolism. The macroembolism was supported by the findings of both the cerebral angiography and the diffusion-weighted images. This is the first report that describes a macroembolism detected as embolic signals and the sudden decline of MCA velocity during carotid stenting. TCD can noninvasively detect both microembolism and macroembolism during carotid stenting.

Section II

Coronary Arteries

29

Systolic Obliteration of the Left Anterior Descending Coronary Artery

Michael A. Fifer, MD; Joon S. Lee, MD; Adolph M. Hutter, Jr, MD; Mortimer J. Buckley, MD

From the Departments of Medicine (Cardiac Unit) (M.A.F., J.S.L., A.M.H.) and Surgery (Surgical Cardiovascular Unit) (M.J.B.), Massachusetts General Hospital and Harvard Medical School, Boston, Mass.

(*Circulation*. 1993;88:2437.)

A 67-year-old man who had undergone aortic valve replacement with a porcine heterograft for aortic stenosis 16 years earlier presented with dyspnea on exertion and fatigue. He did not have angina. Physical examination indicated severe aortic regurgitation. Cardiac catheterization demonstrated right atrial pressure of 5 mm Hg; pulmonary arterial pressure, 44/16 mm Hg; pulmonary capillary wedge pressure, 14 mm Hg; left ventricular pressure, 200/26 mm Hg; and aortic pressure, 140/40 mm Hg. Cardiac output was 5.7 L/min, and cardiac index was 2.9 L min^{-1} m^{-2}. Left ventricular ejection fraction was normal. Supravalvar aortography confirmed the presence of severe aortic regurgitation. Coronary arteriography was normal except for the finding illustrated in the Figure 1.

Repeat aortic valve replacement was performed 2 days after cardiac catheterization. An edge of the pericardium, which was not closed after the first operation, was observed to overlie the mid-to-distal left anterior descending coronary artery. During systole, torsion of the heart resulted in tensing of the pericardium in such a manner as to compress the artery. After the pericardium was freed from the surface of the heart, the left anterior descending coronary artery was observed to be a normal epicardial vessel without an intramyocardial segment.

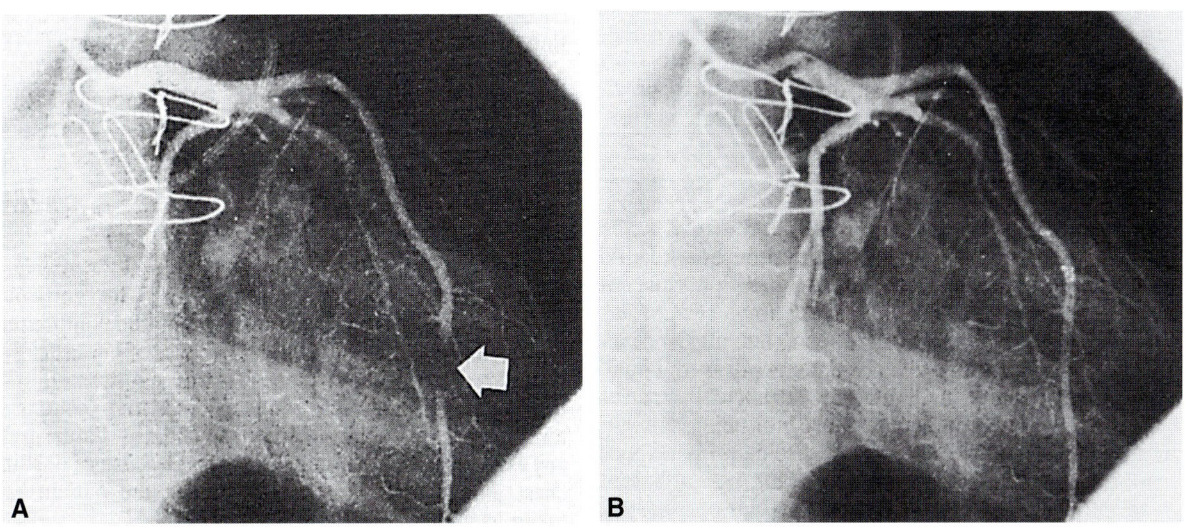

Figure 1. Systolic **(A)** and diastolic **(B)** frames within one cardiac cycle from the left coronary arteriogram. There is obliteration of a segment of the mid-to-distal left anterior descending coronary artery (arrow) in systole, with normal lumen caliber in diastole. The bioprosthetic valve and sternal wires are seen.

30

Multiple Coronary Emboli from a Calcified Rheumatic Aortic Valve

Ranjit Suri, MD; Robert M. Jeresaty, MD

From St Francis Hospital and Medical Center and University of Connecticut School of Medicine, Hartford, Conn.

(*Circulation*. 1994;90:623–624.)

A 51-year-old woman with known rheumatic aortic and mitral valve disease developed progressive exertional angina. Cardiac catheterization demonstrated severe aortic stenosis, mild aortic insufficiency, moderate mitral stenosis, and normal left ventricular function. Cardiac catheterization was not associated with chest pain or electrocardiogram (ECG) changes suggesting coronary embolism during the procedure. Coronary arteriography (Fig. 1A) showed two bizarre intraluminal filling defects (arrows) narrowing the proximal left anterior descending coronary artery (LAD) and a large circumflex marginal (LCx) branch by about 80%. The patient underwent an aortic valve replacement, open mitral commissurotomy, and aortocoronary bypass grafting to the LAD and LCx (Dr S. Chawla). Figure 1B shows the intraluminal calcium embolus (arrow) as seen through the wall of the marginal branch. This was removed by direct arteriotomy; however, attempts at removing the proximal LAD embolus with a Fogarty catheter were unsuccessful. Otherwise, the coronary arteries appeared perfectly normal. Figure 1C shows the calcified aortic valve and the arrow points to the calcium emboli removed from the LCx branch. The patient has done well after surgery.

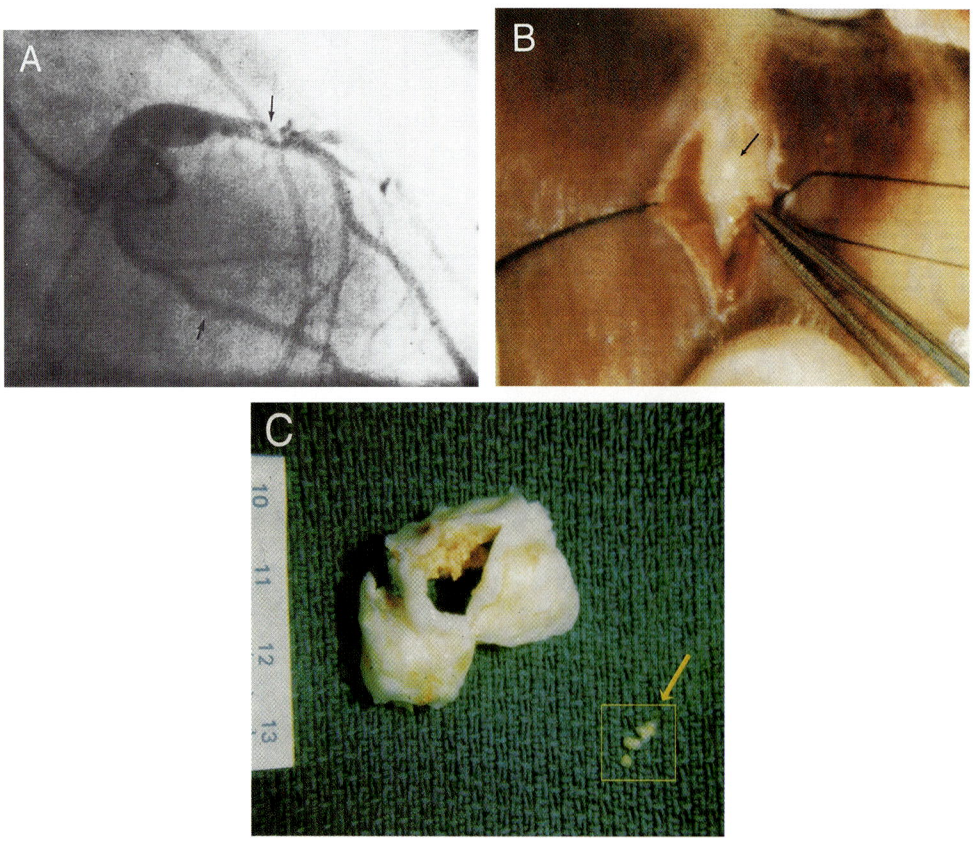

Figure 1.

31 Circumflex Artery Aneurysm

Kamthorn S. Lee, MD; Pieter M. Vandervoort, MD
From the Department of Cardiology, Cleveland Clinic Foundation, Cleveland, Ohio.

(*Circulation*. 1995;92:672.)

The patient was a 71-year-old man who had a known circumflex artery aneurysm and coronary artery bypass surgery in 1982. The aneurysm was left intact because of difficulty in surgical removal at that time. Recently, because of symptoms of angina pectoris, he underwent coronary arteriography, which demonstrated occlusion of saphenous venous grafts and patency of the left internal thoracic arterial graft.

The patient then had an aortocoronary bypass and mitral valve replacement (for mitral regurgitation) at our institution. At surgery, the circumflex artery aneurysm was found to measure 6 × 8 cm in the superior aspect of the atrioventricular grove. This aneurysm was not excised because of technical difficulty.

This case illustrates the appearance of an arterial aneurysm by multiple modalities: transesophageal echocardiography, magnetic resonance imaging (MRI), selective coronary angiography, and direct visualization.

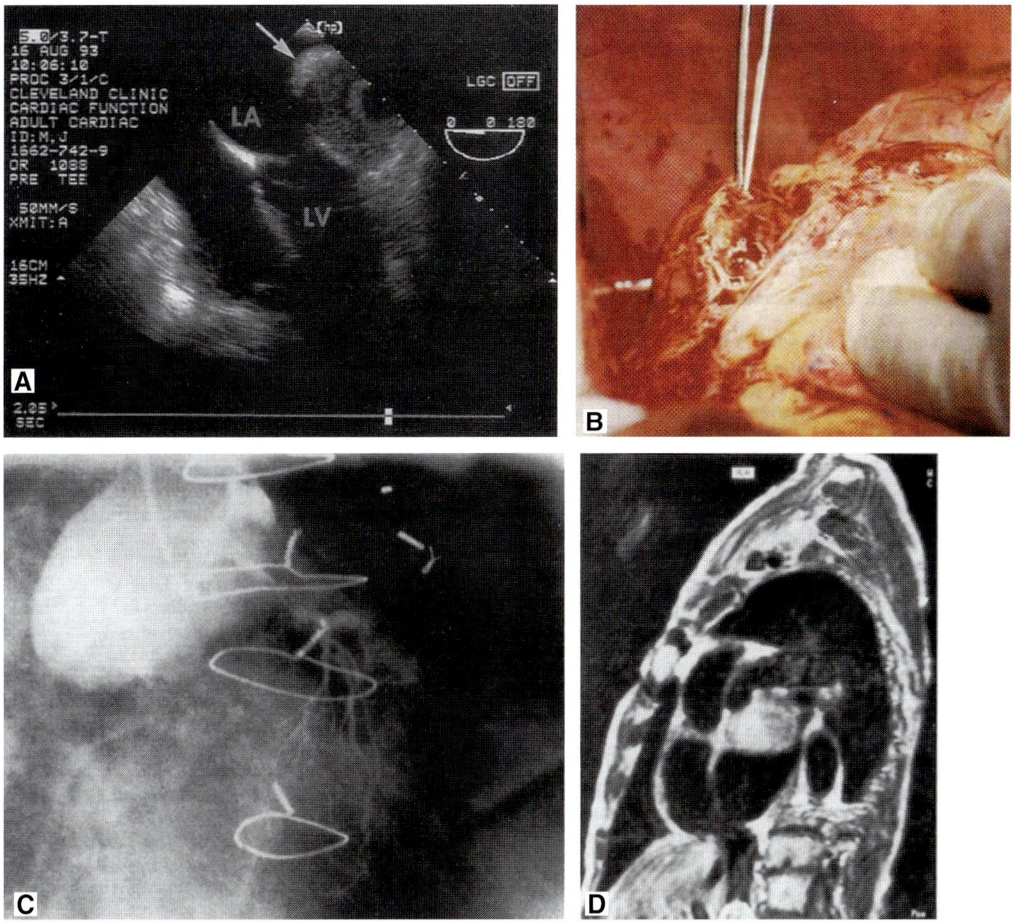

Figure 1. A, Transesophageal echocardiogram: transverse view of the circumflex artery aneurysm. LA indicates left atrium; LV, left ventricle. Arrow points to the circumflex artery aneurysm. **B,** Circumflex artery aneurysm seen by direct visualization. **C,** Right anterior oblique view of the circumflex artery aneurysm at angiography. **D,** Sagittal view of the aneurysm by MRI.

32 Improvement of Myocardial Perfusion after Transmyocardial Laser Revascularization and Coronary Artery Bypass Graft Surgery

Ami E. Iskandrian, MD; James D. Sink, MD; William VanDecker, MD

From Allegheny University of the Health Sciences, MCP–Hahnemann School of Medicine, Philadelphia, Pa.

(*Circulation*. 1998;98:728–729.)

A 69-year-old man with severe angina had severe three vessel disease by coronary angiography. At the time of coronary revascularization, he had left internal mammary artery implantation to the left anterior descending artery, a vein graft to the diagonal branch, and a vein graft to the marginal branch of the left circumflex artery. Transmyocardial laser revascularization was performed in the territory of the right coronary artery (because of poor distal runoff) with a xenon chloride excimer laser (under an investigational device exemption sponsored by United States Surgical Corp). The postoperative course was uneventful. The patient experienced improvement of symptoms.

The patient had an exercise treadmill test by the Bruce protocol before and ≈3 months after surgery. Before surgery, he developed angina during exercise with ST-segment depression at 75% of maximum predicted heart rate. After surgery, he exercised to 87% of maximum predicted heart rate with no angina or ST-segment depression.

Before surgery, exercise single photon emission computed tomography (SPECT) ^{99m}Tc-sestamibi myocardial images revealed extensive reversible perfusion defects consistent with three vessel ischemia. After surgery, the exercise SPECT perfusion images were almost normal (Fig. 1). The improvement in the perfusion pattern during exercise was equally remarkable in the vascular area treated with laser and the vascular territories treated with bypass surgery.

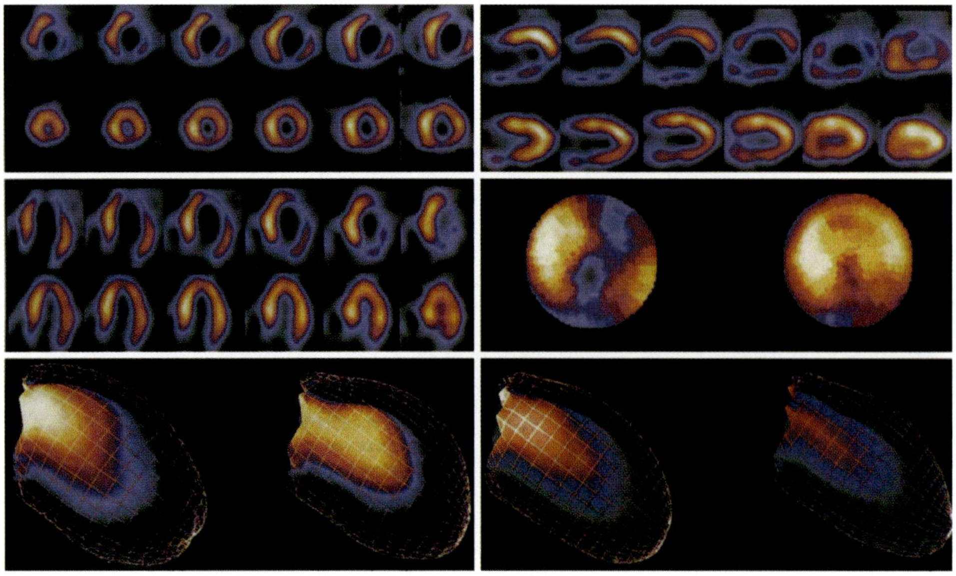

Figure 1.

33

Plaque Types

Bruce J. Kimura, MD; Robert J. Russo, MD, PhD; William F. Penny, MD
From the Division of Cardiovascular Medicine, UCSD Medical Center, San Diego, Calif.

(*Circulation*. 1996;94:3382.)

The accompanying figure illustrates differences in plaque composition, as detected by intravascular ultrasound, in a 57-year-old man with a markedly positive exercise stress test.

The coronary angiogram (left anterior oblique projection) demonstrates a tight 95% stenosis in the left anterior descending artery after the bifurcation of a diagonal branch (B), as well as a mild 50% stenosis in the middle portion of the vessel (C). Intravascular ultrasound imaging was performed at both sites with a 3.5F, 30-MHz catheter. Figure 1B, the proximal lesion has concentric morphology and multiple echogenic regions characteristic of "hard" plaque. Calcific deposits are seen as bright areas with acoustic shadowing (dark arrows). The branching diagonal is noted (Br). Figure 1C, the distal lesion shows an eccentric atheroma with a large echolucent region (white arrow) representative of a necrotic lipid pool in "soft" plaque. In both images, the catheter position within the lumen (+) and the guidewire artifact (gw) can be seen; intermarker distance is 1 mm. Catheter-based revascularization was performed on the proximal lesion only.

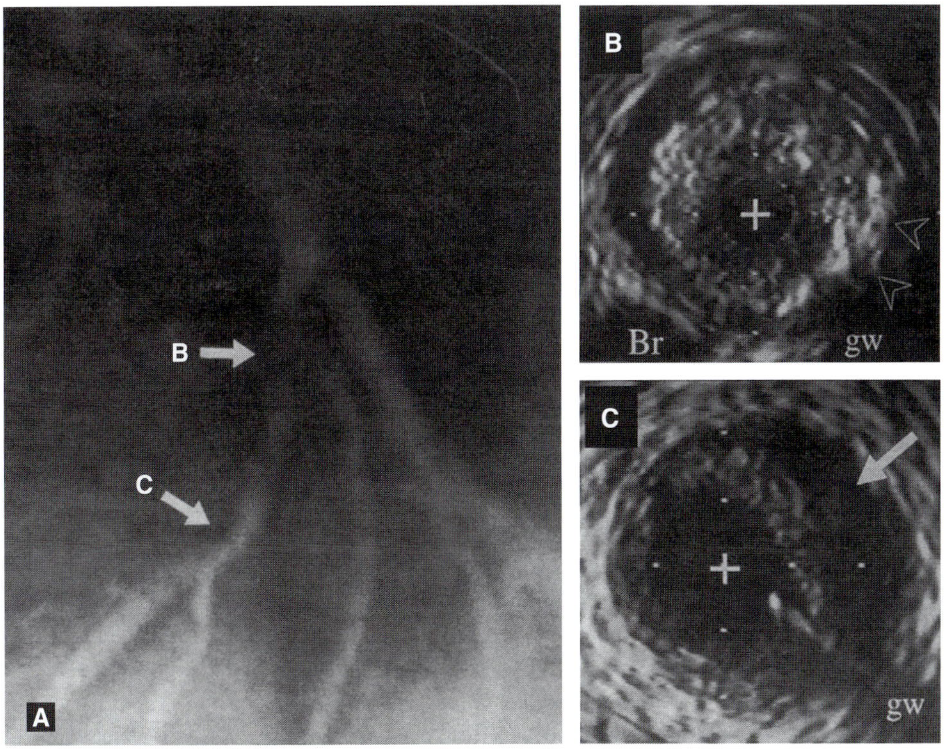

Figure 1.

34 Kawasaki Disease: Coronary Aneurysms in Mother and Son

Elchanan Bruckheimer, MBBS; Ziad Bulbul, MD; Paul McCarthy, MD; Joseph A. Madri, MD; Alan H. Friedman, MD; William E. Hellenbrand, MD

From the Section of Pediatric Cardiology, General Pediatrics (P.M.), and Department of Pathology (J.A.M. and W.E.H), Yale University School of Medicine, New Haven, Conn.

(*Circulation*. 1998;97:410–411).

A 33-year-old woman developed shock and died 16 hours after labor with moderate hemorrhage. Her autopsy revealed (Fig. 1) large (>1.5 cm), calcified aneurysms of the proximal right (RCA), left main (LCA), and left anterior descending coronary arteries (Ao indicates aorta). Plain radiographs (Fig. 2) demonstrated the calcification. Histology showed no atherosclerotic changes or active arteritis, and the aorta and other large vessels were normal. When the patient was 16 years old, she had had a prolonged undiagnosed febrile illness with peripheral edema and desquamation, lymphadenopathy, and rash. The combination of this previous illness and extensive and solely coronary artery disease suggests Kawasaki disease (KD). This woman's son, the product of that pregnancy, was admitted 5 years later with classic KD. Treatment with high-dose aspirin and single-dose intravenous gamma globulin was initiated on day 5 of illness, with defervescence within 36 hours. Four weeks after discharge, two-dimensional echocardiography showed 4-mm dilatation of the proximal right coronary artery with a long fusiform aneurysm of 5- to 6-mm diameter more distally. The left main coronary artery was dilated to 6 mm, and there was a long fusiform aneurysm of the left anterior descending branch of 6-mm diameter. Figure 3, Parasternal short-axis view showing the aortic valve (Ao) with a dilated left main coronary artery (LCA). Figure 4, Parasternal long-axis view with cranial angulation showing the dilated left main coronary artery and a fusiform aneurysm of the proximal left anterior descending branch (LAD). These findings were present for 6 months and then resolved completely. Coronary artery aneurysms due to KD occurring in a parent and child have not been reported previously.

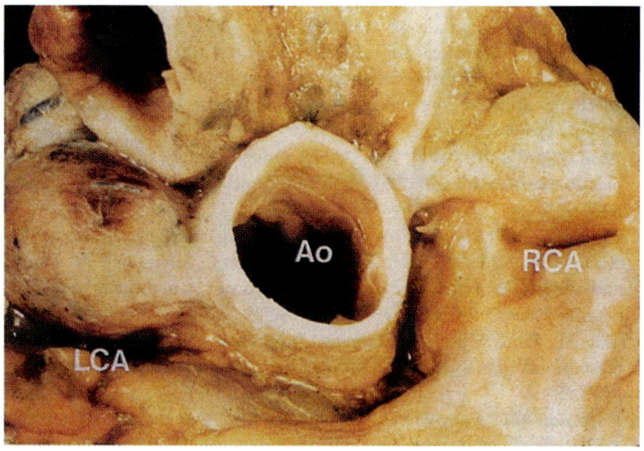

Figure 1.

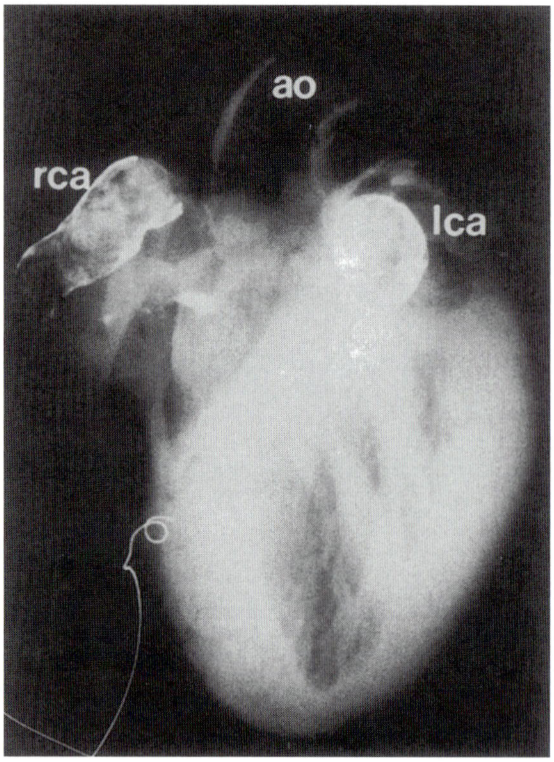

Figure 2.

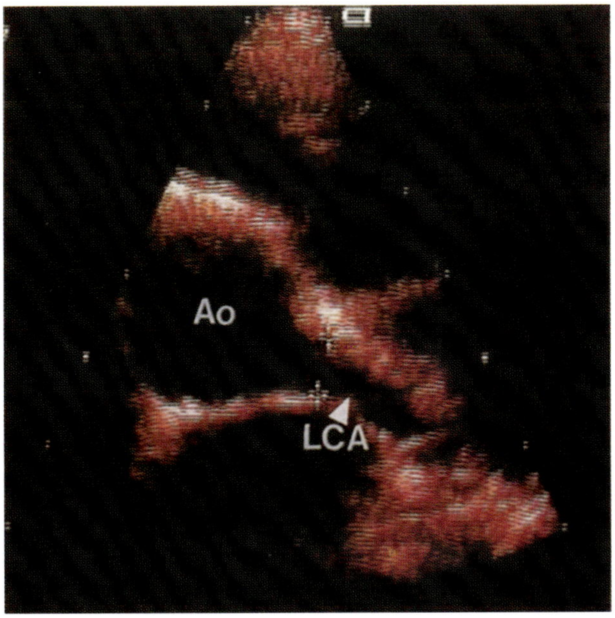

Figure 3.

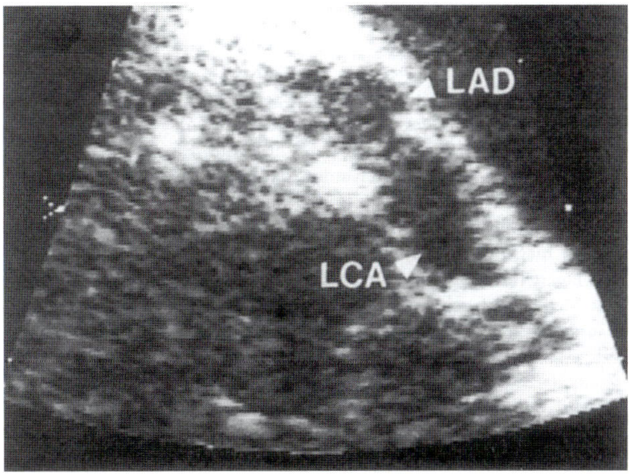

Figure 4.

35 Sudden Death due to Rupture of Coronary Aneurysm in a 26-Year-Old Man

Masahiko Satoda, MD; Hirotaka Tatsukawa, MD; Shuji Katoh, MD

From Asahi University, the Division of Cardiology, Murakami Memorial Hospital, Hashimoto-cho, Gifu, Japan.

(*Circulation*. 1998;97:705–706.)

A 26-year-old man, previously in good health, was transferred to the emergency unit of our hospital on July 19, 1995; however, he was dead on arrival. He was an employee of a machine industry with no history of chest pain or palpitation, and at company checkups, no abnormalities were pointed out except for marked left hilar calcification on chest radiograph in June 1991 (Fig. 1); moreover, when he was 1 year old, he suffered from an acute self-limited febrile illness with diffuse erythematous macular rash followed by membranous desquamation of the fingertips and notable conjunctival infection resembling Stevens-Johnson syndrome or mucocutaneous lymph node syndrome that occurred 2 years after the first description of Kawasaki disease. About half an hour before admission, he had suddenly lost consciousness while playing catch during the noon break. Despite cardiopulmonary resuscitation, he died, and an autopsy was performed immediately.

A small, fresh hematoma was seen on the epicardial surface close to the proximal left anterior descending coronary artery (Fig. 2A). The true lumen was heavily calcified and stenotic, and the pseudolumen was coated internally with a smooth intimal membrane (Fig. 2B). A postmortem angiogram (Fig. 3) revealed that the saccular aneurysm communicated with the true lumen. The circumflex artery was also depicted, suggesting that there was no thrombotic occlusion of the left descending artery, and secondary strangulation of the true lumen due to the aneurysm rupture might have evoked an anteroseptal acute myocardial infarction (Fig. 3).

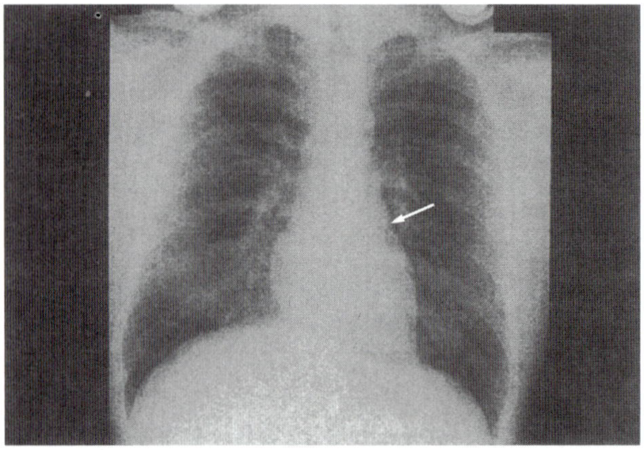

Figure 1. Chest radiograph showing small left hilar calcification (arrow).

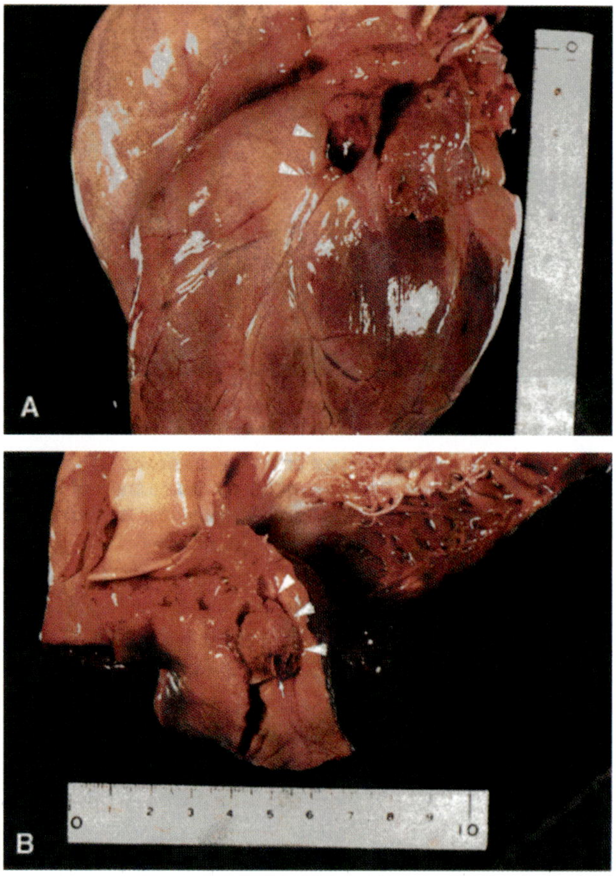

Figure 2. A, Anterior surface of left ventricle showing small, dark-colored hematoma around proximal left descending coronary artery (arrowheads). **B,** When epicardium was removed, true lumen (arrow) was revealed to be heavily calcified and stenotic; saccular aneurysm was depicted posteriorly (arrowheads).

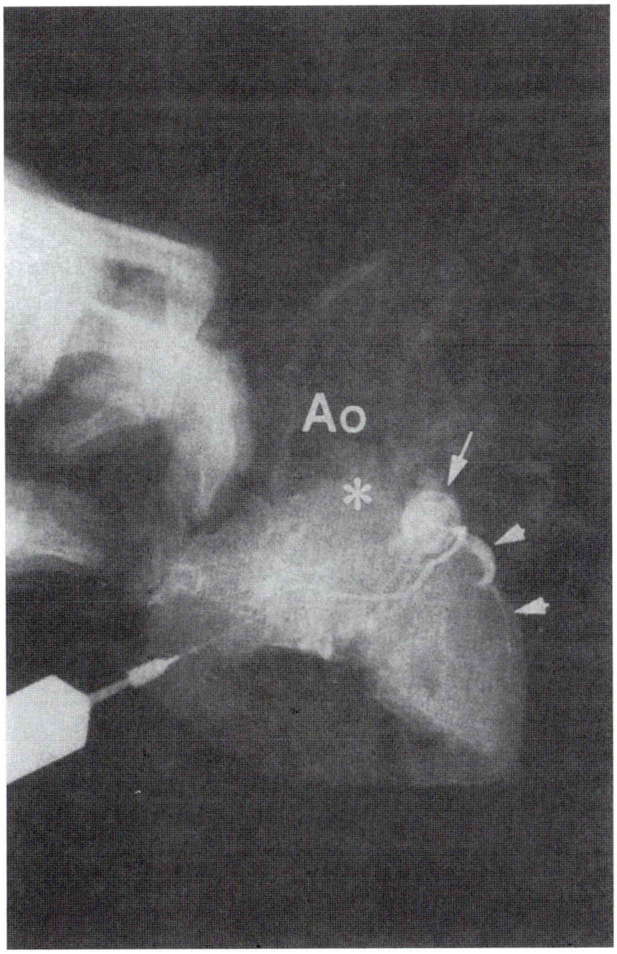

Figure 3. Postmortem angiogram; radiographic contrast agent was injected retrogradely into left anterior descending coronary artery. Saccular aneurysm was depicted (arrow), then medium disclosed tributary of circumflex artery (arrowheads), showing that there was no complete obstruction of true lumen of left anterior descending coronary artery. Ao indicates ascending aorta; asterisk, left sinus of Valsalva and left main trunk.

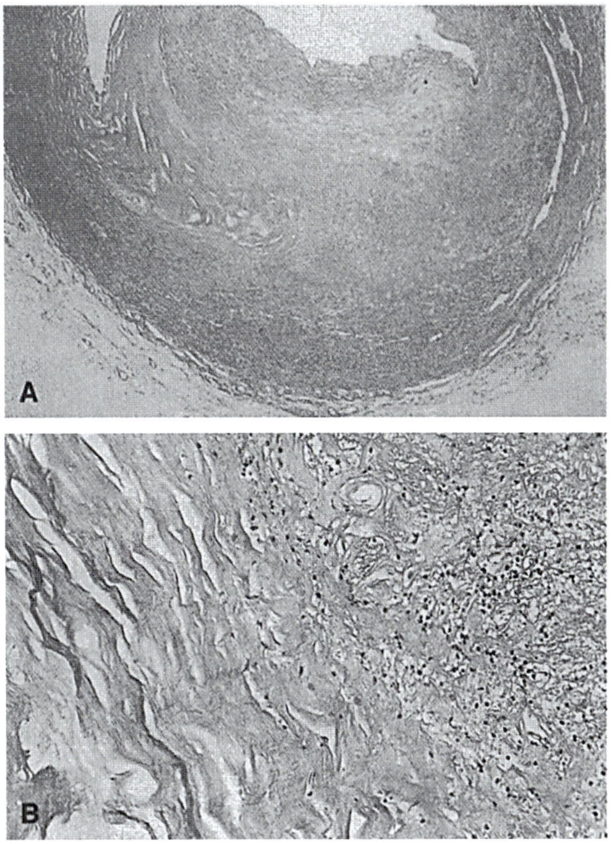

Figure 4. A, Photomicrographs of small epicardial coronary artery showing marked intimal thickening and destruction of intimal lamina, but no inflammatory infiltration was seen in this section (magnification ×60; hematoxylin and eosin stain). **B,** Photomicrograph of epicardial coronary artery near aneurysm showing inflammatory cell infiltration into adventitia. Predominant cells are lymphocytes and plasma cells (magnification ×400).

Histologically, diffuse intimal thickening was seen throughout the epicardial artery, and leukocyte infiltration into the adventitia and vasa vasorum was seen around the aneurysm, indicating persistent mild vasculitis of the artery (Fig. 4). Rupture of a coronary aneurysm is more common in the acute or subacute phase of Kawasaki disease, but to the best of our knowledge, our report is the first case in the literature of mucocutaneous lymph node disease of aneurysm rupture due to persistent vasculitis at the healed stage more than 10 years after disease onset. Further discussion is needed, including therapeutic options for non-aspirin-treated patients.

36 Discordance between Coronary Angiography and Intracoronary Ultrasound

Ted Feldman, MD; Thomas N. Levin, MD

From the University of Chicago Hospital, Cardiology Section, Hans Hecht Hemodynamics Laboratory, Chicago, Ill.

(*Circulation*. 1998;97:1208.)

A 57-year-old woman presented with typical angina. Thallium stress testing showed anteroapical reversible ischemia. Coronary angiography demonstrated only a mild stenosis (open black arrow) of the mid-left anterior descending coronary artery (LAD). She was treated medically and did not improve. Intravascular ultrasound examination was used to further evaluate this ambiguous coronary stenosis.

Figure 1 shows the angiogram of left coronary system and six ultrasound images acquired at various locations within LAD, shown by white arrows. A 7F diagnostic catheter (solid short white arrow) provides a reference diameter of 2.2 mm.

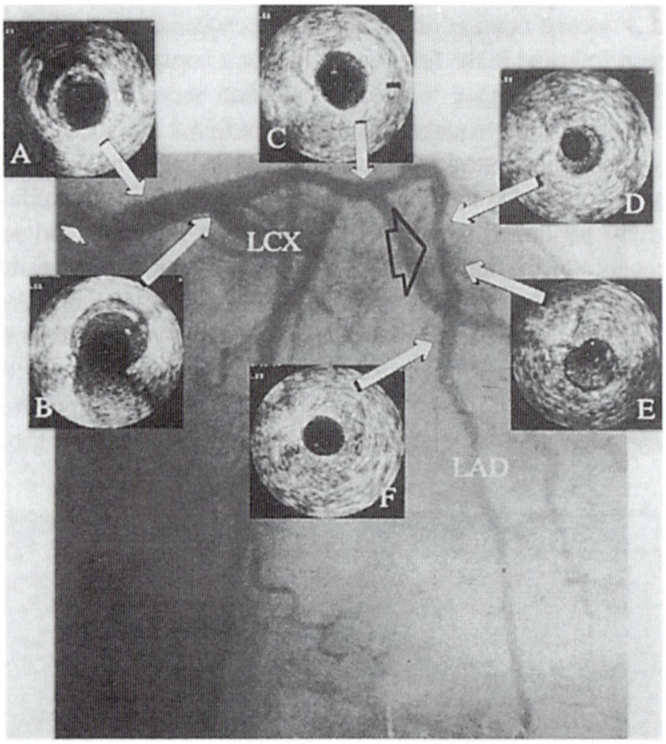

Figure 1. **A,** Image from mid-left main coronary artery. Vessel lumen is compromised by a crescentic fibrous plaque extending from 7 o'clock to 2 o'clock position. **B,** Bifurcation of left main artery into LAD and left circumflex (LCX). **C,** Proximal reference vessel. Lumen diameter is ≈3 × 3 mm. Black hash mark at 3 o'clock position shows a 1-mm calibration. **D,** Entry into this indeterminate lesion has only a small rim of echolucent lumen around ultrasound catheter. A near circumferential plaque fills rest of lumen. **E,** Tightest point seen by intravascular ultrasound demonstrates white echodense plaque surrounding ultrasound catheter, almost obliterating vessel lumen. **F,** Distal reference artery beyond stenosis shows a widely patent vessel with minimal atherosclerosis.

37 Pectus Excavatum with Inferior Ischemia in Right Lateral Position

Thomas A. Heitzer, MD; Helmut Wollschlager, MD
From the Medizinische Klinik III, Kardiologie, Universität Freiburg, Germany.

(*Circulation*. 1998;98:605–606.)

A 56-year-old woman with pectus excavatum presented with a 2-year history of increasing chest pain only while she was lying on her right side. The electrocardiogram (ECG) showed ST-segment elevation in inferior leads (Fig. 1A) when the patient was in the right lateral position and became normal when she turned onto her back. A computed tomography (CT) of the thorax (Fig. 1B) showed the funnel-chest deformity and severe sternal depression, with close contact to the proximal part of the ascending aorta. Coronary angiography showed no coronary artery disease or any abnormality in supine position (Fig. 1D), but revealed proximal compression of the right coronary artery only when the patient lay on her right side (Fig. 1C).

Surgical treatment with repair of the chest deformity was successfully performed and made the patient angina free.

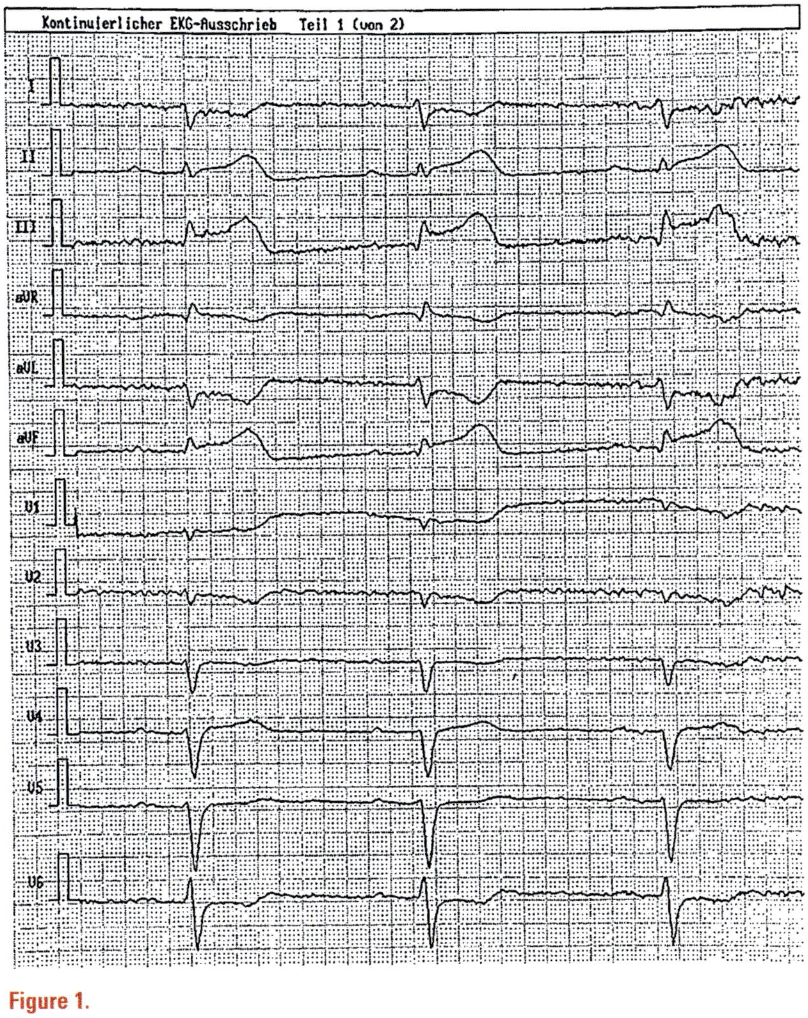

Figure 1.

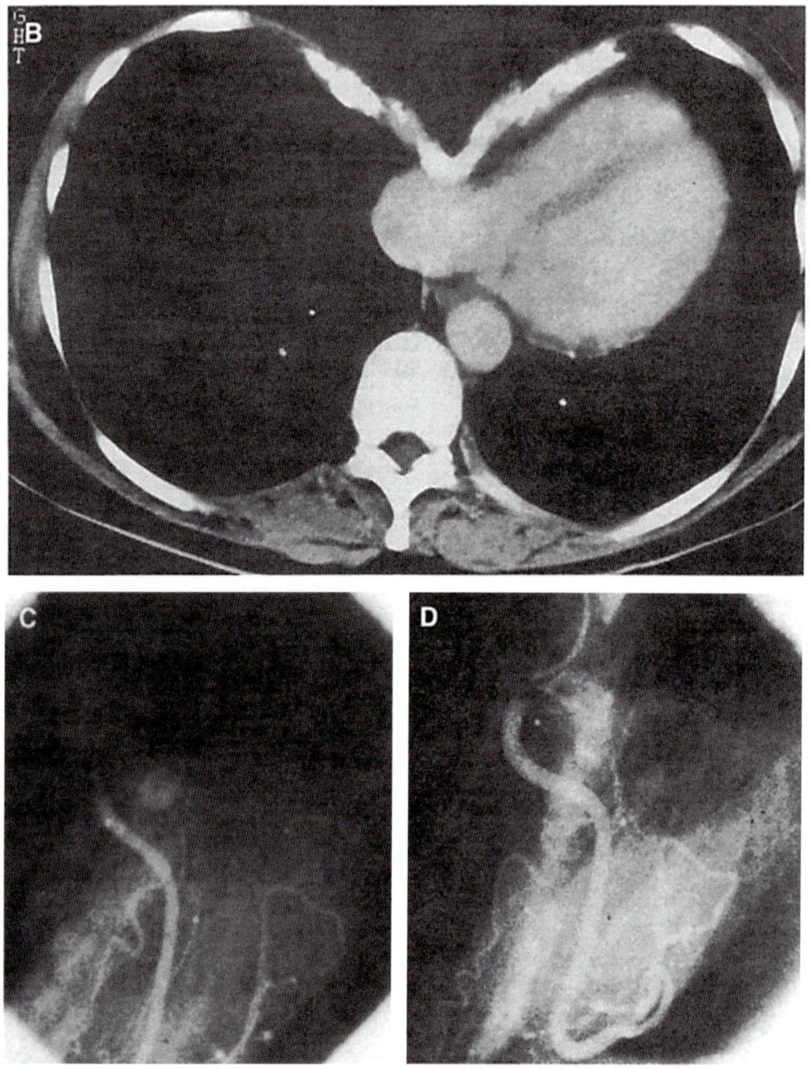

Figure 1. *(continued)*

38 Angiographic and Ultrasonic Evidence of Plaque Rupture Causing Myocardial Infarction

Hani S. Al-Sergani, MBBS; Philip J. Fitzpatrick, MD; Sergio Waxman, MD

From the Cardiovascular Division, Beth Israel Deaconess Medical Center, Harvard Medical School, Boston, Mass.

(*Circulation*. 1998;98:1348.)

A 60-year-old man with no prior cardiac history presented to the emergency room with 1.5 hours of substernal chest pain. An electrocardiogram (ECG) revealed ST-segment elevation in leads V_2 to V_6. Acute anterolateral myocardial infarction was diagnosed, and thrombolytic therapy in the form of tetradecanoylphorbol acetate (tPA) was administered, with resolution of the chest pain and ST-segment elevation. Because of postinfarct angina, he underwent urgent cardiac catheterization. Coronary angiography (Fig. 1A) revealed a focal linear intraluminal filling defect in the middle portion of the left anterior descending coronary artery (arrow). Intravascular ultrasound of the corresponding area (Fig. 1B) demonstrated the presence of an eccentric lesion with a hypoechoic crescentic area within the plaque (large arrow) and an overlying cap (small arrow). The hypoechoic area within the lesion partially filled with contrast material and probably represents the site of a lipid pool in a plaque that ruptured. On the basis of the ultrasound findings, the angiogram showed the eccentric lesion filling with contrast material beneath a fibrous cap. A 4 mm intracoronary Palmaz-Schatz stent was placed successfully, with no residual stenosis. The patient had a full recovery and was discharged home on day five of hospitalization.

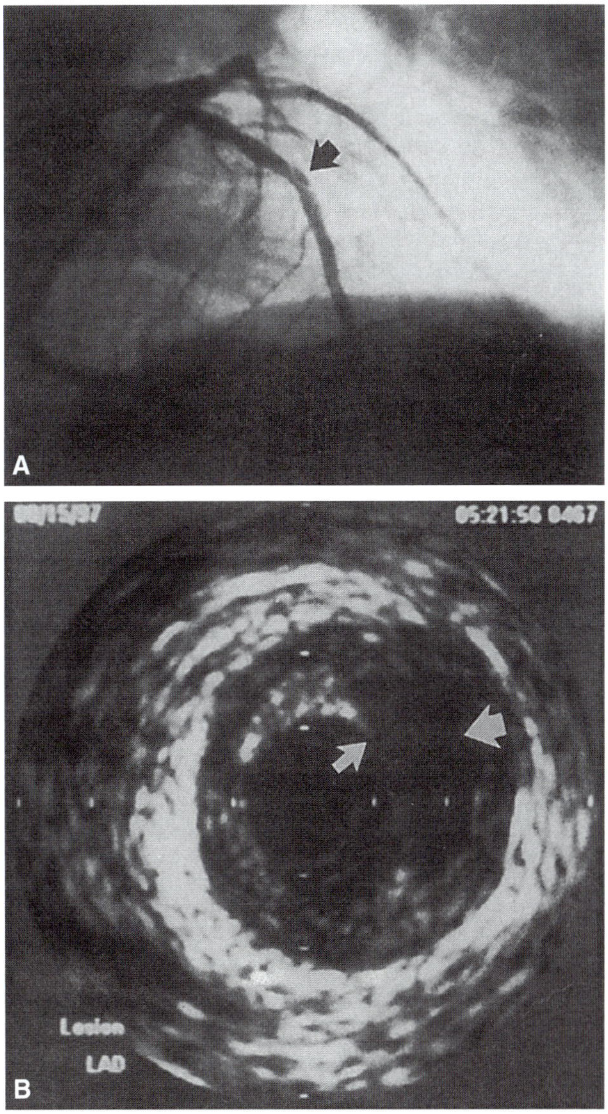

Figure 1.

39

Progress in Device Technology

Victor Parsonnet, MD

From the Department of Surgery and the New Jersey Pacemaker and Defibrillator Evaluation Center, Newark Beth Israel Medical Center, Newark, NJ.

(*Circulation*. 1998;98:1456.)

Advances in implantable device technology over the past few years can be seen in these illustrations. Figure 1 shows a 1997-model implantable cardioverter-defibrillator (ICD) in front of an older version. Beside it is a modern single-chamber pacemaker in front of an older mercury-zinc-cell model. Table 1 shows their relative weights. These devices are now small enough to permit implantation of both in the same pectoral position (Fig. 2). The implanted devices in this case were not the same as the one in the photograph but were of similar vintage. Tomorrow's dual-chamber pacemakers and ICDs will surely be contained in the same "can" and will be smaller still.

TABLE 1. Comparison of Pulse-Generator Weights

	Early Model	1997 Model		Percent Early-Model Weight
	Weight (g)	Weight (g)	Percent Reduction in Weight	
ICD	270	96	64	35
Pacemaker	150	13	150	9

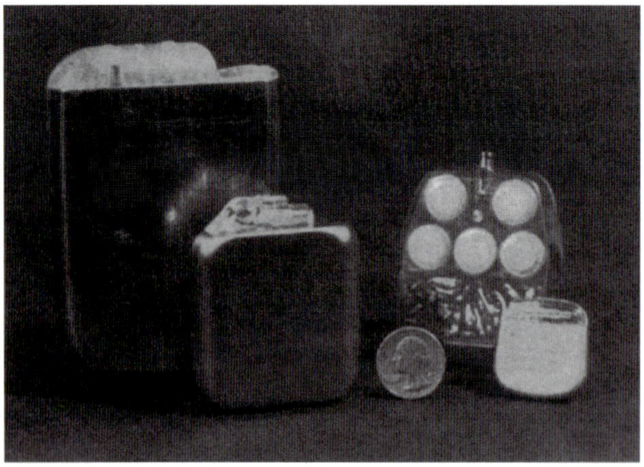

Figure 1.

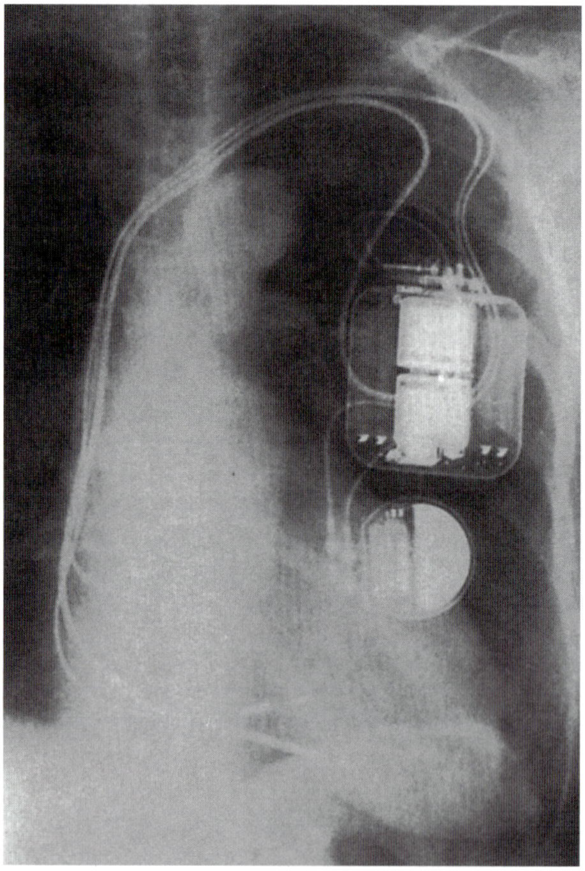

Figure 2.

40 Spontaneous Postpartum Coronary Dissection

Felix H. Lee, MD; Alan C. Yeung, MD; Michael B. Fowler, MB, FRCP; Peter J. Fitzgerald, MD, PhD
From the Division of Cardiovascular Medicine, Stanford University School of Medicine, Stanford, Calif.

(*Circulation*. 1999;99:721.)

A 32-year-old 15-day-postpartum G3P2 woman presented with sudden cardiac arrest due to an acute anterolateral wall myocardial infarction. An emergent coronary angiogram revealed a mild 30% distal left main tapering, severe diffuse compromise of the left anterior descending coronary artery (LAD) as well as the diagonal lumen, and normal left circumflex (LCx) and right coronary arteries. Three days later, the patient developed chest pain with 3 mm inferolateral ST-segment elevations by electrocardiogram (ECG). A second emergent coronary angiogram revealed a new second obtuse marginal occlusion that did not respond to intracoronary nitroglycerin, verapamil, or adenosine. This lesion was successfully treated with percutaneous transluminal coronary angioplasty with a 2.5 mm balloon. The patient was supported with an intra-aortic balloon pump. Intravascular ultrasound evaluation (Fig. 1) revealed a dissection originating at the bifurcation of the LAD and the LCx along the nonmural plane of the vessel. Both retrograde extension into the mid left main coronary artery and anterograde extension into the LAD and involvement of the LCx origin were present. Three months later, the patient has remained asymptomatic and has demonstrated serial improvement in her ejection fraction by transthoracic echocardiogram.

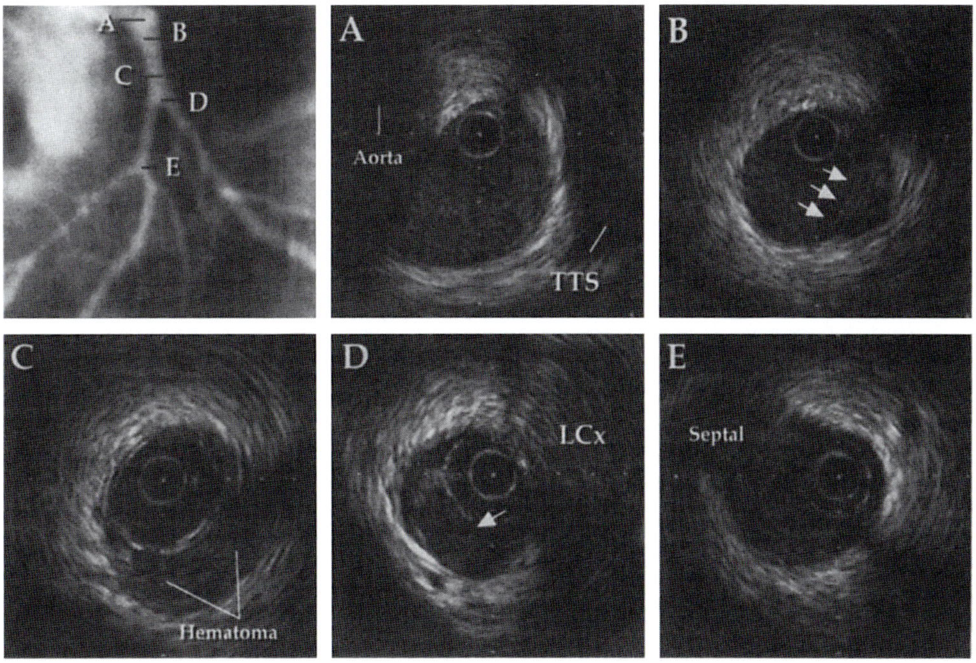

Figure 1. A, Intravascular ultrasound image in proximal aorta demonstrating transthoracic sinus (TTS) as it anatomically defines coronary nonmural surface, opposite mural surface (this plane of dissection contributed to extensive circumferential expansion as well as diffuse distal extension into both LCx origin and entire length of LAD); **B,** Mid left main: retrograde extent of dissection plane and hematoma is demonstrated by arrows; **C,** Distal left main demonstrating hematoma as it arcs around true lumen; **D,** LAD and LCx bifurcation: arrow demonstrates intimal tear of origin with involvement of LCx origin; **E,** Proximal LAD: hematoma continues distally to involve first septal branch.

41

Left Anterior Descending Coronary Artery Stenosis Detected by Subsecond Spiral Computed Tomography

Teruhito Mochizuki, MD; Kenya Murase, PhD; Yasushi Koyama, MD; Hiroshi Higashino, MD; Junpei Ikezoe, MD

From the Department of Radiology, Ehime University School of Medicine (T.M., K.M., J.I.), and the Departments of Cardiology (Y.K.) and Radiology (H.H.), Ehime-Imabari Hospital, Japan.

(*Circulation*. 1999;99:1523.)

A 50-year-old man with angina pectoris was hospitalized for coronary angiography. He was diagnosed with angina pectoris from the typical symptom (angina on exercise), positive exercise ECG (depressed ST-T in leads I, aVL, and V_1 through V_3), and positive exercise ^{201}Tl single photon emission computed tomography (CT) (decreased ^{201}Tl perfusion in anteroseptal wall on exercise and significant redistribution on the 4-hour delayed scan). The coronary angiogram (CAG) depicted left anterior descending coronary artery (LAD) stenoses (75% stenosis in segment 6 and 50% stenosis in segment 7) (Fig. 1A). Plain CT depicts no calcification of the LAD, and contrast-enhancement CT depicts LAD stenoses concordant with the CAG (Figs. 1A and 1B).

To demonstrate coronary arteries, we used 3-mm-thick, 2-mm-per-rotation table speed (0.8 second per rotation), and 0.1 pitch overlapping reconstruction. Because a half-scan helical reconstruction algorithm was applied, time resolution (full width-half maximal) to obtain one transaxial slice was 0.4 second. This protocol allowed clear images of the coronary artery with less motion artifact. Clear images were obtained mainly in the end-diastolic and end-systolic phases. This image (quality and resolution) supports the potential use of subsecond spiral CT in the evaluation of coronary artery disease.

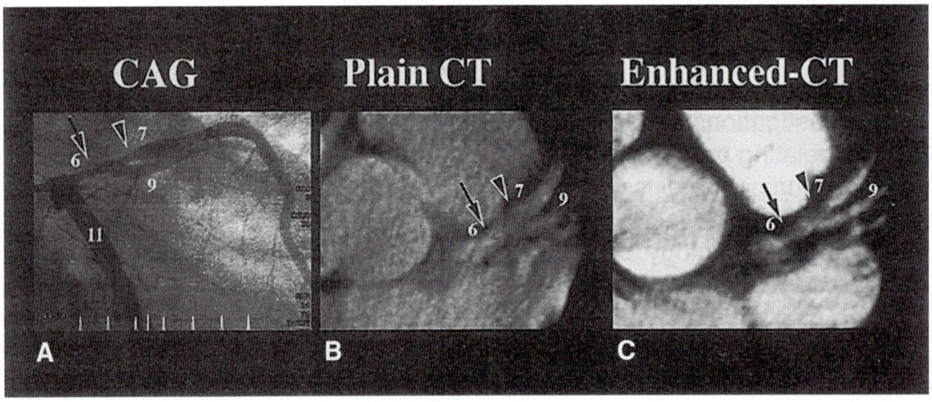

Figure 1. CAG **(A)** and plain and contrast-enhancement CT **(B** and **C)** of 50-year-old man with angina pectoris. Coronary angiogram depicts LAD stenoses (75% stenosis in segment 6 [arrow] and 50% stenosis in segment 7 [arrowhead]). Plain CT depicts left coronary arteries, and no calcification is observed. Contrast-enhancement CT depicts LAD stenoses concordant with CAG.

42 Chronic Coronary Artery Dissection Presenting as Heart Failure

Robert E. Hobbs, MD; Amy P. Scally, MD; Walter A. Tan, MD, MS

From the Department of Cardiology, The Cleveland Clinic Foundation, Cleveland, Ohio.

(*Circulation*. 1999;100:445.)

The patient was a 31-year-old man with a past history of polycythemia vera, *enlarged heart* (1992), transient ischemic attack (1995), and decompensated heart failure (1997). He was referred for evaluation and management of suspected dilated cardiomyopathy. An electrocardiogranm (ECG) demonstrated Q waves in the anterolateral leads. Cardiac catheterization was performed.

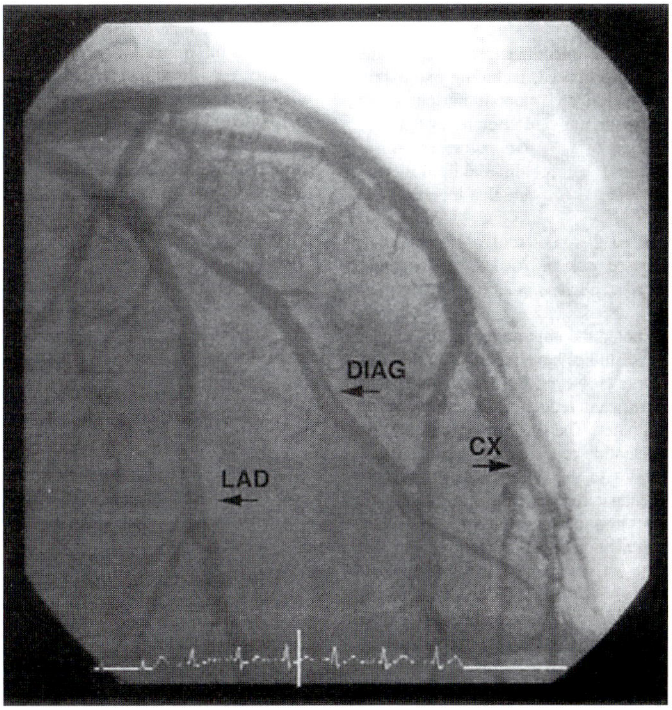

Figure 1. Posteroanterior cranial view of the left coronary artery. Note the radiolucent linear streaks in the left anterior descending coronary artery (LAD), diagonal branch (DIAG), and left circumflex branch (CX), consistent with chronic coronary artery dissection. The left ventriculogram revealed a dilated left ventricle with severe impairment in contractility.

43

Aortocoronary Bypass Surgery in a Patient with Aortic Calcification

Friedrich D. Knollmann, MD; Joachim Knörig, MD

From Charité, Campus Virchow-Klinikum, Strahlenklinik (F.D.K.) and Deutsches Herzzentrum Berlin, Klinik für Herz-, Thorax-, und Gefäßchirurgie (J.K.), Berlin, Germany.

(*Circulation*. 1999;100:1131.)

A 61-year-old woman was referred for aortocoronary bypass surgery. At cardiac catheterization, calcifications of the ascending aorta were noted. To assess the exact extent of aortic calcification, we performed an electrocardiogram (ECG)-gated electron-beam computed tomography (EBCT) study of the thoracic aorta. Figure 1 displays a three-dimensional (3-D) volume-rendering reconstruction of the EBCT data set, with thresholds set to display calcium-density voxels only. The aortic root is completely encased in calcifications, which extend to the aortic arch. The course of the three main coronary artery territories is outlined by calcific plaques. Bypass surgery was successfully completed after cannulation of the ascending aorta at a plaque-free spot in the aortic arch and occlusion of the aorta by a transventricular balloon technique for initiation of extracorporeal circulation. Complete myocardial revascularization was achieved by a left internal mammary artery bypass to the left anterior descending coronary artery and a venous Y-graft from the brachiocephalic artery trunk to the right coronary artery and the obtuse marginal branch.

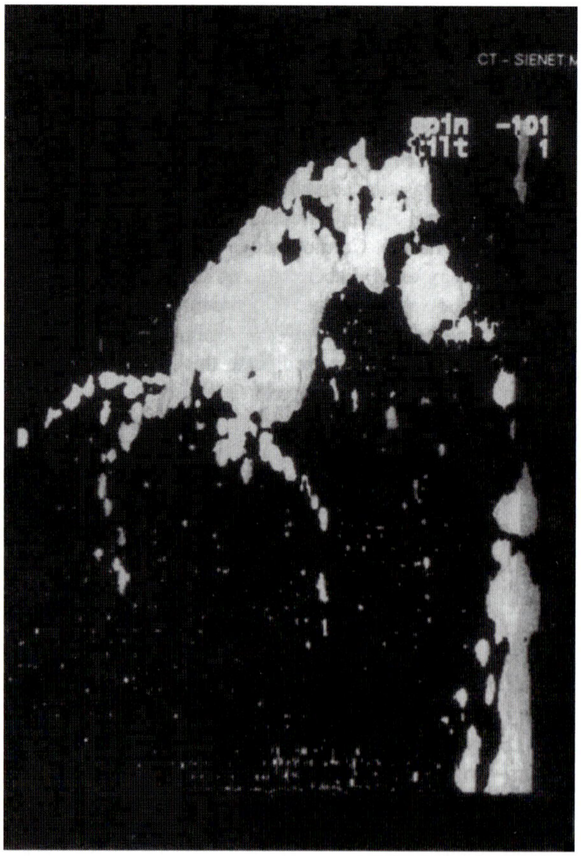

Figure 1.

44 Abciximab-Associated Pseudothrombocytopenia

Michael B. Holmes, MD; Samer Kabbani, MD; Matthew W. Watkins, MD; Robert W. Battle, MD; David J. Schneider, MD

From The University of Vermont College of Medicine, Burlington.

(*Circulation*. 2000;101:938–939.)

A 60-year-old woman was transferred for coronary angiography after a non-Q-wave myocardial infarction. She was treated with aspirin, metoprolol, unfractionated heparin, and abciximab administered as a weight-based bolus followed by infusion. A complete blood count in blood anticoagulated with ethylenediaminetetraacetic acid (EDTA) (purple-top Vacutainer) was obtained shortly after her arrival in the catheterization laboratory, 4 hours after the abciximab bolus. The reported platelet count had decreased from 440,000/mL to 21,000/mL. Examination of the peripheral blood smear revealed prominent clumping of the platelets (Fig. 1A). Repeat analysis performed in the catheterization laboratory in blood anticoagulated with citrate (blue-top Vacutainer) demonstrated a true platelet count of 320,000/mL associated with a normal appearance of the peripheral smear (Fig. 1B). She subsequently underwent angiography without delay or complications.

Pseudothrombocytopenia is an artifactual clumping of platelets in vitro without clinical significance. Most frequently, EDTA alters the conformation of the platelet surface glycoprotein IIb such that a neoepitope is exposed that is recognized by autologous antibodies. The incidence of pseudothrombocytopenia in the general population is ≈0.1%. The incidence of pseudothrombocytopenia was 1.1% in patients receiving abciximab as a bolus plus infusion in the evaluation of 7E3 for the prevention of ischemic complications (EPIC) trial, whereas the incidence of true acute thrombocytopenia was 2.7%. Thus, pseudothrombocytopenia is an important etiology of thrombocytopenia to consider in patients receiving abciximab.

Evaluation of the automated platelet count and peripheral smear in blood anticoagulated in citrate can distinguish pseudothrombocytopenia from heparin-induced thrombocytopenia and true thrombocytopenia related to abciximab. The distinction is critical because with pseudothrombocytopenia, thrombotic or hemorrhagic risk is not increased, antithrombotic and antiplatelet therapy can be continued, and invasive procedures can be performed.

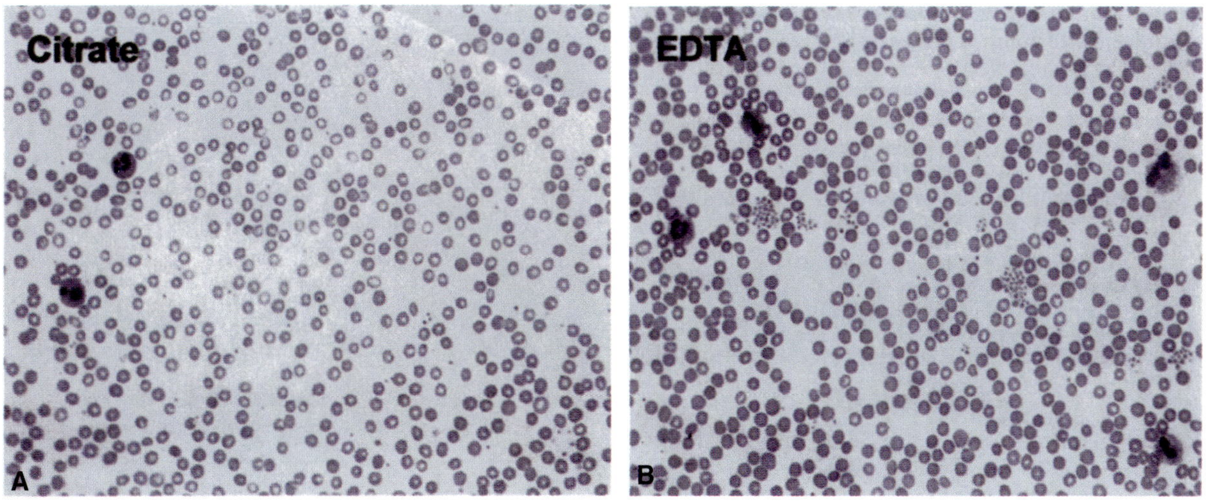

Figure 1. A and **B**

45

Contrast-Enhanced Magnetic Resonance Angiogram of Coronary Artery Bypass Graft Aneurysm

Nicholas H. Bunce, MD; Raad H. Mohiaddin, MD; Maher D. Dandal, MD; J. Simon R. Gibbs, MD; Dudley J. Pennell, MD

From the Magnetic Resonance Unit, Royal Brompton Hospital (N.H.B., R.H.M., D.J.P.), and Charing Cross Hospital (M.D.D., J.S.R.G.), London, UK.

(*Circulation*. 2000;102:3148.)

A 49-year-old man presented with a 4-hour history of central chest pain. Seventeen years earlier, he had suffered a myocardial infarction with subsequent coronary artery bypass surgery. The admission electrocardiogram (ECG) showed a left bundle branch block pattern, and chest x-ray showed bilateral mediastinal enlargement (Fig. 1). An echocardiogram (Fig. 2) identified a left-sided aneurysm measuring 7 cm that was located anterior to the aorta; the aneurysm was compressing the main pulmonary artery. He had a second right-sided aneurysm measuring 6 cm. A gadolinium contrast-enhanced magnetic resonance (MR) angiogram was performed to establish the anatomy. Maximum-intensity-projection reformatting of the angiogram demonstrated an aneurysm of the graft to the left anterior descending artery (Fig. 3) and an aneurysm of the graft to the right coronary artery (Fig. 3). Surgical resection of the aneurysms and quadruple-bypass grafting were successfully performed 2 months later. The man has returned to normal activities.

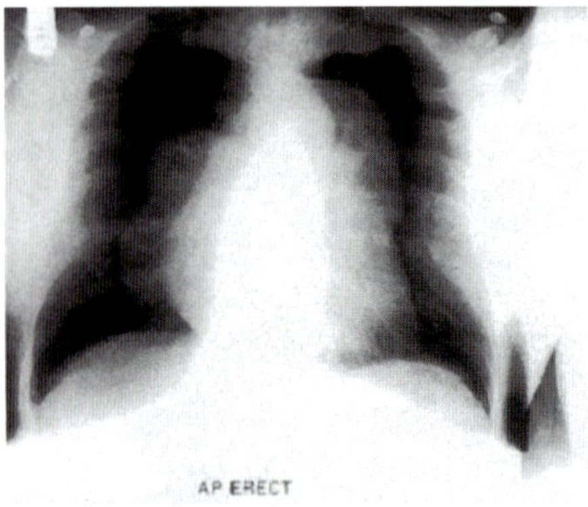

Figure 1. Anteroposterior chest x-ray on admission shows bilateral mediastinal enlargement.

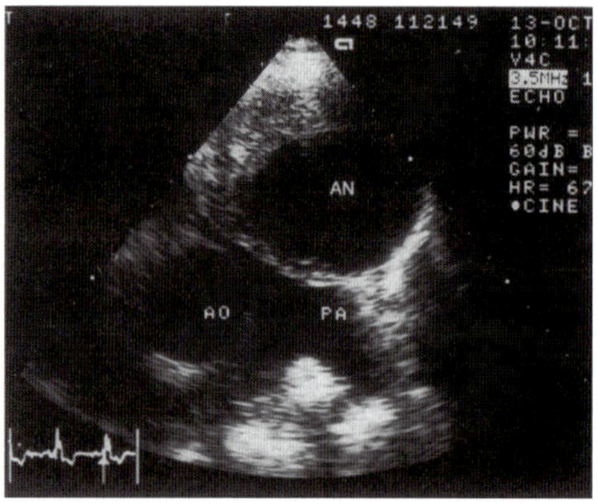

Figure 2. Transthoracic echocardiography shows aneurysm (AN) anterior to aorta (AO) that is compressing main pulmonary artery (PA).

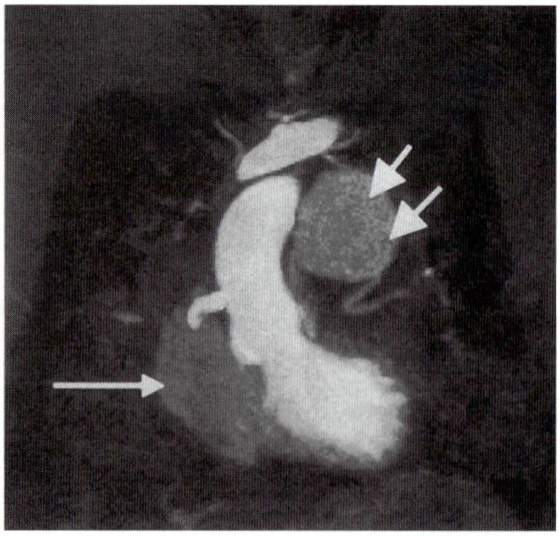

Figure 3. Maximum-intensity projection of gadolinium-enhanced MR angiogram shows aneurysm of graft to left anterior descending coronary artery (short arrows) and second aneurysm of graft to the right coronary artery (long arrow).

46

Visualization of Tissue Prolapse between Coronary Stent Struts by Optical Coherence Tomography: Comparison with Intravascular Ultrasound

Ik-Kyung Jang, MD; Guillermo Tearney, MD, PhD; Brett Bouma, PhD

From Massachusetts General Hospital, Harvard Medical School, Boston, Mass.

(*Circulation.* 2001;104:2754.)

A 65-year-old man underwent cardiac catheterization for unstable angina pectoris. The coronary angiogram revealed a significant stenosis of the right coronary artery, which was treated with a 3 × 16 mm NIR stent. A postintervention coronary angiogram showed excellent results, and intravascular ultrasound (IVUS); 30 MHz, Ultracross, Boston Scientific) showed a well-deployed stent (Fig. 1A). A 3.2 F optical coherence tomography (OCT) catheter, advanced to the same site, showed well-apposed stent struts (Fig. 1B). In addition, tissue prolapse between the stent struts (12 to 3 o'clock in Fig. 1B) was clearly visualized. The tissue prolapse occurred mainly in an area with a lower OCT signal intensity (vessel wall visualized between the stent struts), which is suggestive of a plaque with decreased collagen content. A retrospective review of the IVUS study showed an area of possible tissue prolapse at the corresponding location (1 o'clock in Fig. 1A).

OCT is an optical analog of IVUS with a high resolution (10 μm vs. 100 pm of IVUS). Recently, our laboratory developed a catheter-based intracoronary OCT system. The OCT image (Fig., B) was acquired during the first application of this technology in humans. This new imaging modality may be useful in improving the outcome of coronary intervention and may also help identify vulnerable coronary plaques.

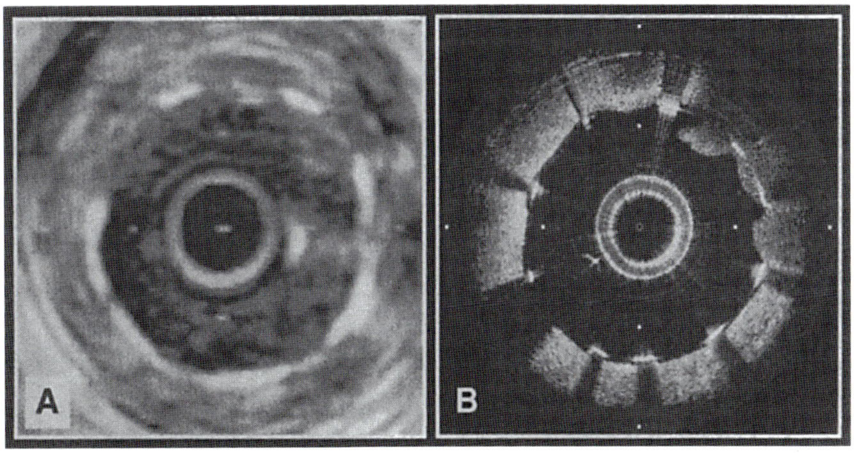

Figure 1. IVUS **(A)** and OCT **(B)** images of the stented right coronary artery are shown. Although IVUS showed a well-deployed stent, the detailed structure around the stent struts is not well visualized. In addition, OCT clearly visualized tissue prolapse between the stent struts (12 to 3 o'clock). The tissue prolapse occurred mainly in an area with lower OCT signal intensity, which is suggestive of a plaque with large lipid content.

47 Regression of a Donor Atheroma after Cardiac Transplantation: Serial Observations with Intravascular Ultrasound

Hiroshi Tsutsui, MD; Paul Schoenhagen, MD; Jon D. Klingensmith, MS; D. Geoffrey Vince, PhD; Steven E. Nissen, MD; E. Murat Tuzcu, MD

From the Department of Cardiology, Cleveland Clinic Foundation, Cleveland, Ohio.

(*Circulation*. 2001;104:2874.)

A 42-year-old man received a cardiac transplantation in October 1995 for dilated cardiomyopathy. He had no history of hyperlipidemia or coronary artery disease. The heart donor was a 41-year-old woman with a history of hypertension. The first intravascular ultrasound (IVUS) study was obtained 14 days after cardiac transplantation, and the last follow-up examination was performed 5 years later. Figures 1 and 2 show a hypoechoic atheroma in the proximal left anterior descending artery that was transmitted from the donor. At this site, serial IVUS imaging demonstrates apparent spontaneous regression of the donor atheroma (Fig. 1 and Fig. 2). The presence of prominent perivascular landmarks confirms the identical location of IVUS images from both time points. Of note, the regression in atheroma volume is accompanied by new calcification, a process that is thought to represent plaque stabilization. These changes show a dramatic regression in a transmitted donor atheroma after cardiac transplantation and suggest the potential for antiatherosclerotic therapy to regress atherosclerosis in the natural course of native coronary artery disease.

Acknowledgment

Dr. Tsutsui was partially supported by a research grant from the Japanese Association for the Advancement of Medical Equipment, which is affiliated with the Ministry of Health and Welfare of Japan.

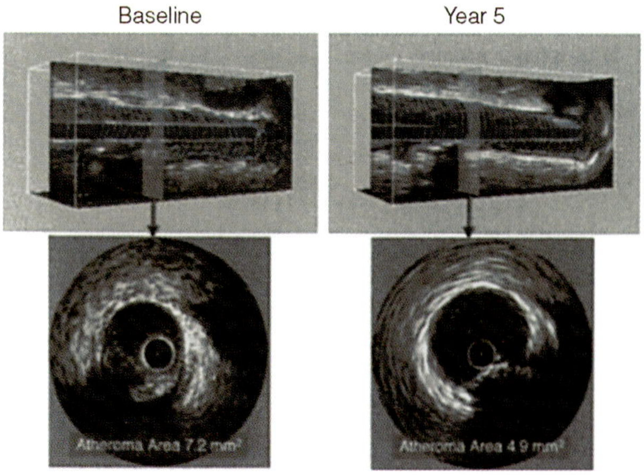

Figure 1. Reconstructed three-dimensional (3-D) IVUS images and IVUS still images. The blue lines on the 3-D images show the lumen area in each slice. Baseline study is shown on left; images 5 years after transplantation are shown on right.

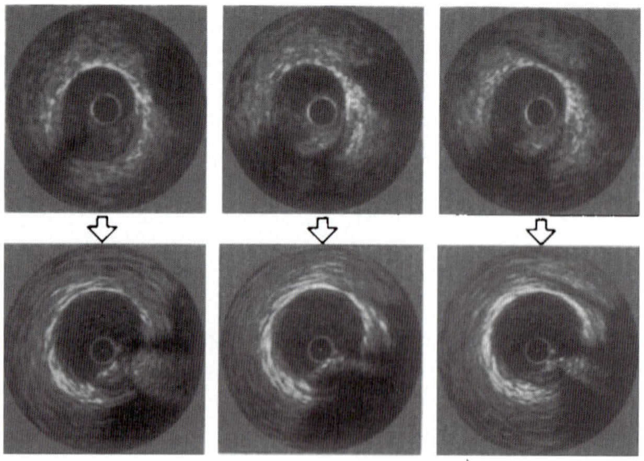

Figure 2. Sequential IVUS still images matched for the two IVUS examinations. Baseline study is shown on top; images 5 years after transplantation are shown on bottom.

48 Postmortem Three-Dimensional Reconstruction of the Entire Coronary Arterial Circulation Using Electron-Beam Computed Tomography

Brian R. Rah, MD; Richard J. Katz, MD; Alan G. Wasserman, MD; Jonathan S. Reiner, MD

From the Division of Cardiology (B.R.R., R.J.K.), the Department of Medicine (A.G.W.), and the Cardiac Catheterization Laboratory (J.S.R.), George Washington University Medical Center, Washington, DC.

(*Circulation*. 2001;104:3168.)

A 50-year-old man died suddenly while exercising on a treadmill at a local health club. He had no known previous cardiac history. During autopsy, a radio-opaque silicone compound was injected into the coronary arteries. The explanted heart was then imaged by electron-beam computed tomography (EBCT) using 3-mm slices. A complete three-dimensional (3-D) reconstruction was then obtained using commercially available software (Accuimage Diagnostics). Figure 1 shows the heart rotated into the equivalent of an angiographic left anterior oblique projection. This view reveals a completely occluded proximal right coronary artery. A significant narrowing involving a diagonal artery is also visible. Figure 2 corresponds to an angiographic right anterior oblique projection. The distal right coronary arterial circulation is supplied by collaterals from the left circumflex artery, and there is significant narrowing at the origin of the posterior descending coronary artery.

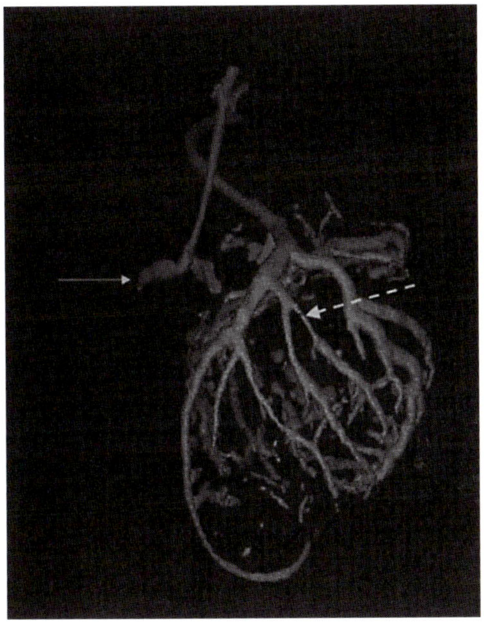

Figure 1. Angiographic equivalent of a left anterior oblique projection revealing a completely occluded proximal right coronary artery (solid arrow) and a significant narrowing involving a diagonal artery (dashed arrow).

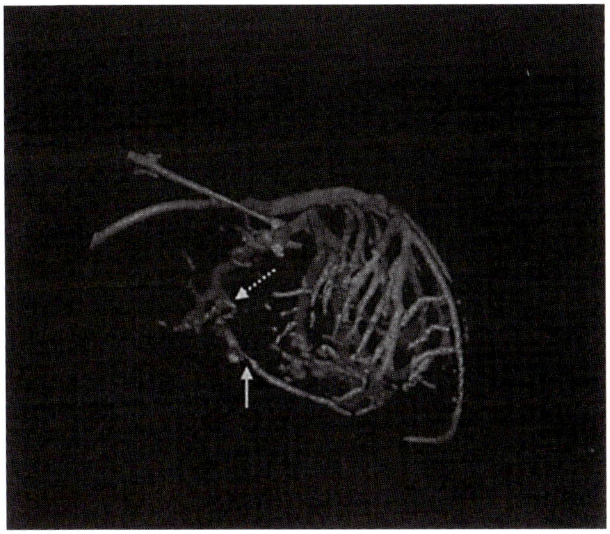

Figure 2. Angiographic equivalent of a right anterior oblique projection. The distal right coronary arterial circulation is supplied by collaterals from the left circumflex artery (dashed arrow). A significant narrowing can also be seen at the origin of the posterior descending artery (solid arrow).

49

Visualization of the Ruptured Plaque by Magnetic Resonance Imaging

Frank Wiesmann, MD; Matthew D. Robson, PhD; Jane Francis, DCR; Steffen E. Petersen, MD; C. Paul Leeson, PhD, MRCP; Keith M. Channon, MD, MRCP; Stefan Neubauer, MD, MRCP

From the Department of Cardiovascular Medicine, John Radcliffe Hospital, University of Oxford, UK.

(*Circulation*. 2003;108:2542.)

DOI: 10.1161/01.CIR.0000083603.61183.BB

A 61-year-old man at risk of generalized arteriosclerosis due to heavy long-term smoking (60 pack-years) but no other risk factors was enrolled in a research study of atherosclerosis by noninvasive vascular magnetic resonance imaging (MRI). The patient reported an episode of amaurosis fugax of the right eye 4 months before the scan but had no other clinical symptoms.

MRI of the neck vessels revealed a pronounced bilateral increase in wall thickness of internal carotid arteries as well as of the common carotid and vertebral arteries on both sides (Figs. 1A and 1B). Immediately below the carotid bifurcation, the right common carotid artery showed significant thickening of the vessel wall with an appearance consistent with two atherosclerotic plaques (Fig. 1B). On enlargement of the region of interest, both plaques showed a dark, lipid-rich core covered by a thin fibrous cap (Fig. 1C). One lesion was suggestive of a ruptured plaque showing discontinuity of the fibrous cap (arrow). However, there was no evidence of significant luminal narrowing.

Vascular ultrasound confirmed these findings with evidence of irregular atheroma around the carotid bifurcation (Fig. 2). Bilateral Doppler recordings displayed velocities within normal range.

This case likely represents a ruptured carotid plaque leading to an episode of amaurosis fugax.

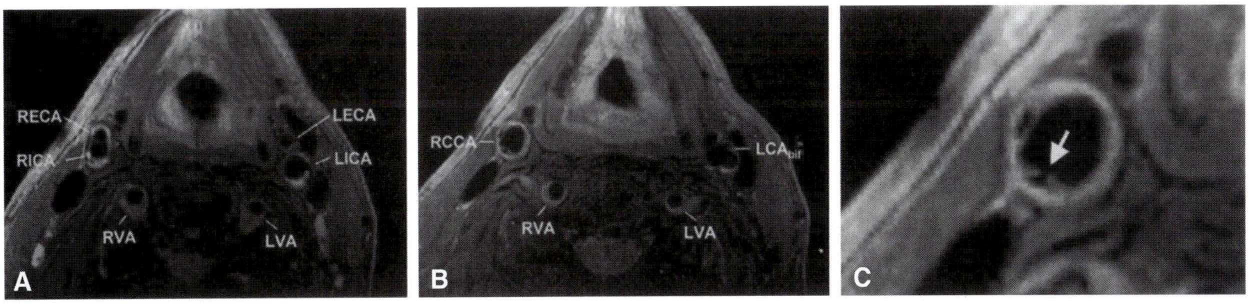

Figure 1. Magnetic resonance T2-weighted turbo spin-echo images in transverse orientation revealing increased wall thickness of the carotid and vertebral arteries. **A,** Note the pronounced thickening of the posterior arterial wall in both the right and left internal carotid artery. **B,** Significantly thickened vessel wall in the left carotid bifurcation (LCA_{bif}). Also shown are two arteriosclerotic lesions in the right common carotid artery (RCCA) with dark lipid core and thin fibrous cap. **C,** Close-up of right common carotid artery suggestive of plaque rupture with discontinuity of the thin fibrous cap (arrow). Electrocardiogram (ECG)-gated MRI (double-inversion recovery turbo spin-echo) was performed on a 1.5-T clinical scanner by use of a paired surface coil phase array for signal reception. Imaging parameters were the following: TR, 2 cardiac cycles; TE, 81 ms; field of view, 12 cm; in-plane resolution, 0.47×0.47 mm^2; and slice thickness, 3 mm. RECA indicates right external carotid artery; RICA, right internal carotid artery; LECA, left external carotid artery; LICA, left internal carotid artery; RVA, right vertebral artery; and LVA, left vertebral artery.

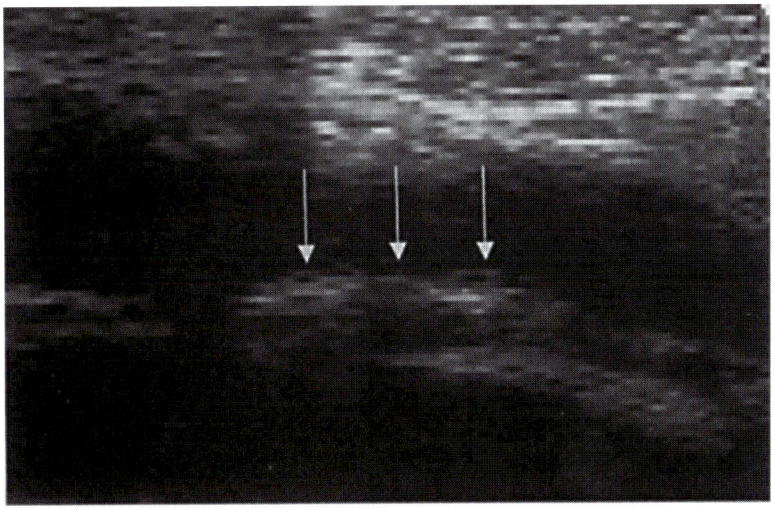

Figure 2. Ultrasound image of the right carotid bifurcation showing irregular atheroma (arrows).

50 Transplant Vasculopathy: Evaluation with Multidetector Computed Tomography

Sibyll Goetze, MD; Gardar Sigurdsson, MD; Neil L. Greenberg, PhD; Hilal Yamani, MD; Mario J. Garcia, MD
From the Department of Cardiovascular Imaging, The Cleveland Clinic Foundation, Cleveland, Ohio.

(*Circulation.* 2004;110:e80–e81.)
DOI: 10.1161/01.CIR.0000140671.80741.E1

A 43-year-old man was admitted with progressive fatigue, shortness of breath, and orthopnea. He received an orthotopic heart transplant 13 years ago, which was complicated by multiple episodes of rejection. His last catheterization 2 years before presentation demonstrated moderate transplant vasculopathy. More recently, a nuclear perfusion scan showed a myocardial scar in the mid to basal anterior and anterolateral walls, but no reversible stress-induced ischemia. On admission, the ECG showed normal sinus rhythm with a rate of 95 beats per minute, complete right bundle-branch block, inferior Q waves, and lateral ST- and T-wave abnormalities. A transthoracic echocardiogram revealed a left ventricular ejection fraction of 40%. A 16-slice multidetector computed tomographic (MDCT) scan of the heart was performed after the injection of 100 cc nonionic iodinated contrast medium. The examination demonstrated diffusely thickened coronary vessel walls with severe narrowing of the left main trunk, a totally occluded left circumflex artery, and a severely diseased right coronary artery (Fig. 1A and 1B). Left heart catheterization demonstrated 80% stenosis of the left main trunk (Fig. 2) and confirmed the MDCT findings of severe three-vessel disease. The patient underwent coronary artery bypass grafting to the left anterior, left circumflex, and right coronary arteries, as well as tricuspid valve repair. At the time of his operation, diffuse thickening of the left coronary artery consistent with transplant vasculopathy was noted. He was discharged from the hospital 6 days after his surgery. This case demonstrates that valuable information can be gained from the evaluation of the coronaries by MDCT, which can not only reveal the presence of severe luminal narrowing, but can also depict the morphology of the vessel walls.

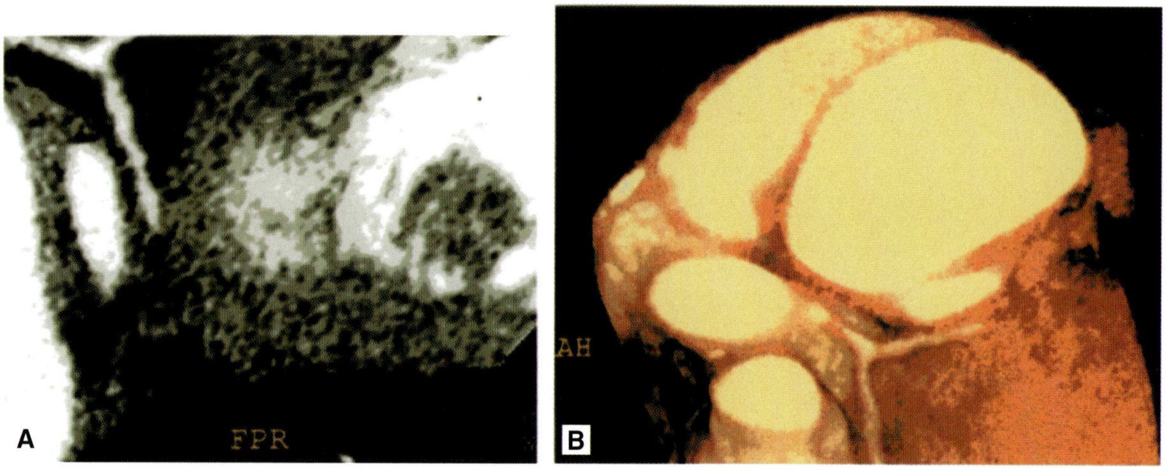

Figure 1. **A** and **B,** Multidetector computed tomographic image (**A,** multiplanar reconstruction; **B,** three-dimensional rendering technique) demonstrating severe stenosis of the lumen and thickening of the wall of the left main trunk as well as an occluded left circumflex artery. During the MDCT examination, the patient's heart rate ranged from 90 to 108 beats per minute (average 95 beats per minute).

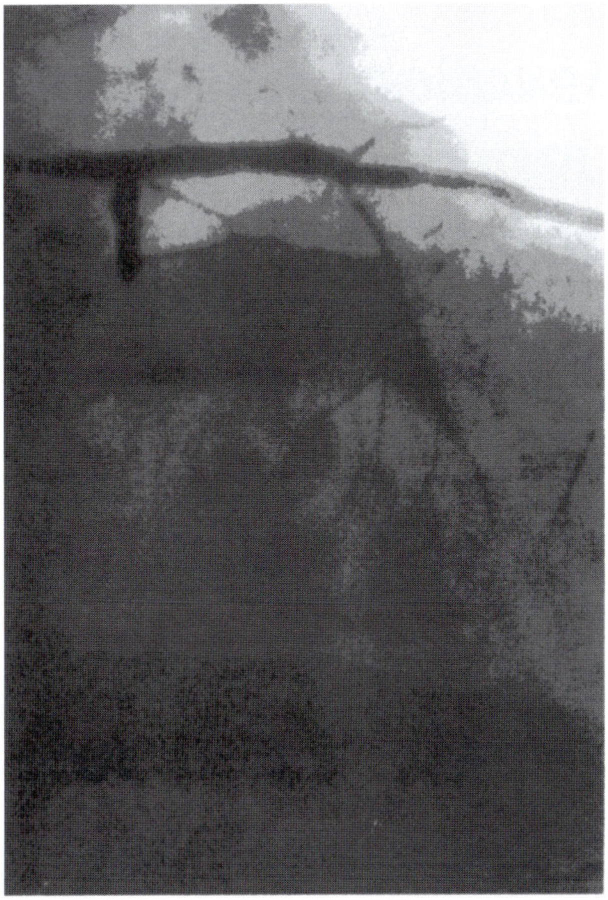

Figure 2. Conventional angiography demonstrating severe stenosis of the left main coronary artery and occlusion of the circumflex artery.

51 ST Elevation During Open Heart Surgery: Floating Air Bubble in Saphenous Vein Graft

Ken-ichi Komukai, MD; Keiji Hirooka, MD, PhD; Manabu Taneike, MD; Yoshinori Yasuoka, MD; Hiroyoshi Yamamoto, MD; Katsuji Hashimoto, MD, PhD; Wakatomi Chin, MD; Yukihiro Koretsune, MD, PhD; Hideo Kusuoka, MD, PhD; Yoshio Yasumura, MD, PhD

From the Cardiovascular Division, Osaka National Hospital, Osaka, Japan.

(*Circulation*. 2005;111:e374.)

DOI: 10.1161.CIRCULATIONAHA.104.474874

A 58-year-old man with severe mitral regurgitation and silent myocardial ischemia underwent mitral valvuloplasty and coronary artery bypass graft (CABG). Preoperative coronary angiography revealed a total occlusion of the left circumflex coronary artery. The right coronary artery supplied the collateral flow to the posterior descending branch of the left circumflex coronary artery. The saphenous vein graft (SVG) was anastomosed to this branch after valvuloplasty. Just before closure of the chest wall, the electrocardiogram (ECG) showed severe ST-segment elevation in leads II, III, and aVF (Fig. 1A). Despite continuous infusion of nitroglycerin and initiation of nicorandil, ST-segment elevation did not recover; therefore, an intra-aortic balloon was inserted. As soon as the operation was finished, the patient was taken to the catheterization laboratory, and emergency coronary catheterization was performed. His native coronary arteries showed no changes compared with preoperative findings. Interestingly, a floating air bubble was demonstrated in the distal part of the anastomosed SVG (Figs. 2A, 2B, and 2C). As the bubble traveled to the distal part of the SVG, the ST-segment was

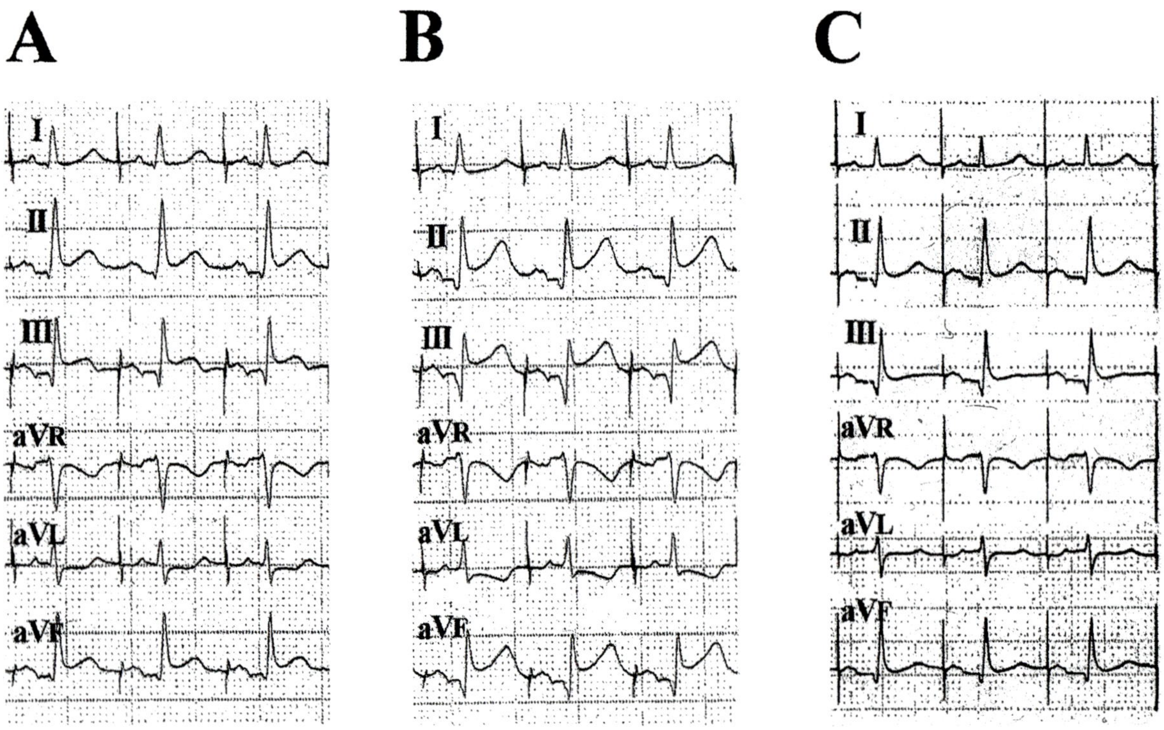

Figure 1. Monitor ECG showing changes in ST segment. **A,** Before catheterization, ST-segment elevation in leads II, III, and aVF. **B,** As bubble traveled to distal part of SVG, ST segment was further elevated. **C,** After distal aspiration, ST-segment elevation was recovered.

further elevated (Fig. 1B). A 6F AL-1 guiding catheter for coronary angioplasty was then positioned at the ostium of the SVG, and a 0.014-inch guidewire was advanced into the posterior descending branch through the SVG. The tip of the thrombectomy catheter (Thrombuster; Kaneka Medix Corp) was placed at the distal SVG (Fig. 2D) and pulled back, aspirating blood and the bubble. Immediately after this maneuver, brisk blood flow was restored (Fig. 2E), with restoration of ST-segment elevation (Fig. 1C).

Coronary air embolism is a potential complication of cardiopulmonary bypass surgery, especially open heart surgery. Nevertheless, it is unusual for emergency coronary catheterization to demonstrate a floating air bubble in the coronary artery. Air embolism can be fatal if not treated promptly. Distal air aspiration with a thrombectomy catheter is a quick and effective maneuver for rescuing the distal circulation in cases of air embolism associated with cardiac surgery or catheterization.

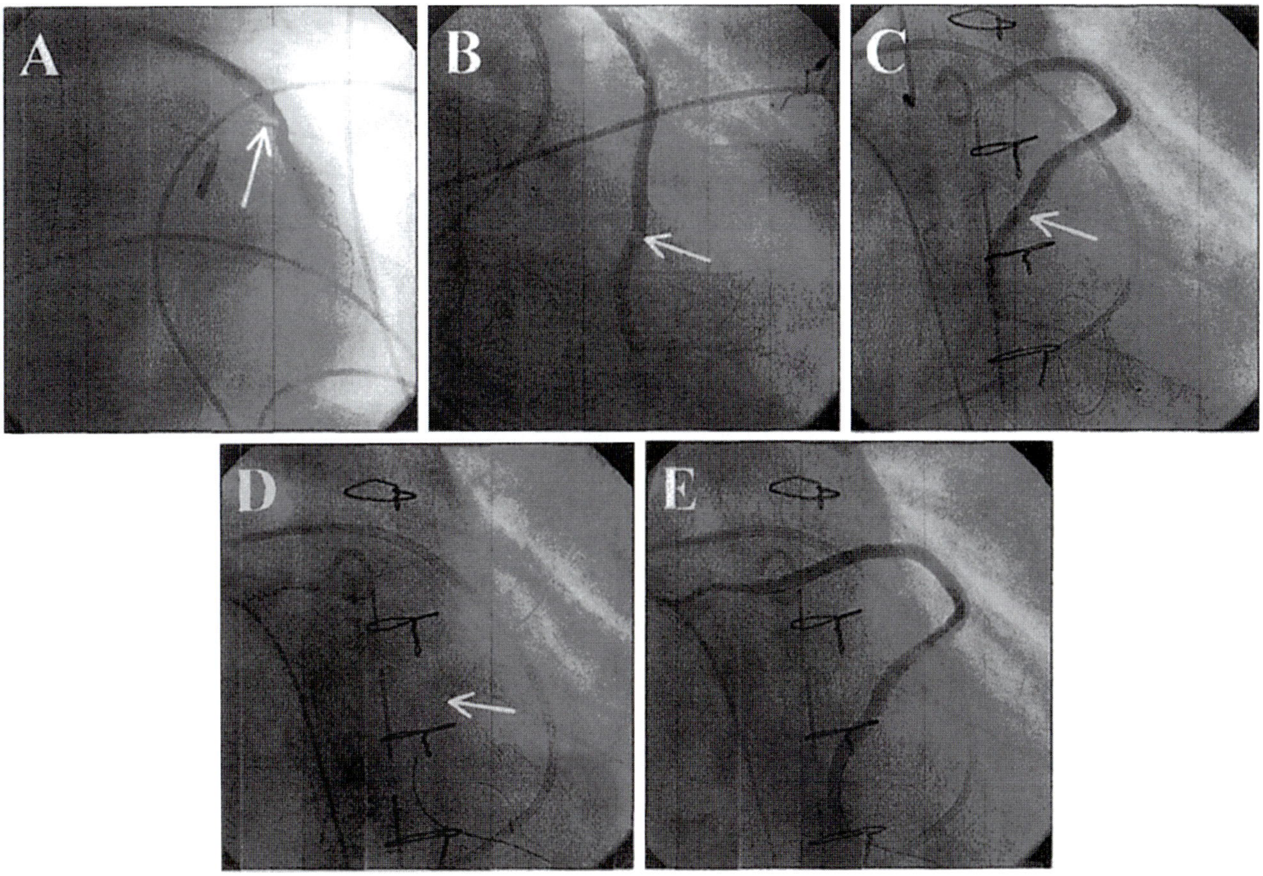

Figure 2. Floating air bubble (arrows in A through C; **A,** left anterior oblique projection; **B,** straight caudal projection; **C,** right anterior oblique projection) in distal part of SVG. **D,** Tip of thrombectomy catheter aspirating blood and bubble. **E,** Air bubble had disappeared.

52 Giant Coronary Artery Aneurysms in Kawasaki Disease

Christian Lilje, MD; James J. Joyce, MD

From the Department of Pediatrics (C.L., J.J.J.), Section of Pediatric Cardiology, Tulane University Health Sciences Center, New Orleans, La, and the Pediatric Cardiovascular Center (J.J.J.), University of Florida Health Sciences Center, Jacksonville, Fla.

(*Circulation*. 2005;111:C440.)

DOI: 10.1161.CIRCULATIONAHA.104.491811

A 5-month-old boy presented with a 3-week history of intermittent high-grade fevers and previous treatment for a presumptive pneumonia. Retrospectively, a strawberry tongue, bilateral conjunctival injections, and a cervical lymph adenopathy had initially been present. His physical examination was remarkable for a grade 1/6 systolic ejection murmur at the left midsternal border. The electrocardiogram (ECG) showed sinus tachycardia and nonspecific J-point elevations in the lateral chest leads. Echocardiography displayed a pericardial effusion and giant coronary artery aneurysms (Fig. 1). An area suspicious for dissection (Fig. 2, arrow) was found to be a markedly dilated but intact conal branch of the right coronary artery by biplane aortography (Fig. 3, arrow). The fever resolved after a single dose of intravenous immunoglobulin. Aspirin and warfarin were started to prevent coronary thrombus formation. The subsequent clinical course has thus far been uneventful, without any signs of myocardial ischemia.

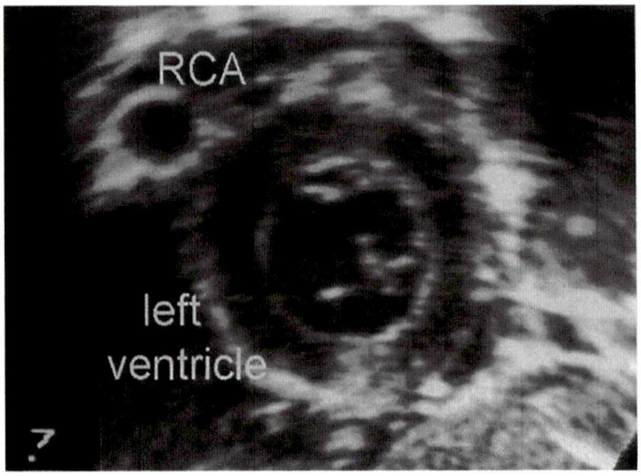

Figure 1. Echocardiography, subcostal short-axis view. Right coronary artery (RCA) is grossly dilated and echogenic.

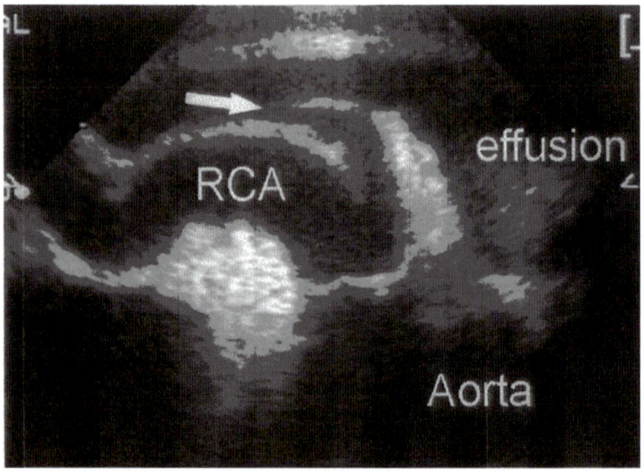

Figure 2. Echocardiography, parasternal short-axis view. In presence of pericardial effusion, proximal part of RCA is suspicious for dissection (arrow). Imaging plane is off axis of nondilated RCA ostium.

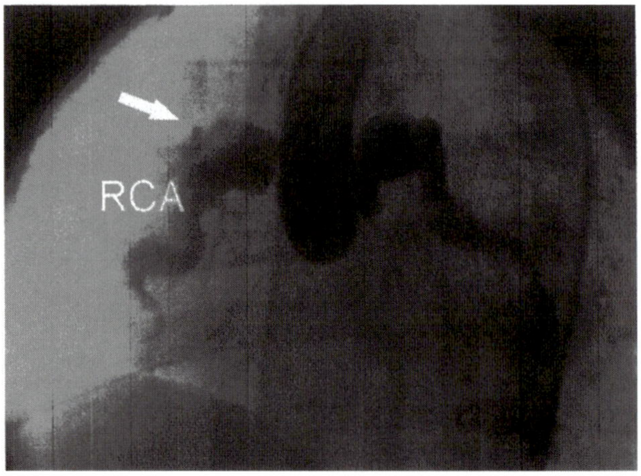

Figure 3. Aortography and nonselective coronary arteriography, lateral projection. Diffuse long-segment aneurysmal dilation of both main coronary arteries. Area suspicious for dissection (arrow) is dilated but intact conal branch of RCA.

53 Anomalous Coronary Anatomy

Scott C. Turner, DO; D. Scott Gantt, DO; Dan Giebel, MD

From Texas A&M University Health Science Center and College of Medicine, Scott & White Hospital and Clinic, Scott, Sherwood and Brindley Foundation, Temple Tex.

(*Circulation.* 2005;111:e441.)

DOI: 10.1161.CIRCULATIONAHA.104.493031

A 67-year-old woman was admitted with chest pain. She was subsequently found to have an abnormal myocardial perfusion study that showed possible ischemia at the basal to midanterior wall and normal left ventricular function. She had a history of a stent to her right coronary artery in 2001. She reported, "They told me I had an artery in a strange place," but none of her medical records were available at the time of catheterization. Her angiogram revealed anomalous coronary anatomy (Fig. 1). The image demonstrates three main coronary arteries from a common cusp. To the best of our knowledge, this particular combination of anomalies has not been reported previously.

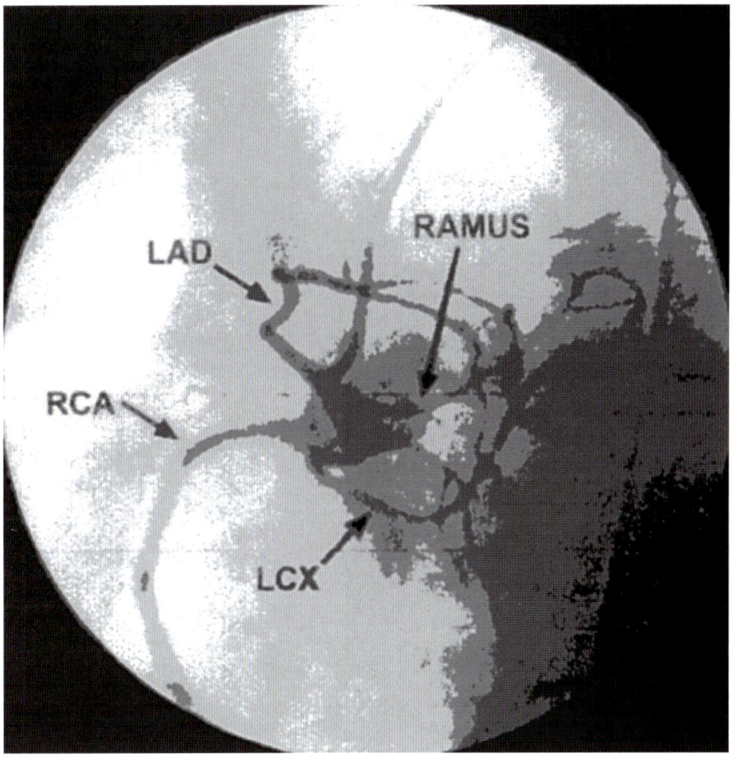

Figure 1. Angiogram showing anomalous coronary anatomy. RCA indicates right coronary artery; LAD, left anterior descending coronary artery; and LCX, left circumflex.

Section III

Intracardiac Masses

54

An Unusual Case of Right-Sided Heart Failure

Carlos M. Gaos, MD; Patrick J. Hogan, MD; Susan Wilansky, MD
From the Department of Cardiology, St. Luke's Episcopal Hospital, Houston, Tex.

(*Circulation*. 1993;88:1)

A 57-year-old man with a history of coronary artery disease and chronic obstructive pulmonary disease was admitted to another hospital with progressive dyspnea, ascites, edema, and mild jaundice. He was transferred to St. Luke's Episcopal Hospital for further evaluation. Biplane transesophageal echocardiography (TEE) revealed an extensive tumor mass in the right atrium and left atrium (Fig. 1A) with obstruction of the superior vena cava. TEE-guided biopsy of the superior vena cava mass revealed histology of large-cell lymphoma (B-cell type). At 6-month follow-up, after appropriate chemotherapy, repeat TEE showed almost total resolution of the tumor bulk, with only a small residual mass seen in the right atrium (Fig. 1B).

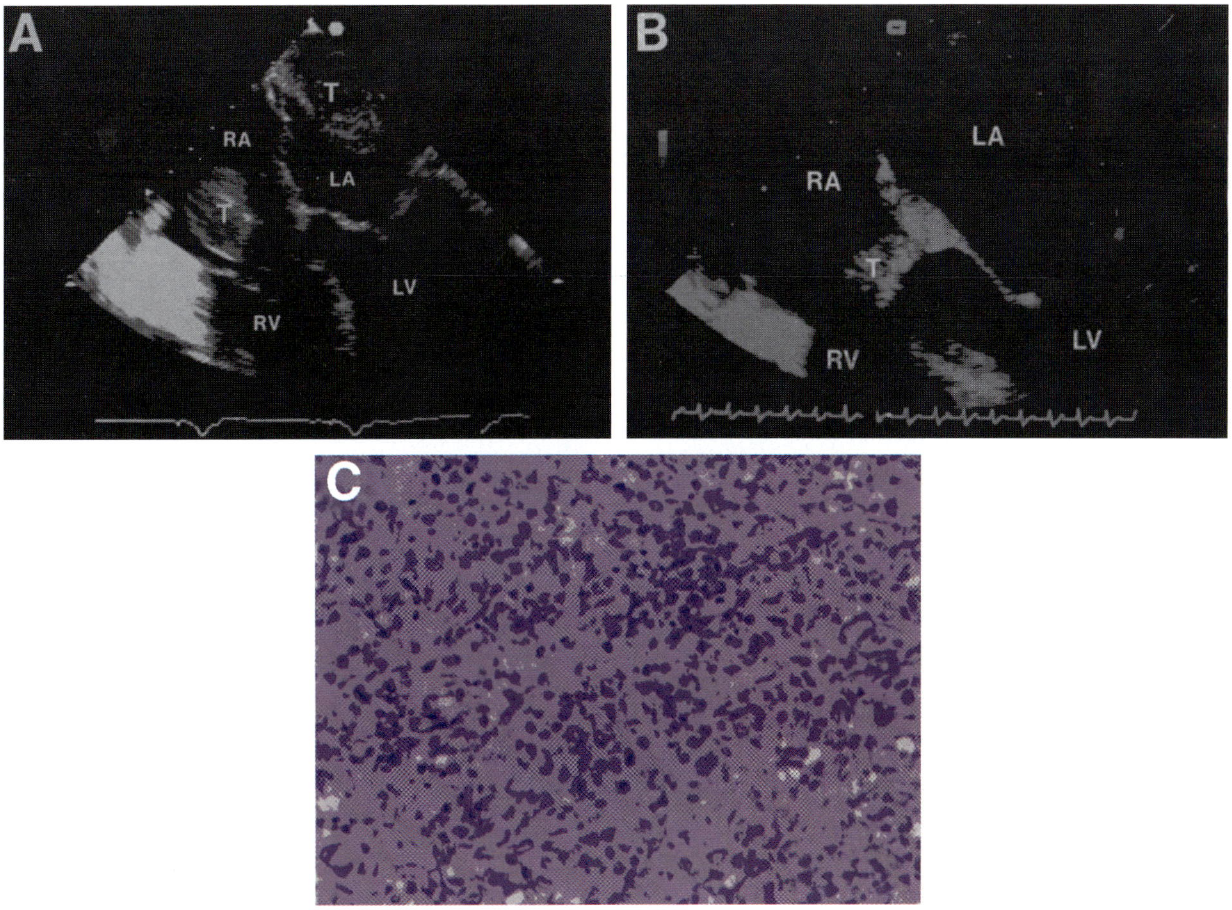

Figure 1. Transesophageal echocardiographic images in the horizontal plane; four-chamber view. **A** shows extensive tumor (T) mass in the right and left atria (LA). **B** is a transesophageal echocardiographic image in the same plane and view as A in the patient 6 months after chemotherapy for lymphoma. Note the small residual tumor mass (1 × l.2 cm) in the right atrium (RA). **C** is a photomicrograph of section of large cell lymphoma obtained with bioptome. Immunocytochemistry documented the lymphoma as B-cell type. RV, right ventricle; LV, left ventricle.

55 A Heavily Calcified Left Atrial Myxoma

James M. Beattie, MBChB, FRCP

From the Department of Cardiology, Birmingham Heartlands Hospital, Birmingham, B9 5SS, UK.

(*Circulation*. 1993;88:2972.)

A mildly demented 83-year-old woman presented with palpitation and ischemic cardiac pain. Penetrated posteroanterior (Fig. 1A) and lateral radiographs (Fig. 1B) revealed a calcified mass within the cardiac silhouette, which was later confirmed by echocardiography to be a calcified left atrial myxoma attached along the limbus of the fossa ovalis. This tumor is noteworthy for the extent of calcification that was evident on routine radiographic examination. This may be present to a lesser extent in up to 15% of myxomata examined by fluoroscopy. A similar proportion exhibits calcification on histological section with occasional foci of metaplastic bone. The advanced age of the patient at presentation is also uncommon, although 12% of left atrial myxomata in the Armed Forces Institute of Pathology (AFIP) series presented after the age of 70 years. A conservative approach was agreed upon, and the patient died of a stroke 2 years later after having survived general anesthesia for right hip arthroplasty.

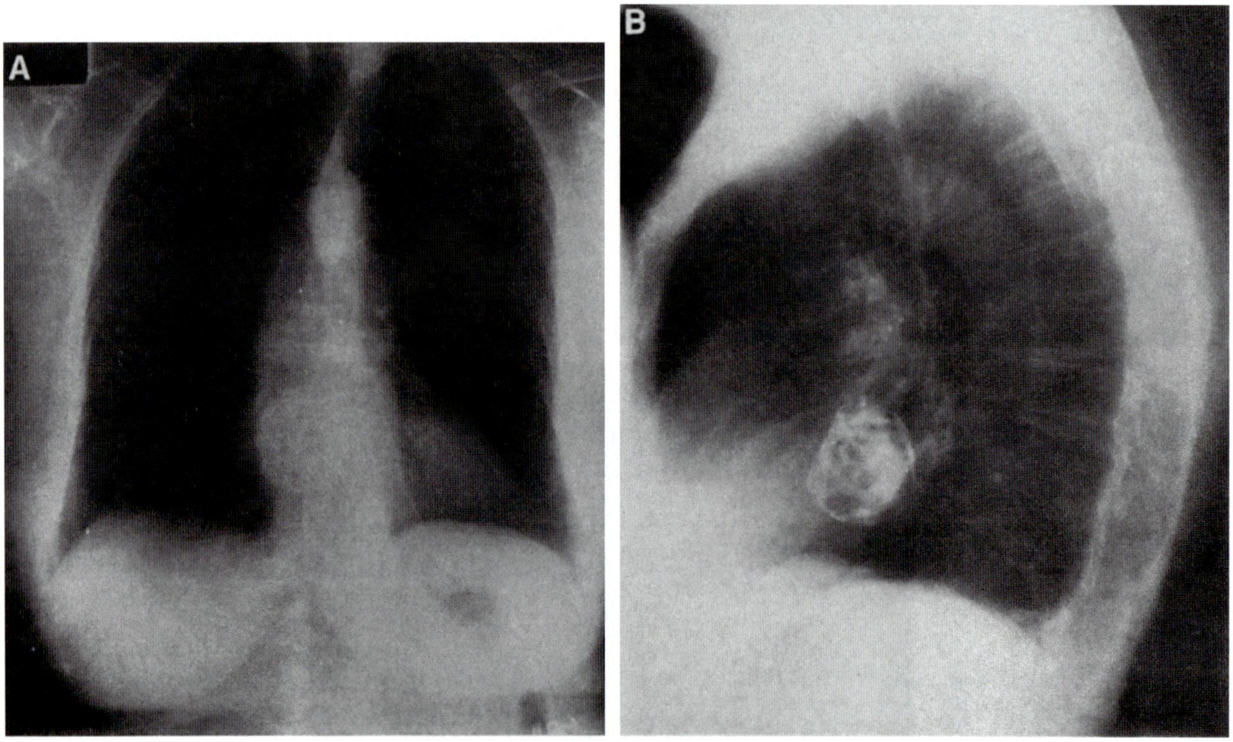

Figure 1. Penetrated posteroanterior **(A)** and lateral **(B)** radiographs showing the heavily calcified 5 × 5 × 4 cm intracardiac mass.

56

Papillary Fibroelastoma as an Unusual Source of Repeated Pulmonary Embolism

Johannes Waltenberger, MD; Stefan Thelin, MD

From the Ludwig Institute for Cancer Research and Department of Medicine (J.W.) and the Department of Thoracic Surgery (S.T.), Uppsala University, Uppsala, Sweden.

(*Circulation*. 1994;89:2433.)

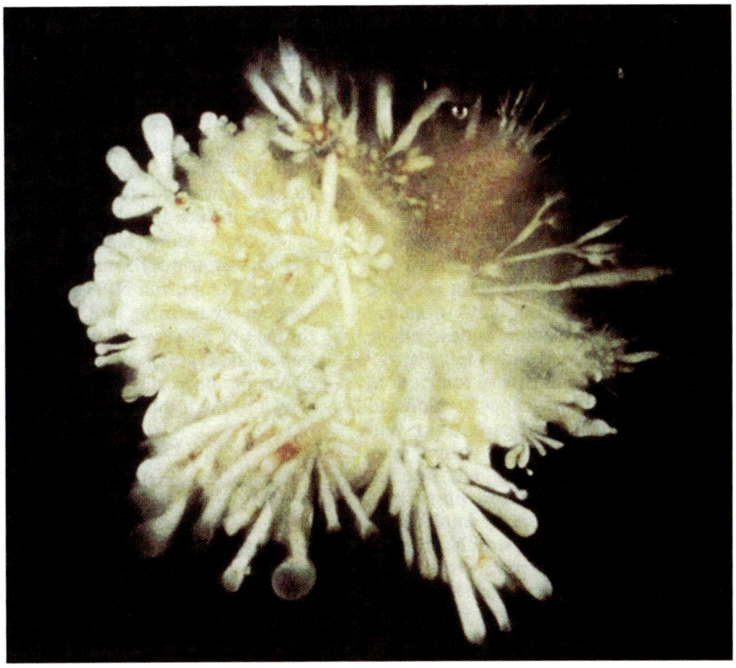

Figure 1. Papillary fibroelastoma of the heart. This tumor was excised from the right heart of a 66-year-old patient who presented with a history of repeated episodes of respiratory distress and fever. The diagnosis of recurrent pulmonary embolism was made, open heart surgery was performed, and the tumor was classified by additional histopathological evaluation. No signs or symptoms were reported during the first 18 months after surgery, strongly suggesting the papillary fibroelastoma as the embolic source. The diameter of the tumor measured 10 mm. The specimen was carefully washed in phosphate-buffered saline and photographed immediately after excision.

57 Cardiac Rhabdomyomas in Tuberous Sclerosis (Bourneville Disease)

Humberto Guerrero, MD; Pablo Campos, MD; Carlos Harrison, MD

From the Departments of Cardiology (H.G.G., C.H.G.) and Dermatology (P.C.M.) of Hospital Aranda de la Parra, Leon, Guanajuato, Mexico.

(*Circulation*. 1994;90:3113–3114.)

This report describes the case of a 14-year-old boy with moderate mental retardation who had had seizures since infancy. At birth, it was noticed that he had hypochromatic ash leaf-shaped macules in the trunk. Two years later, facial and ungual lesions appeared (Figs. 1 and 2). When he was 7 years old, a diagnosis of tuberous sclerosis (Bourneville disease) was made. At 13 years of age, a cranial computed axial tomographic scan and echocardiogram revealed characteristic lesions related to Bourneville disease (Figs. 3 and 4). The patient has never had cardiac symptoms, and physical examination and ECG are normal.

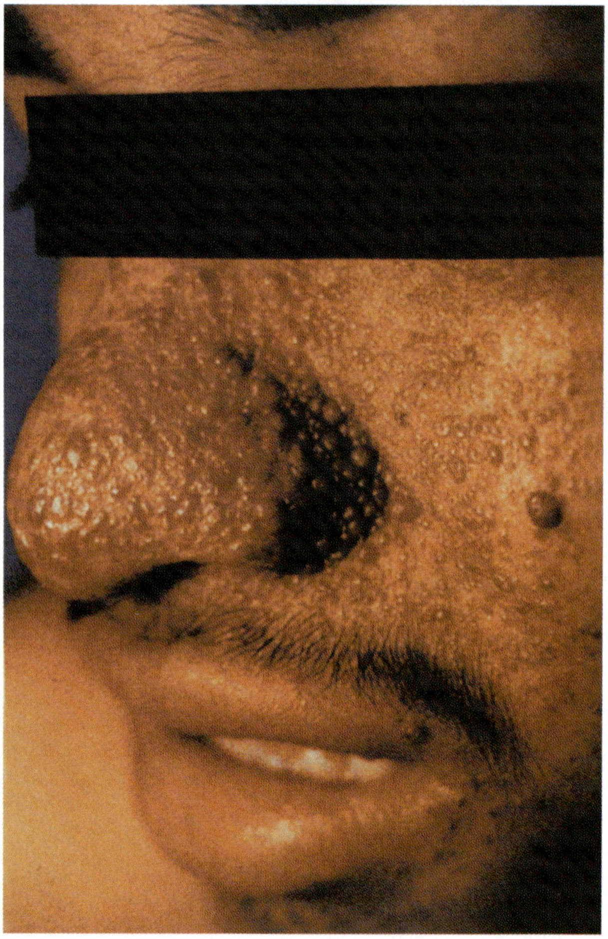

Figure 1. Photograph showing facial angiofibromas involving cheeks, nose, and chin, with relative sparing of the upper lip.

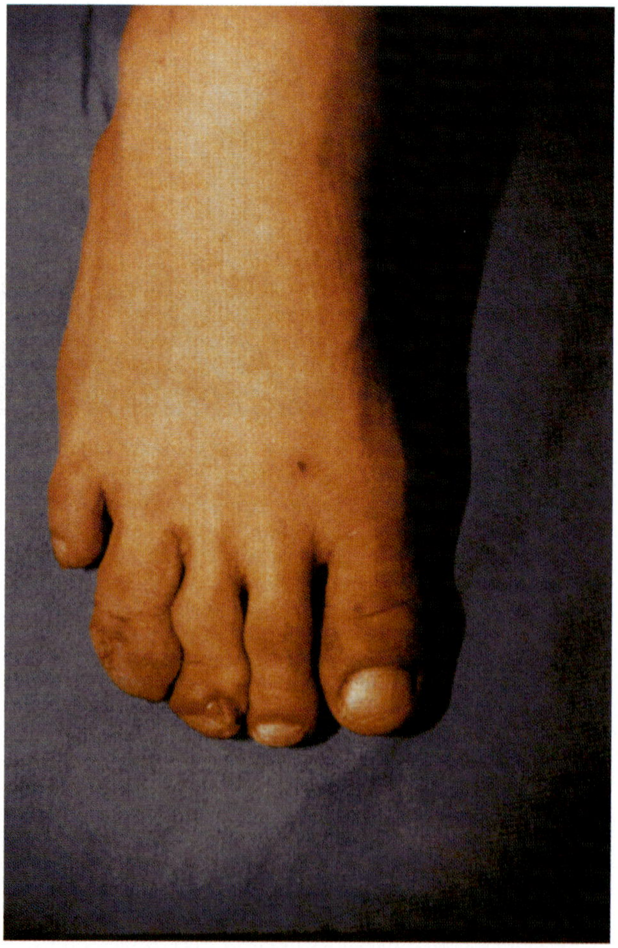

Figure 2. Photograph showing fibromas of nails.

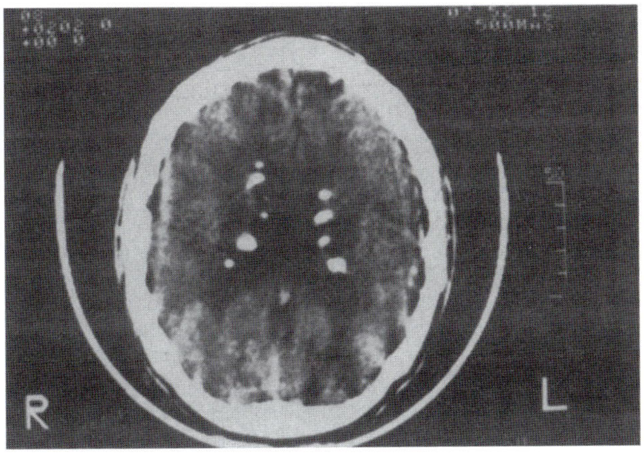

Figure 3. Cranial computed axial tomographic scan showing calcified subependymal glial nodules in the lateral walls of the lateral ventricles.

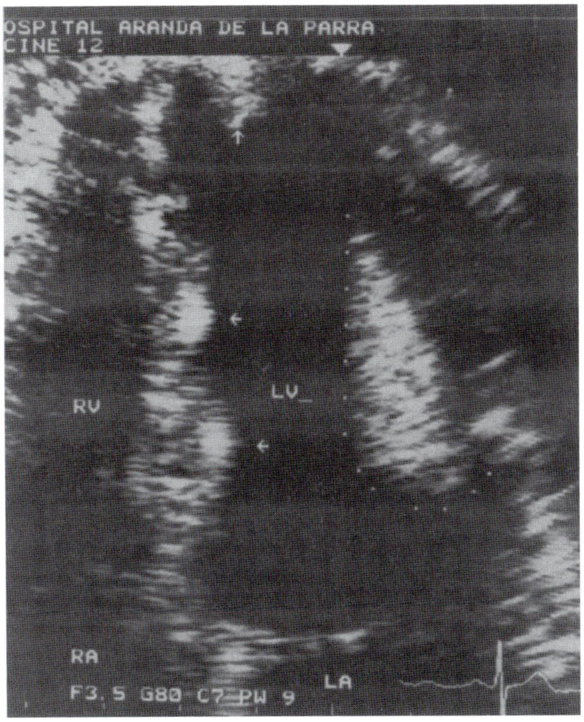

Figure 4. Echocardiogram in apical four-chamber view with several medium-size (0.8- to 1-cm) intracardiac masses (probably rhabdomyomas) in the left ventricle located in the apex and interventricular septum. There is also a large mass (3.5 × 1 cm) attached to the lateral wall of the left ventricle.

58 Permanent Pacemaker Wire Vegetation in the Right Atrium

Prasad Chalasani, MD; David H. Montgomery, MD; George L. Chang, MD; Wacin Buddhari, MD; Joel M. Felner, MD

From the Division of Cardiology, Emory University School of Medicine, Atlanta, Ga.

(*Circulation*. 1995;92:148.)

A 64-year-old patient presented with methicillin-sensitive staphylococcal bacteremia 4 weeks after intravenous implantation of a ventricular pacemaker. The patient continued to have positive blood cultures despite antibiotic therapy with nafcillin. Multiple pulmonary abscesses were noted on chest radiograph and computed tomography (CT) scan of the chest. A transesophageal echocardiogram revealed the images presented in Figures 1 and 2. This patient was managed with pacemaker wire removal through venotomy followed by a course of antibiotics. At the time of pacemaker removal, infection of the pacemaker pocket was also noted, and cultures revealed the same organism.

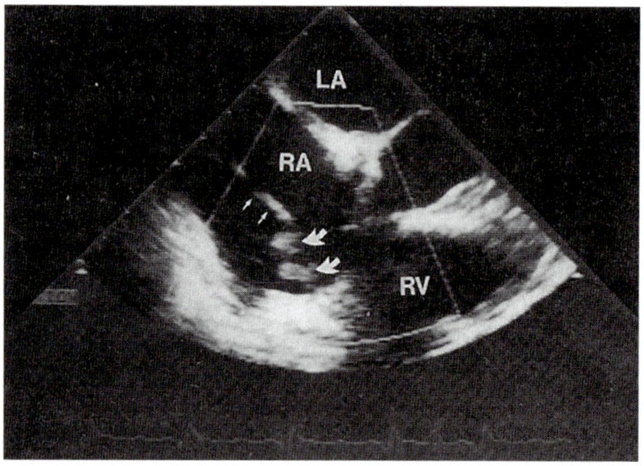

Figure 1. Transesophageal echocardiogram shows the right atrium (RA) with two large masses (bold arrows) attached to the pacemaker (small arrows). LA indicates left atrium; RV, right ventricle.

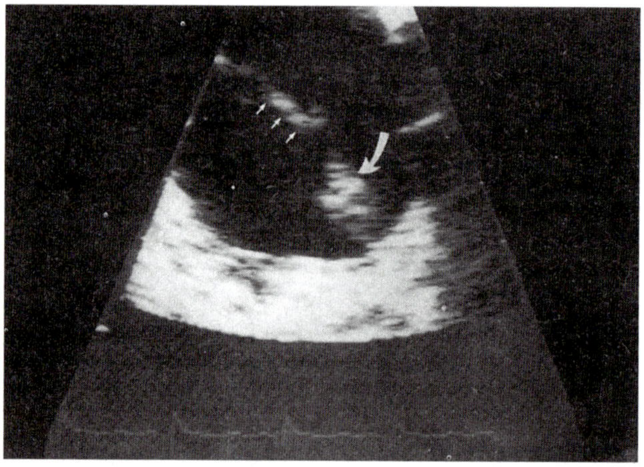

Figure 2. Transesophageal echocardiogram: Magnification of right atrium shows a large mass (bold arrow) attached to the pacemaker wire (small arrows).

59 Impending Paradoxical Embolus

Barry P. Rosenzweig, MD; Lawrence Glassman, MD; Itzhak Kronzon, MD
From the Departments of Medicine and Surgery (L.G.), New York University School of Medicine, NY.

(*Circulation*. 1996;93:387.)

The diagnosis of paradoxical embolization typically requires evidence of acute systemic arterial occlusion, systemic venous thrombosis, and a pathway for the thromboembolus to bypass the pulmonary vasculature. However, even when all of these findings are present, they cumulatively represent only a "smoking gun" from which a diagnosis is inferred. It is rare that one captures the actual process of paradoxical embolization "red-handed."

These transthoracic and transesophageal echocardiographic images demonstrate a thrombus traversing the patent foramen ovale of a 76-year-old woman (Fig. 1). She had presented with syncope, and a ventilation-perfusion lung scan revealed a segmental abnormality strongly suggestive of pulmonary embolus. Emergency surgery confirmed the echocardiographic diagnosis and may have saved her the devastation of systemic arterial occlusion. The thrombus that was extricated from the atria and the patent foramen ovale is shown in Figure 2.

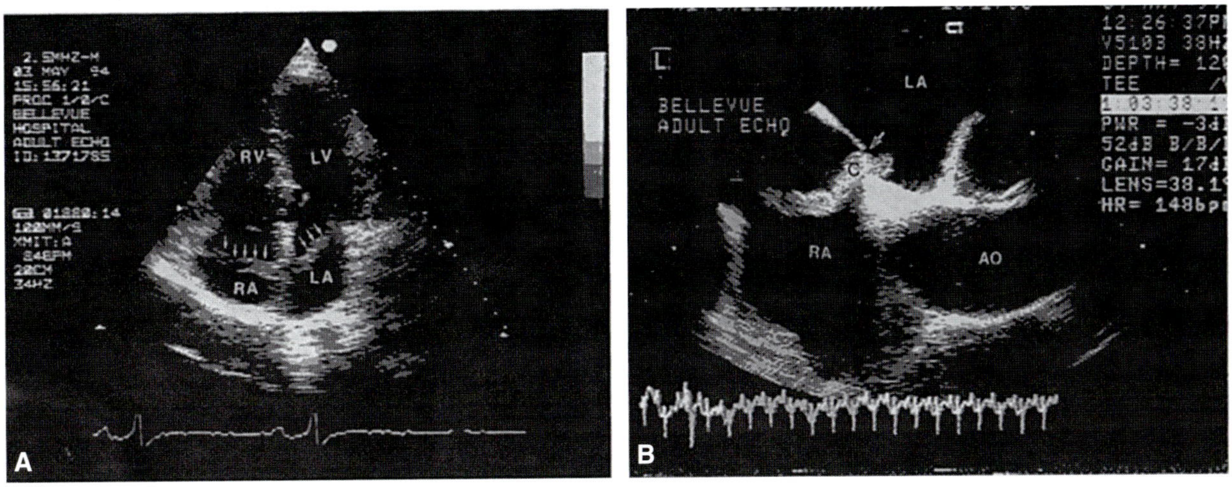

Figure 1. A, Transthoracic echocardiographic image obtained from the apical view. A long thrombus (arrows) is seen within both atria apparently traversing the interatrial septum in its midportion. In real time, its ends were wildly mobile and even entered the atrioventricular valve orifices during diastole. LA indicates left atrium; LV, left ventricle; RA, right atrium; and RV, right ventricle. **B,** Transesophageal echocardiographic image in the longitudinal plane. A thrombus (C) extends from the right atrium (RA) across the interatrial septum via a patent foramen ovale (arrow) into the left atrium (LA). The full length of the thrombus and its extent into the left atrium as well as its wild motion are lost in this still frame image. AO indicates aorta.

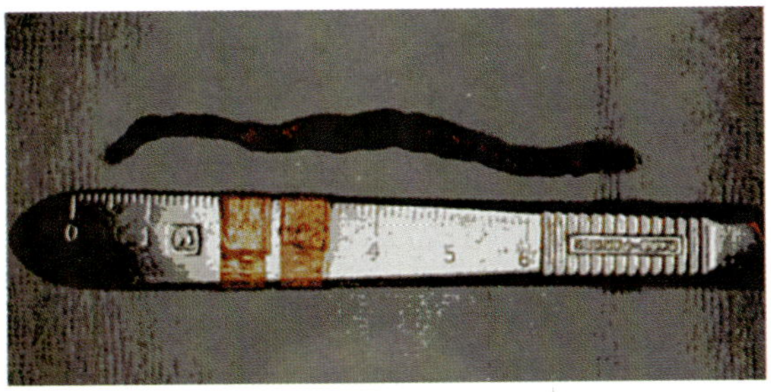

Figure 2. Gross pathological specimen removed from the heart via a right atriotomy. This elongated thrombus traversed a patent foramen ovale and was freely mobile in both atria.

60 Superior Vena Caval Thrombosis

Thomas C. Mathew, MD; Eddison K. Ramsaran, MD; Jayashri R. Aragam, MD
From the Division of Cardiology, Saint Vincent Hospital, Worcester, Mass.

(*Circulation*. 1996;93:1767.)

A 56-year-old man presented with dyspnea and chest discomfort following gastrectomy for metastatic adenocarcinoma. Transthoracic echocardiography showed a mass in the right atrium (RA); he subsequently underwent transesophageal echocardiography using a biplane probe. Imaging done in the horizontal plane (Fig. 1) showed a mass (arrows) in the RA; vertical plane imaging (Fig. 2) revealed a serpentine mass (arrows) originating in the superior vena cava (SVC) and extending into the RA, consistent with thrombus. AO indicates aorta; IVC, inferior vena cava; and LA, left atrium.

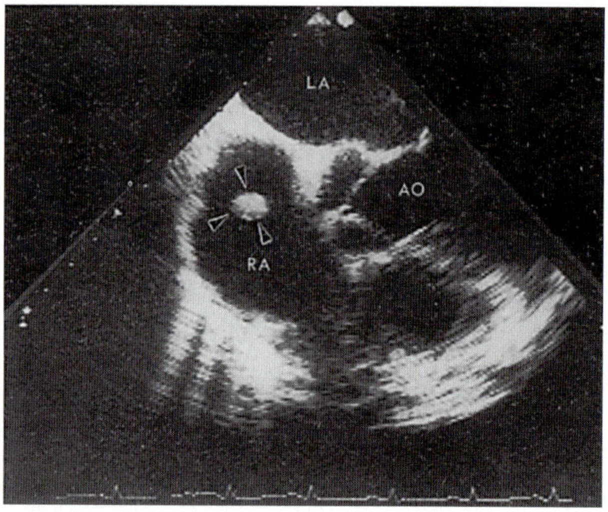

Figure 1. Horizontal plane imaging.

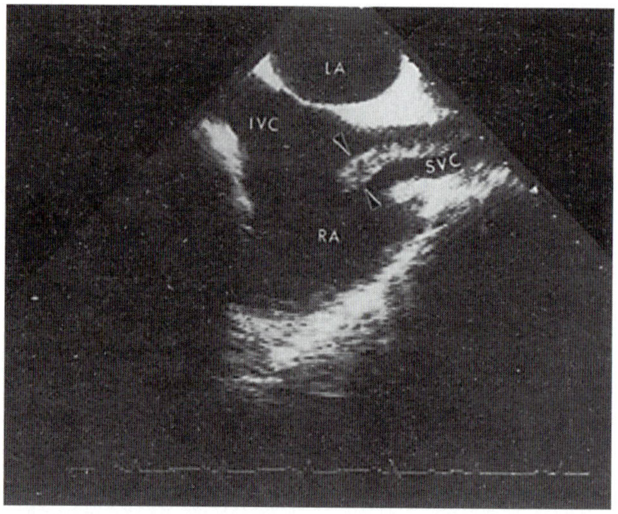

Figure 2. Vertical plane imaging.

61

Left Ventricular Thromboembolism

Dean G. Karalis, MD; John J. Ross, Jr, RCVT, RDCS; Joseph L. Neri, DO

From Allegheny University Hospital, Hahnemann Division, Philadelphia, Pa.

(*Circulation.* 1998;97:498.)

Left ventricular thrombi can occur after acute myocardial infarction or in patients with chronic left ventricular dysfunction. Stasis of blood within areas of akinesis or dyskinesis is thought to be the mechanism by which thrombi form. Cardioembolic stroke is the most feared complication of left ventricular thrombi.

A 37-year-old man with progressive heart failure after myocardial infarction was found to have severe left ventricular dysfunction and a left ventricular posterobasal pseudoaneurysm. The patient underwent patch repair of the pseudoaneurysm and coronary artery bypass graft surgery. Intraoperative transesophageal echocardiography was used to image the heart throughout the surgical procedure. After separation of the patient from cardiopulmonary bypass, left ventricular function remained severely depressed, and a protruding and mobile thrombus was observed to form at the left ventricular apex, a site distinct from the aneurysm repair. The left ventricular thrombus took only several minutes to develop and then embolized from the heart into the peripheral arterial circulation (Fig. 1). Surprisingly, the patient suffered no neurological sequelae. The patient was discharged home without complications on chronic anticoagulation therapy with warfarin.

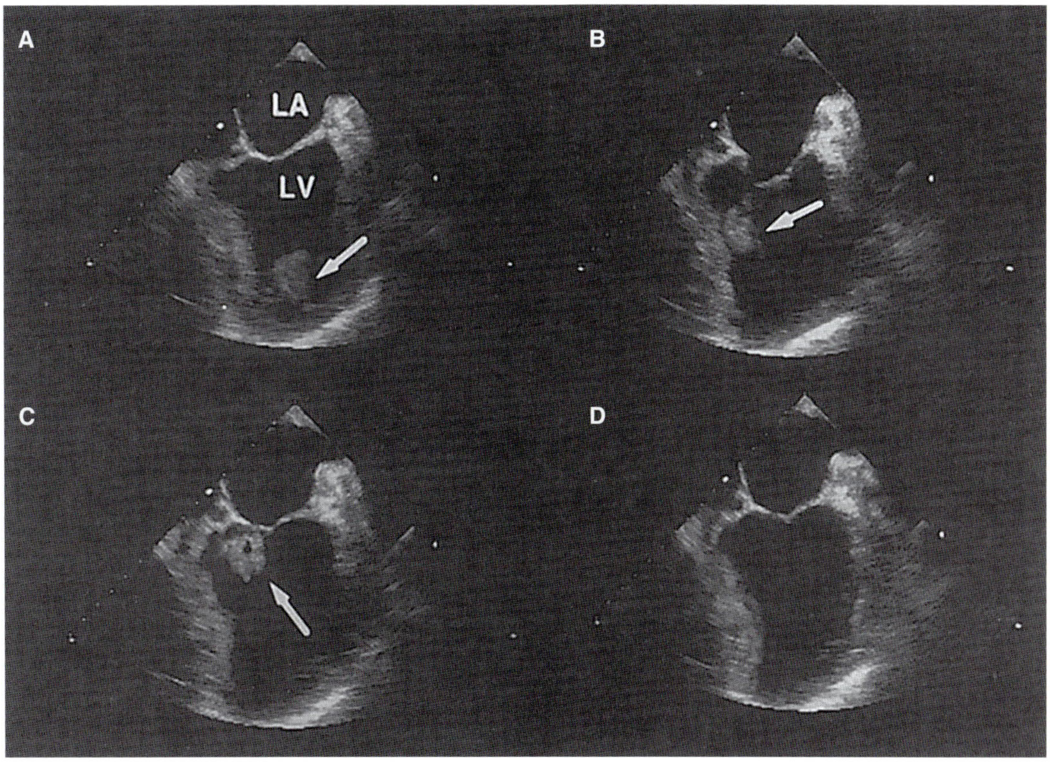

Figure 1. Serial transesophageal echocardiographic images as left ventricular thrombus embolized into peripheral arterial circulation. **A,** A protruding and mobile thrombus is seen at left ventricular (LV) apex. **B,** Thrombus has embolized and is now floating free in LV cavity. **C,** Thrombus is now below aortic valve in LV outflow tract. **D,** Thrombus has embolized distally out of heart into peripheral arterial circulation. LA indicates left atrium.

62

Primary Malignant Fibrous Histiocytoma of the Heart Treated with Orthotopic Heart Transplantation

Henry A. Harlamert, MD; Jonathan S. Moulton, MD; William Lewis, MD

From the Department of Pathology and Laboratory Medicine (H.A.H., W.L.) and the Department of Radiological Services (J.S.M.), University of Cincinnati (Ohio) College of Medicine.

(*Circulation.* 1998;97:703–704.)

A 24-year-old Caucasian man presented with dyspnea and fatigue. Physical examination revealed hepatosplenomegaly. A chest roentgenogram showed small pleural effusions without infiltrates. Ultrasound examination revealed ascites of the abdomen and pelvis and echogenic liver vessels that suggested congestive heart failure. A nuclear magnetic resonance image of the chest (Fig. 1A) showed a 4 × 6 cm mass occupying the right ventricle. The mass filled the apex and obstructed the right ventricular cavity. A computerized tomogram (Fig. 1B) localized the mass to the anterior and inferior right ventricular wall. For treatment, the tumor was debulked to reduce right ventricle obstruction. Histopathologically, the tumor was a malignant fibrous histocytoma. There was no evidence of an extracardiac primary site or distant metastasis. The patient underwent subsequent cardiac transplantation.

The explanted native heart contained the remaining tumor, measuring 6.2 × 3.5 × 8.5 cm, confined to the myocardium. The mass involved primarily the right ventricle and impinged significantly on the right ventricular cavity (Fig. 2). It extended cephalad from the right ventricular apex, involved the tricuspid valve, and penetrated the right atrial wall. Anteriorly, it extended into the interventricular septum and involved the left ventricular free wall and apex. The endocardium overlying the tumor was generally intact, with a few foci of adherent fibrin. Grossly, the tumor was white-to-tan and gelatinous, with a rubbery consistency (Fig. 3). Microscopically, sections showed a myxoid appearance with variable cellularity (Fig. 4). Mitoses were abundant, and abnormal mitoses were seen frequently. Tumor cells were oval and fusiform and had indistinct cell borders and abundant cytoplasm. Immunohistochemical stains of the tumor showed reactivity with antibodies to smooth muscle actin but not with antibodies to S-100 protein, cytokeratin, or desmin.

Primary cardiac sarcomas are rare. The patient is doing well 4 months after surgery.

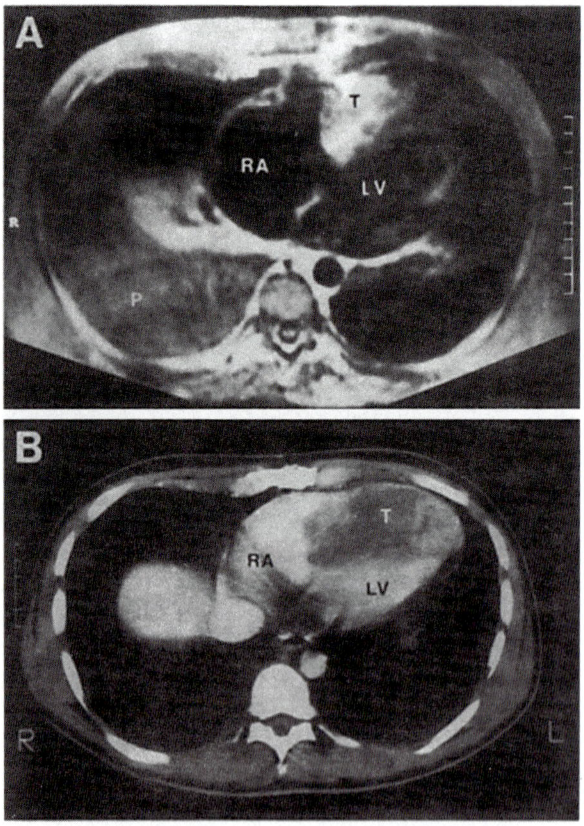

Figure 1. A, Magnetic resonance T1-weighted (T1W) image (after contrast) of chest showing a right ventricular tumor almost completely occluding the outflow tract and a large right pleural effusion. **B,** Computerized tomogram with intravenous contrast enhancement at level of cardiac apex with tumor involving anterior right ventricular wall and interventricular septum. RA indicates right atrium; LV, left ventricle; P, pleural effusion; and T, tumor.

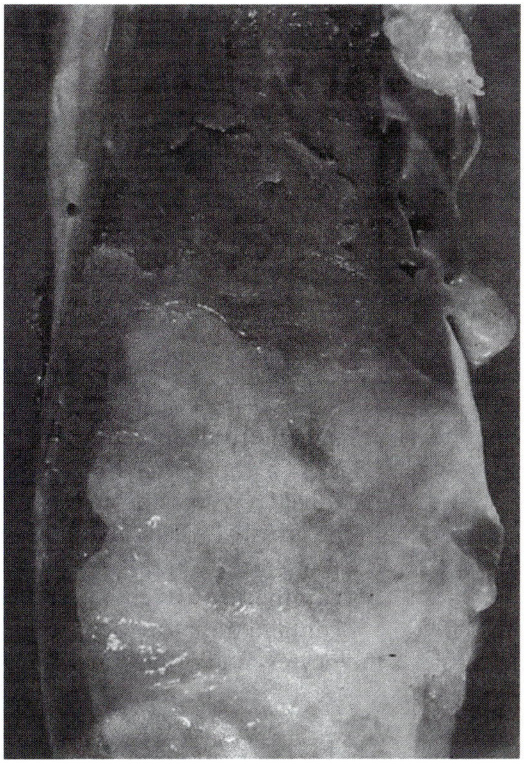

Figure 2. Gross photograph of tumor involving right ventricle, tricuspid valve, and right atrium with severe compression of right ventricular cavity.

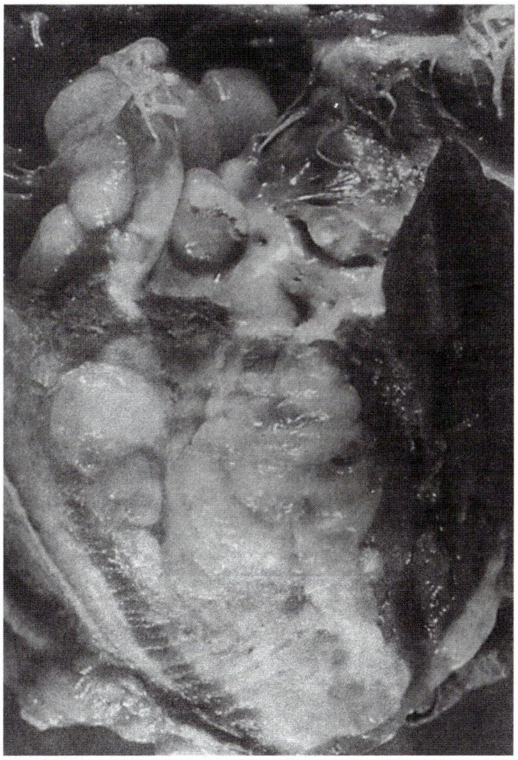

Figure 3. Gross photograph of cut section of tumor showing white-to-tan, gelatinous appearance.

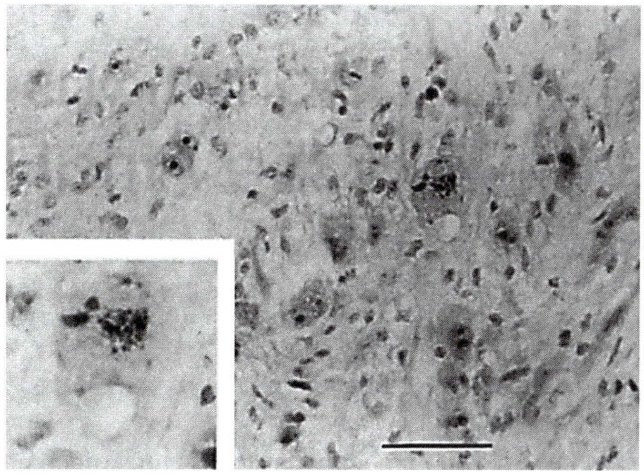

Figure 4. Microscopic section showing pleomorphic, fusiform tumor cells. One large cell contains an atypical mitotic figure (inset). Bar = 50 μm.

63 Lipomatous Hypertrophy of the Atrial Septum

C. Basso, MD; R. Barbazza, MD; G. Thiene, MD
From the Department of Pathology, University of Padua Medical School, Italy.

(*Circulation*. 1998;97:1423.)

A 74-year-old woman with a history of lung tuberculosis, peptic ulcer, diabetes mellitus (type 2), and progressive deterioration of psychomotor activity died after admission to hospital for acute bronchitis.

A basal ECG showed sinus rhythm, heart rate of 88 bpm, and P-wave abnormalities consisting of amplitude >2.5 mm in lead II, duration >100 ms, and "notching" configuration. Lipomatous hypertrophy of the atrial septum was found incidentally at autopsy, with a mass 3 × 2 cm in size.

In vitro nuclear magnetic resonance of a heart specimen showed (Fig. 1A) a round mass of bright intensity similar to epicardial fat within the atrial septum, corresponding to the grossly evident lipomatous accumulation (Fig. 1B).

At histological examination (Fig. 1C), the nonencapsulated mass contained mature adipocytes with intermingled myocytes and mild interstitial fibrosis (Azan stain).

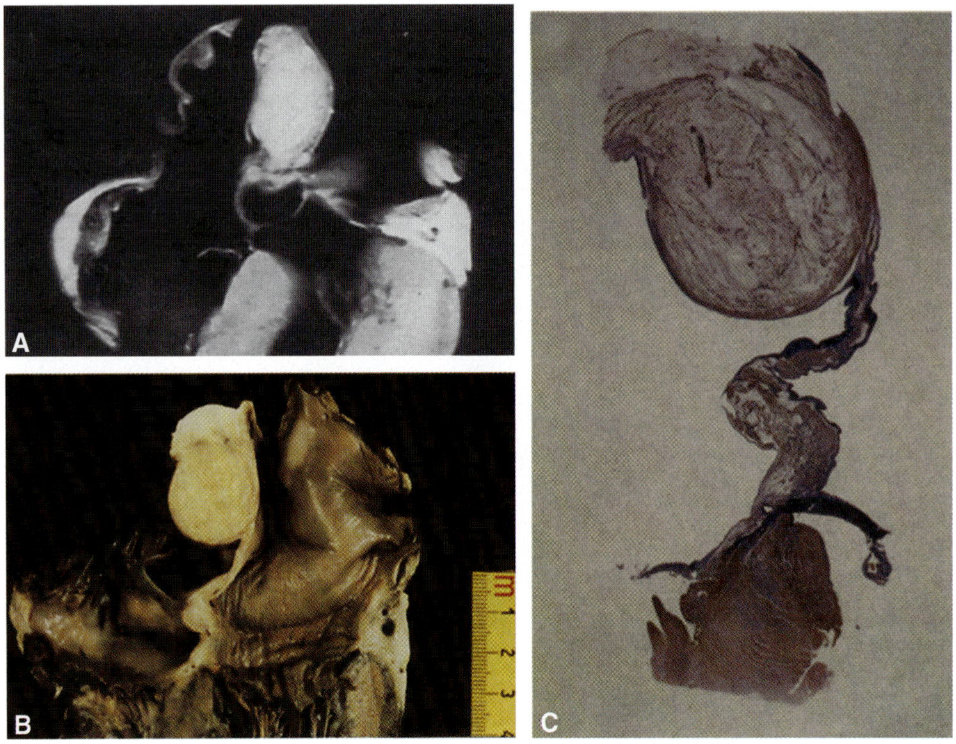

Figure 1.

64

Three-Dimensional Imaging of Atrial Myxoma

René Prêtre, MD; Cédric Vuille, MD; Sophie Diebold-Berger, MD; René Lerch, MD

From the Département de Chirurgie (R.P.), Service de Cardiologie (C.V., R.L.), and Division de Pathologie clinique (S.D.-B.), Hôpitaux Universitaires de Genève, Switzerland.

(*Circulation*. 1998;97:2186–2187.)

A 36-year-old man was admitted for investigation of night sweats and increasing exertional dyspnea. On clinical examination, he was afebrile, with normal blood pressure, regular cardiac rhythm, and no signs of cardiac failure. Auscultation revealed a holosystolic murmur, a diastolic rumbling, and an early diastolic sound (*tumor plop*). Routine blood tests were normal except for a sedimentation rate of 80 mm/hour (normal, <10 mm/hour) and a platelet count at 430,000/L (normal range, 150,000 to 300,000/L).

Echocardiography revealed a voluminous, mobile, and spherical tumor in the left atrium attached to the interatrial septum, suggesting myxoma. There was moderate mitral regurgitation. Size, location, and motion of the tumor were particularly well delineated by transesophageal echocardiography with three-dimensional reconstruction (Fig. 1). The echocardiographic findings were confirmed by MRI (Fig. 2).

The patient underwent resection of the myxoma and repair of the mitral valve under cardiopulmonary bypass and moderate hypothermia. The myxoma was a 7 × 5 × 5 cm tumor attached to the atrial septum, and it was removed with part of the interatrial septum (Fig. 3). The atrial defect was closed with a patch of autologous pericardium. Mitral regurgitation was due to prolapse of the anterior leaflet. Shortening of elongated chordae and ring annuloplasty restored valve competence, as assessed by intraoperative transesophageal echocardiography.

Anatomicopathological analysis (Fig. 4) confirmed the diagnosis of myxoma. The patient had an uneventful recovery and was discharged on warfarin sodium, which was discontinued after 2 months.

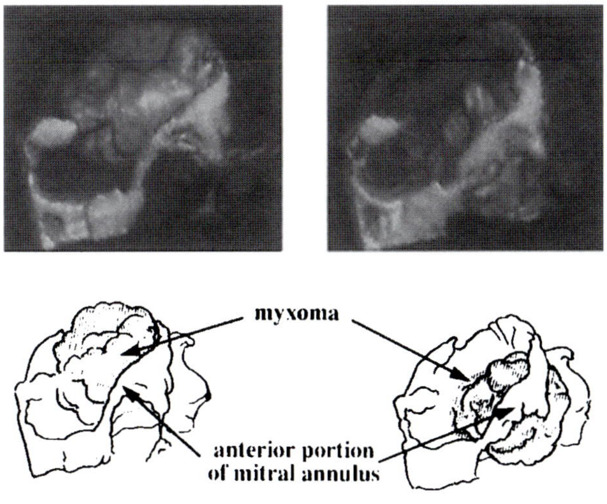

Figure 1. Three-dimensional transesophageal echocardiography showing a left atrial mass attached by stalk to interatrial septum, prolapsing through mitral valve during ventricular diastole.

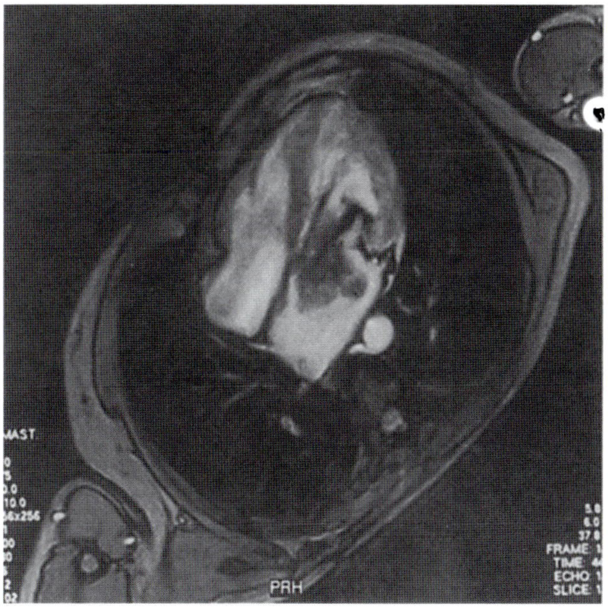

Figure 2. MRI showing mass in left atrium prolapsing through mitral valve during ventricular diastole.

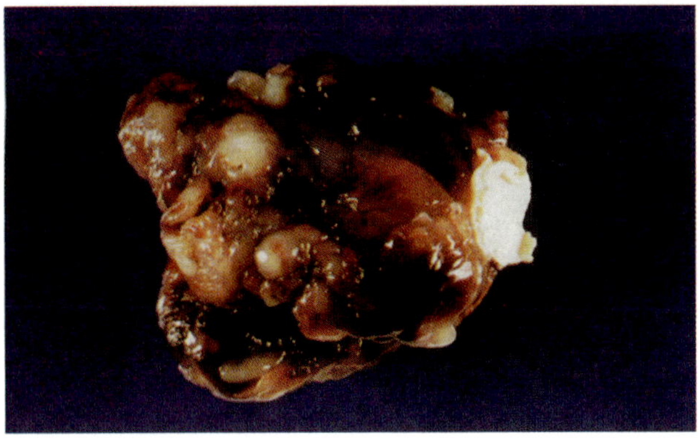

Figure 3. Macroscopic view of surgical specimen. Tumor was resected with a piece of interatrial septum.

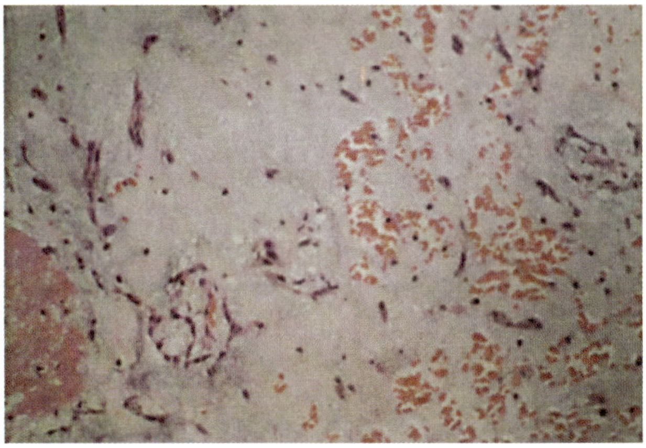

Figure 4. Microscopic examination of tumor showing an abundant stroma of glycosaminoglycan and dispersed, isolated, or clustered polygonal cells consistent with a cardiac myxoma (hematoxylin and eosin, ×400).

65 Left Ventricular Thrombus Detected by Two- and Three-Dimensional Computed Tomographic Ventriculography: A New Application of Helical Computed Tomography

Teruhito Mochizuki, MD; Yasushi Koyama, MD; Hiroaki Tanaka, MD; Junpei Ikezoe, MD; Yun Shen, PhD; Shogo Azemoto, RT

From the Departments of Radiology (T.M., H.T.) and Cardiology (Y.K.), Ehime-Imabari Hospital; the Department of Radiology, Ehime University School of Medicine (J.I.); and GE-Yokogawa Medical Systems (Y.S., S.A.), Japan.

(*Circulation*. 1998;98:933–934.)

A 67-year-old man presented with chest discomfort. At the age of 65 years, he had been hospitalized because of acute anteroseptal myocardial infarction. Coronary angiography and left ventriculography (LVG) were performed to evaluate his present status. The LVG revealed left ventricular (LV) aneurysm. A LV thrombus at the apex was suspected (Fig. 1A). By use of a new application of helical computed tomography (CT) with contrast enhancement, that is, computed tomographic ventriculography (CT-VG), a LV aneurysm and the apical thrombus were demonstrated by both two-dimensional (2-D) and three-dimensional (3-D) CT-VG (Figs. 1B and 1C). In addition, the 2-D CT-VG depicted markedly thinned anteroseptal wall.

CT-VG is a new application of helical CT, which can assess heart function, such as wall motion and systolic thickening in any direction (2-D and 3-D + cine movie) as well as clear morphological information. The 50-rotation raw data were acquired with a single-breath-hold helical CT. Approximately 500 transaxial slices were obtained from the raw data with 0.1 pitch overlapping reconstruction (3 mm thick, 0.08 second, and 0.2 mm slice per frame interval). All 500 transaxial slices, which included different cardiac phases, were reordered to separate different cardiac cycles (end-diastolic, end-systolic, and others) and stored in new files. The separated new files were reformatted to 2-D and 3-D images.

(Figures follow on next page.)

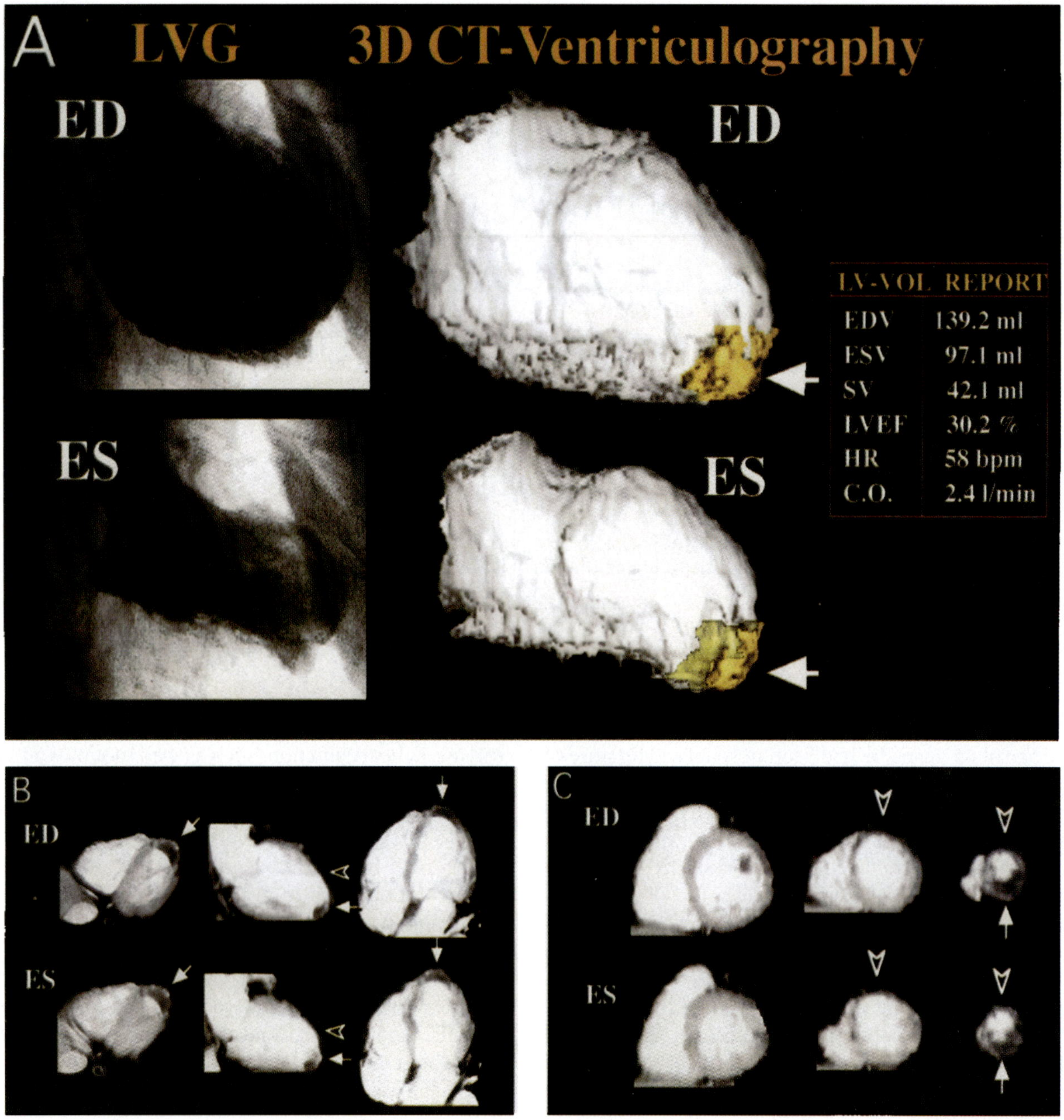

Figure 1. A, LVG depicts LV aneurysm. Thrombus at apex is suspected. CT-VG from same view of LVG clearly demonstrates both LV aneurysm and apical thrombus (yellow mass, arrow). Top, End-diastolic (ED) and bottom, end-systolic (ES) phases. LV volumes were assessed. EDV indicates end-diastolic volume; ESV, end-systolic volume; SV, stroke volume; LVEF, LV ejection fraction; HR, heart rate; and C.O., cardiac output. **B,** 2-D CT-VG in transaxial (left), vertical long-axial (middle), and horizontal long-axial (right) planes. Both ED (top) and ES (bottom) images depict LV thrombus. In vertical long axis, markedly thinned anterior (arrowhead) wall and LV aneurysm are evident. Neither wall motion nor systolic thickening was observed in infarct lesion. **C,** 2-D CT-VG in short-axial plane (left, basal; middle, midventricle; and right, apex). In midventricular and apical short-axial images, markedly thinned anteroseptal wall (arrowhead) is evident. LV thrombus (arrow) at apex is also depicted.

66

Mobile Left Atrial Thrombus Associated with Mitral Stenosis

G.R. Wright-Smith, MBBS; D.J. Burstow, FRACP; R. Seymour, FRACP; C. Smith, FRACS; M.F. O'Brien, FRACS, FRCS

From The Prince Charles Hospital, Brisbane, Queensland, Australia, Departments of Cardiology and Cardiothoracic Surgery.

(*Circulation.* 1998;98:931–932.)

A 68-year-old woman presented with a 6-week history of shortness of breath on exertion. She had longstanding mitral stenosis and atrial fibrillation and was not taking oral anticoagulants.

Thirty years previously, she reportedly had had a stroke and made a full recovery. Transthoracic echocardiography (Fig. 1) demonstrated a freely mobile mass in the left atrium associated with severe mitral stenosis and mild aortic stenosis. The mass bounced around the atrium like a ball in a pinball machine.

At surgery, a large, unattached, completely smooth, circular thrombus (Figs. 2 and 3) was removed, and the patient had a mitral valve replacement and aortic valvotomy.

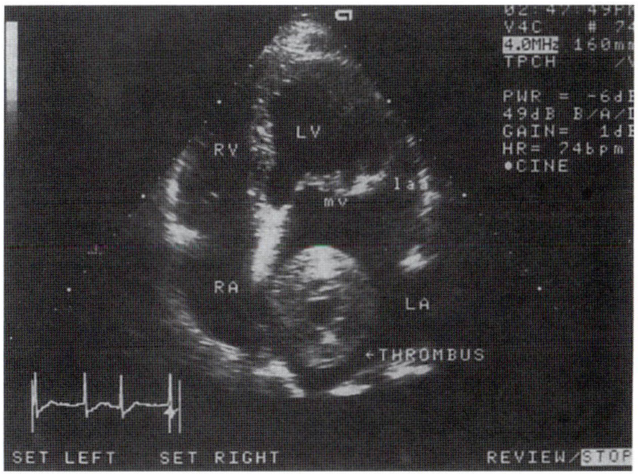

Figure 1. Transthoracic echocardiogram showing a large, ball-shaped mass, with an echolucent center, that was freely mobile within the left atrial cavity. The mitral valve was thickened and calcified, and Doppler hemodynamics demonstrated severe mitral stenosis with a valve area of 0.8 cm^2 and moderate left atrial dilatation.

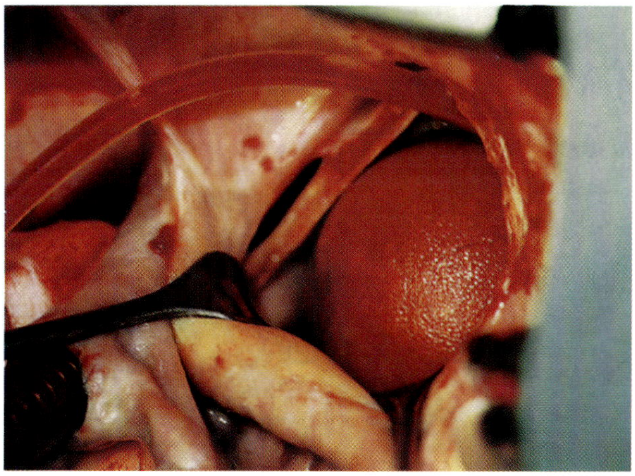

Figure 2. At surgery, the mass was not adherent to the atrial wall and was easily removed from the left atrium.

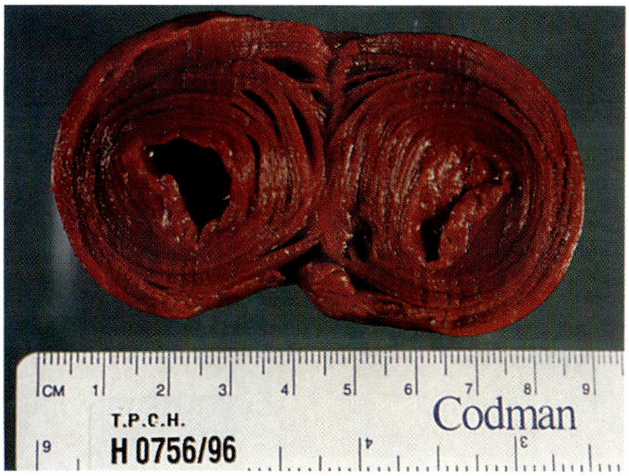

Figure 3. Cut section of the mass revealed laminated thrombus, giving an onionskin appearance with central cavitation.

67 Fungal Whip Beats the Heart

Antonio Rivero Román, MD; Isabel Rodriguez-Bailón, MD; Juan José Gómez-Doblas, MD
From the Virgen de la Victoria University Hospital, Málaga, Spain.

(*Circulation*. 1999;100:1249.)

A 24-year-old man was admitted to the hospital because of fever, cough, and dyspnea of 4 weeks' duration. The patient gave a history of parenteral drug abuse since he was 17 years old and had been diagnosed with human immunodeficiency virus (HIV) infection 4 years before admission. A chest radiograph showed multiple alveolar infiltrates. Four blood cultures were positive for *Candida albicans*.

Different echocardiographic views of the right heart cavities are shown in Figure 1.

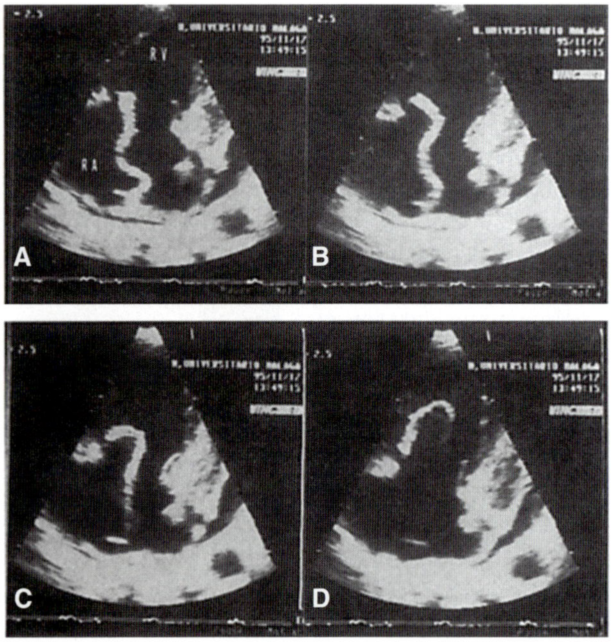

Figure 1. A long, highly mobile, and whiplike structure can be seen attached to the nonseptal leaflet of the tricuspid valve, traveling from the right atrium (RA) to the right ventricle (RV) with each cardiac cycle **(A, B, C,** and **D)** It represents a bizarre form of fungal vegetation that hits the patient's heart with each cardiac beat.

68

Intracardiac Extension of Pelvic Leiomyoma

Himadri Dasgupta, MD; Louis A. Nassef, MD; Christian L. Gilbert, MD; John M. Costello, Jr, MD; Silvia E. Garcia-Mayorca, MD

From the Department of Cardiology and the Division of Cardiothoracic and Vascular Surgery, Geisinger Medical Center, Danville, Pa.

(*Circulation*. 1999;100:2035–2038.)

A 48-year-old woman presented with a pulmonary embolus diagnosed by ventilation-perfusion scan 2 years after removal of a uterine leiomyoma with intravascular extension. Transthoracic echocardiography revealed a dilated inferior vena cava (IVC) containing a mass extending into the right atrium (RA). Transesophageal echocardiography showed a large vacuolated tumor filling the RA (Fig. 1). The IVC was seen to be dilated and partly obstructed by the tumor, causing spontaneous echo contrast in the residual lumen due to the low-flow state (Fig. 2).

The T1-weighted axial MRI images revealed dilatation of the IVC, with tumor extending from the left iliac vein via the IVC into the heart (Fig. 3). The angiogram showed neovascularity filling a pelvic mass (tumor vessels, Fig. 4) via the left hypogastric artery.

Sternotomy with right atriotomy and laparotomy confirmed the presence of a 6-cm pelvic tumor extending into the RA via the IVC (Fig. 5). The nonadherent intracardiac portion of the tumor was removed retrogradely through a longitudinal IVC incision.

Histopathology confirmed the diagnosis of intravascular leiomyoma (Fig. 6).

LA indicates left atrium; TV, tricuspid valve; MV, mitral valve; RV, right ventricle; LV, left ventricle; and HV, hepatic vein.

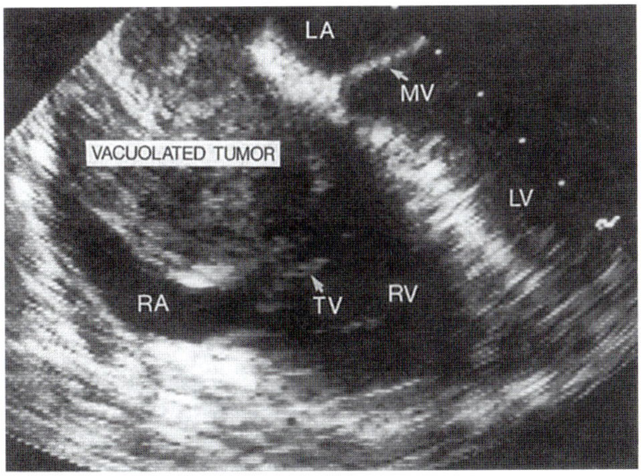

Figure 1.

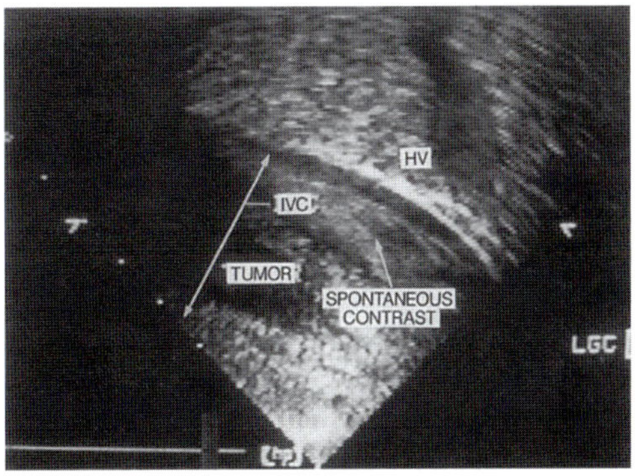

Figure 2.

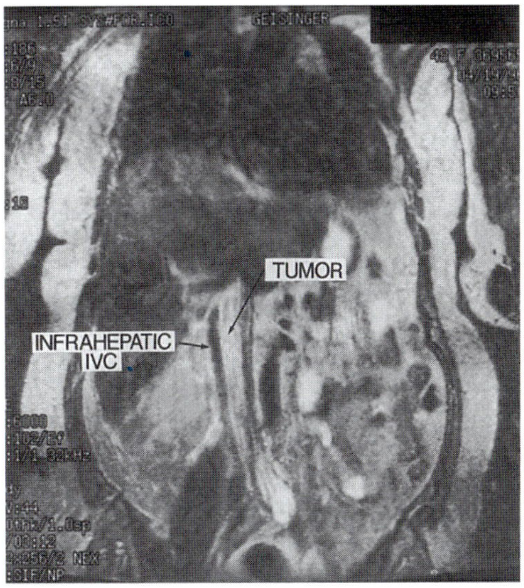

Figure 3.

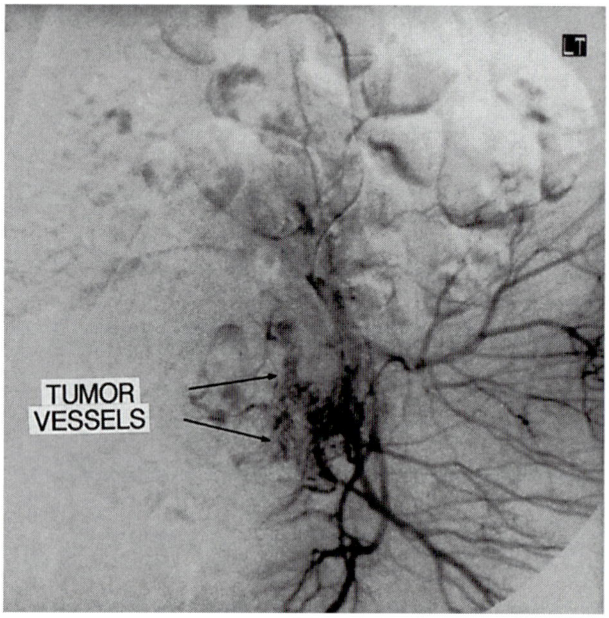

Figure 4.

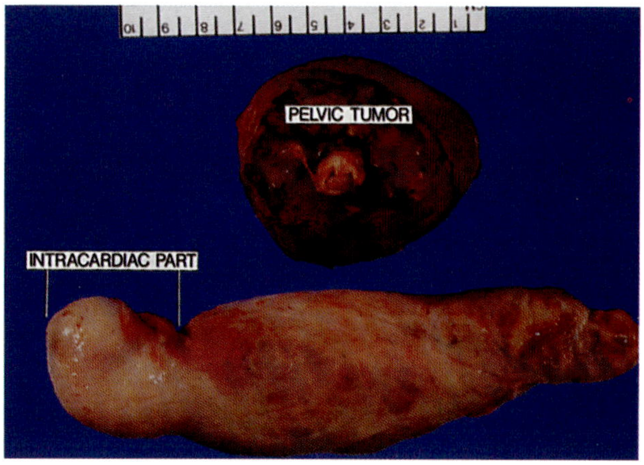

Figure 5.

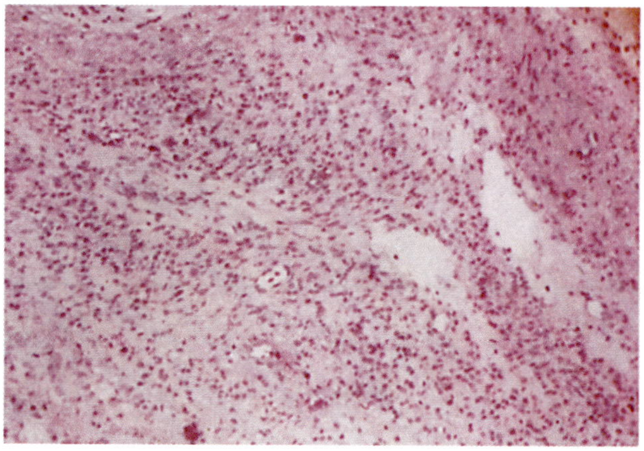

Figure 6.

69

Clostridium perfringens within Intracardiac Thrombus: A Case of Intracardiac Gas Gangrene

Pertha S. Chowdhury, MD; Steven B. H. Timmis, MD; Pamela A. Marcovitz, MD

From the Department of Internal Medicine, Division of Cardiology, William Beaumont Hospital, Royal Oak, Mich.

(*Circulation*. 1999;100:2119.)

A 70-year-old man with ischemic dilated cardiomyopathy and a known right atrial mass, presumed to be thrombus, presented to the hospital with 3 weeks of fevers and chills. One year before this admission, transesophageal echocardiography had demonstrated a 3 × 3 cm mass in the right atrium, extending into the superior vena cava (Fig. 1A). The mass was contiguous with the tip of a Groshong catheter, which was used for home dobutamine infusion. Because of a high operative risk at that time, the patient had declined surgical resection of the right atrial mass. During the present hospital admission, the Groshong catheter was removed after four of six blood cultures grew *Clostridium perfringens*. The presumed source of the bacteremia was the patient's oropharynx, because he had extremely poor dentition. Repeat transesophageal echocardiography demonstrated increased size of the mass with loss of echoes centrally and extensive shadowing posteriorly (Fig. 1B). Computed tomography (CT) of the chest revealed a gas-filled mass in the right atrium, occluding the superior vena cava and extending into the right brachiocephalic vein (Fig. 1C). Given the presence of bacteremia with a known gas-producing organism, it is likely that the thrombus was infected with *C. perfringens*. Considering the extensive nature of the thrombus and the patient's underlying cardiomyopathy, surgical treatment was not feasible, and the patient was placed on long-term antibiotic therapy with penicillin and metronidazole. To the best of our knowledge, this is the first reported case of such a lesion.

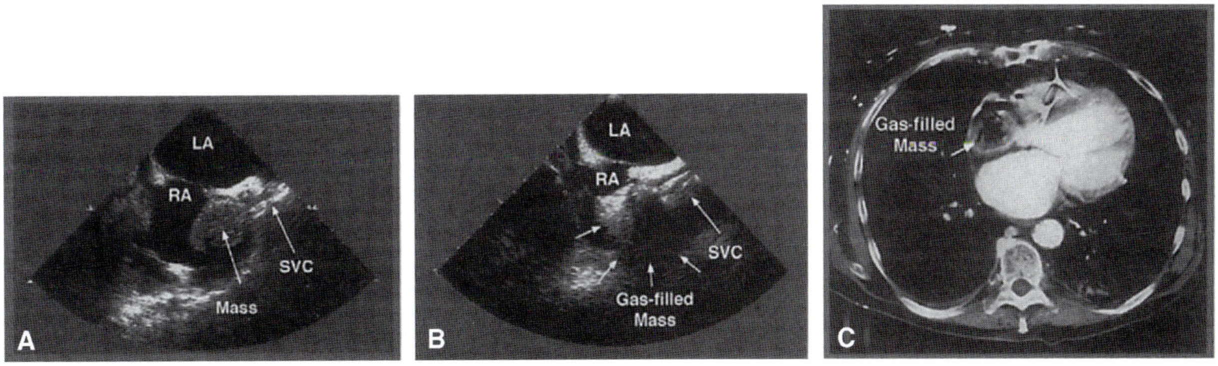

Figure 1. A, Transesophageal echocardiography of left atrium (LA), right atrium (RA), and superior vena cava (SVC) 1 year earlier demonstrates a mass occupying RA, extending into SVC. **B,** Present transesophageal echocardiogram in same view displays right atrial mass with a new central echolucency and posterior shadowing. **C,** CT with intravenous contrast demonstrates that right atrial mass is gas-filled with no contrast opacification.

70 Migration of Intrahepatic Portosystemic Stent into Right Ventricle: An Unusual Cause of Tricuspid Regurgitation

Andre Z. Linka, MD; Rolf Jenni, MD, MSEE

From the Cardiovascular Center, Echocardiography Laboratory, University Hospital, Zurich, Switzerland.

(*Circulation*. 2001;103:161–162.)

A 65-year-old woman with terminal liver disease and portal hypertension secondary to alcohol-induced cirrhosis underwent an elective transjugular intrahepatic portosystemic shunt procedure. A self-expanding, 100 × 80 mm Nitinol (Jomed AG) stent was implanted and extended cranially using an additional 40 × 12 mm Wallstent (Boston Scientific). During the same admission, she was evaluated and accepted for liver transplantation, which was performed 4 days later when an organ was available. In the explanted liver, one patent intraparenchymal stent was described by the pathologist. Three weeks after surgery, she was referred to a rehabilitation facility. The new organ showed good function, but she had a recurrence of ascites that was managed medically, and she returned home 6 weeks after liver transplantation. In the seventh postoperative week, however, the amount of ascites increased, which necessitated the drainage of several liters of peritoneal fluid. About 8 weeks after surgery, she became increasingly dyspneic. A chest radiograph at that time showed no evidence of pleural effusion or consolidation, but, surprisingly, it did reveal a radio-opaque stent-like structure projected over the right ventricle. Doppler echocardiography (Figs. 1 and 2) was performed, and it revealed a stent in the right ventricle caught within the subvalvular tricuspid apparatus, leading to severe tricuspid regurgitation.

The stent was removed at surgery, and the tricuspid valve was reconstructed because the stent had perforated the septal leaflet. She had an uneventful postoperative recovery without recurrence of ascites.

It was concluded that the second Wallstent had dislodged during the perioperative period, most likely during the transplantation itself. In retrospect, the stent was seen on the first postoperative chest radiograph performed on the day of surgery.

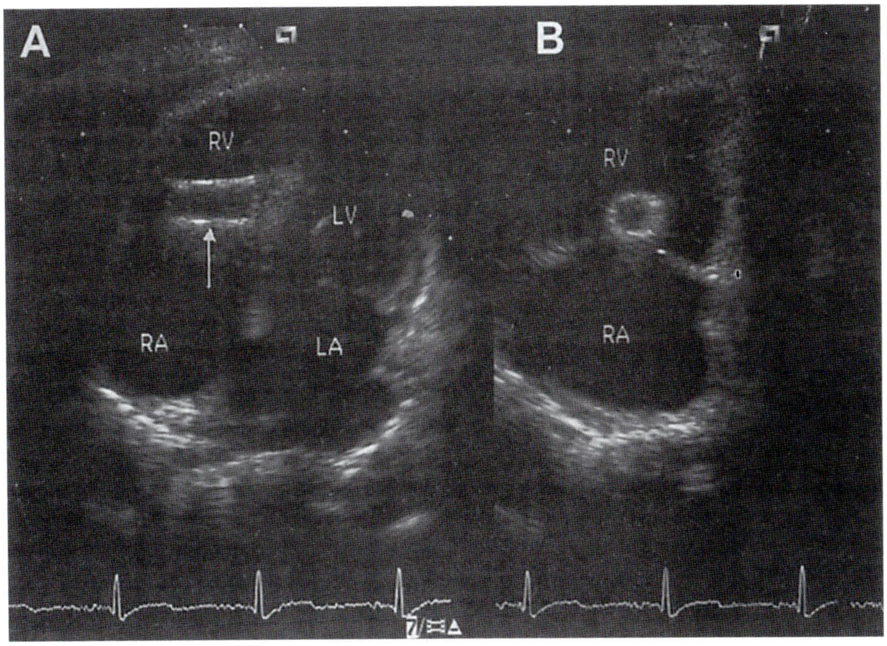

Figure 1. A, Apical four-chamber view by transthoracic echocardiography. Right ventricle (RV) and right atrium (RA) are enlarged. Stent (arrow) is caught horizontally within subvalvular tricuspid apparatus. **B,** View perpendicular to that in A. LV indicates left ventricle; LA, left atrium.

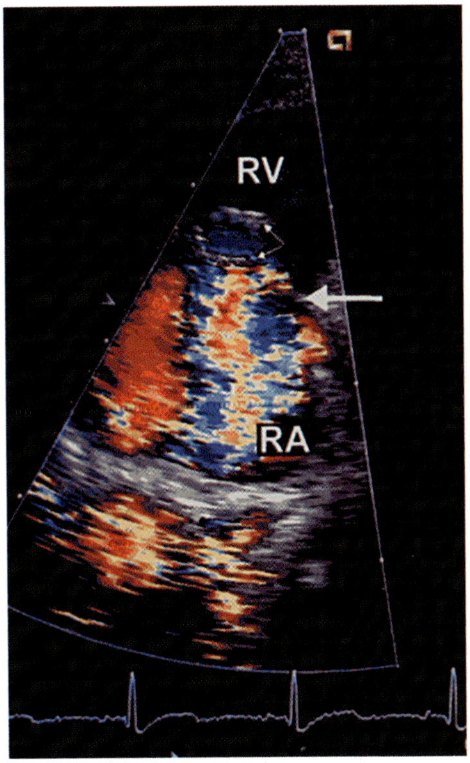

Figure 2. Apical four-chamber color Doppler recording (same view as that shown in Fig 1A) demonstrating a broad and turbulent regurgitant jet in systole extending from tricuspid valve (large arrow) to superior wall of right atrium (RA), indicating severe tricuspid regurgitation. Note perfusion (blue color) of stent (small double arrow). RV indicates right ventricle.

71 Right Ventricular Lead Perforation Presenting as Left Chest Wall Muscle Stimulation

Scott Greenberg, MD; Jennifer Lawton, MD; Jane Chen, MD

From the Cardiovascular Division (S.G., J.C.) and Cardiothoracic Surgery Division (J.L.), Washington University School of Medicine, St. Louis, Mo.

(*Circulation*. 2005;111:e451–e452.)

DOI: 10.1161.CIRCULATIONAHA.104.494732

An 83-year-old man with a history of coronary artery disease and three-vessel coronary artery bypass grafting underwent implantation of a pacemaker (Medtronic EnPulse E2DR01) at an outside facility because he experienced recurrent syncope and an abnormal response to tilt table testing. Active fixation leads were implanted in the right atrium (Medtronic 5076–52) and right ventricle (Medtronic 5076–58). At the time of implantation, all lead parameters were within normal limits, and the right ventricular lead was positioned in the apex. Twelve days after the implantation, the patient developed intermittent left chest muscle twitching. He presented to an outside hospital's emergency department, where chest radiographs revealed that the right ventricular lead was outside the cardiac silhouette (Fig. 1). A transthoracic echocardiogram excluded a pericardial effusion. He was subsequently transferred to our institution, where interrogation revealed visible evidence of left pectoralis major muscle contraction when pacing the right ventricle at 2.5 V and 0.5 ms. Left chest muscle twitching resolved with reprogramming to AAI mode at a rate of 50 bpm.

Chest CT showed the right ventricle electrode tip position to be in the anterior chest wall and confirmed the absence of a pericardial effusion (Fig. 2). The

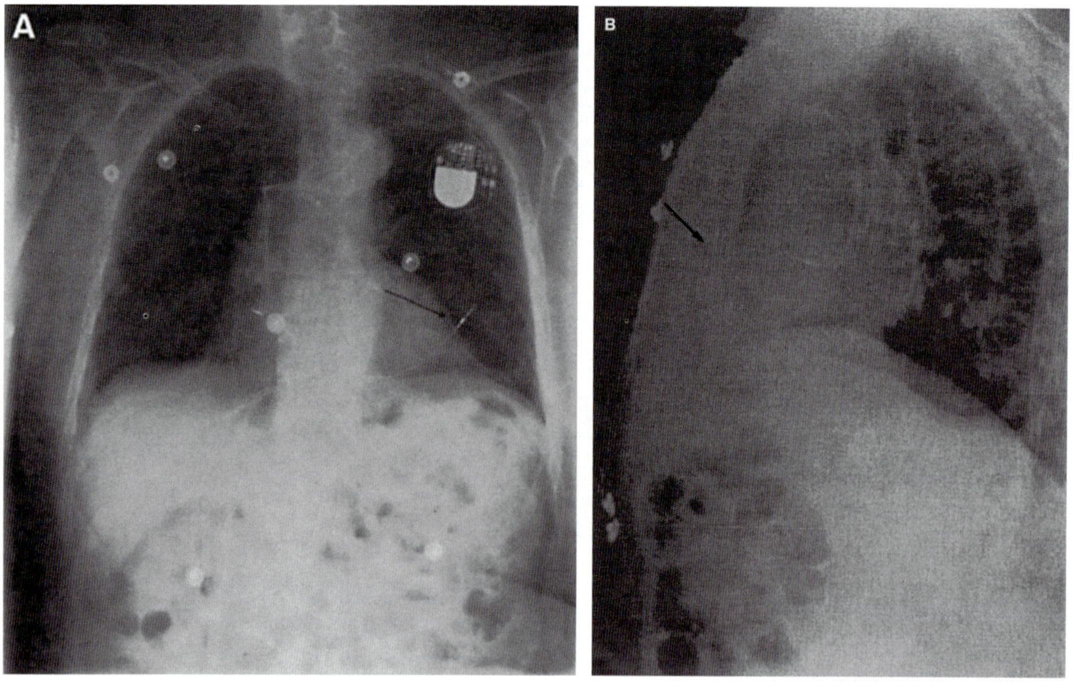

Figure 1. Chest radiographs in the posterior-anterior **(A)** and lateral views **(B)**. A dual-lead transvenous pacemaker is evident. The right ventricular (RV) lead (arrow) appears to penetrate the RV free wall and terminate in the left lung. There is no pneumothorax. Median sternotomy wires and mediastinal clips are noted consistent with previous coronary artery bypass grafting.

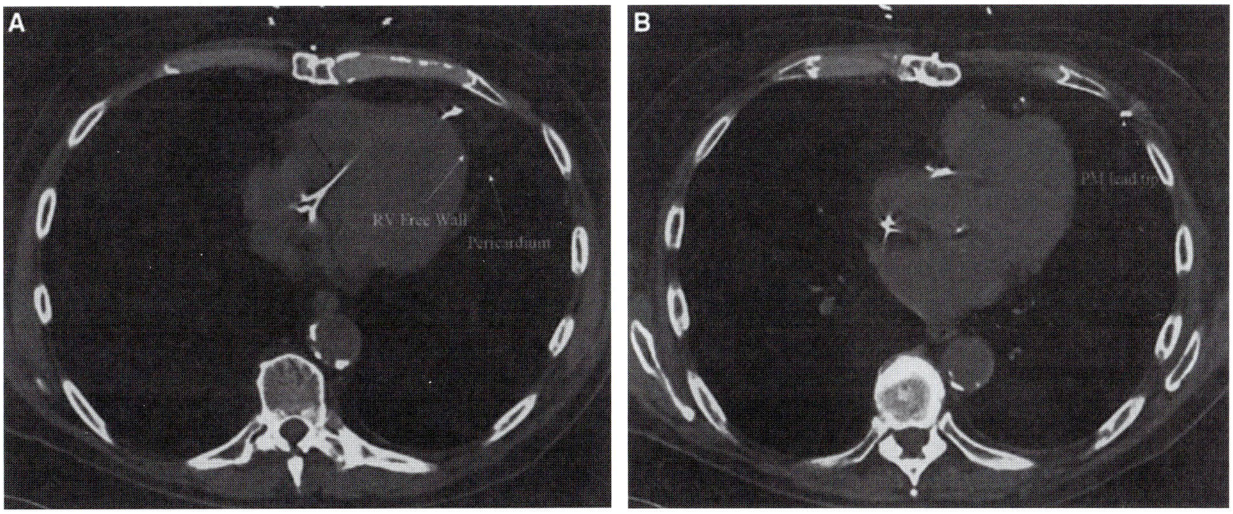

Figure 2. CT scan of the chest without intravenous contrast. Axial images display the pacemaker lead (black arrow) extending through the right ventricular (RV) free wall and epicardial fat pad **(A)** before penetrating the pericardium and terminating in the left anterior chest wall **(B)**. There is no evidence of pericardial or pleural effusion.

patient was taken to the operating room. The right femoral vein and artery were exposed to provide rapid access in the event that cardiopulmonary bypass would be required. Continuous transesophageal echocardiography was used to monitor the pericardial space. The ventricular lead was disconnected from the pacemaker generator. Under fluoroscopic guidance, the surgeon retracted the screw into the lead. Gentle, steady traction resulted in lead extraction in its entirety without complications or the development of pericardial fluid. A new ventricular lead was not implanted at the time. The patient was discharged home and was doing well at his 1-month follow-up examination.

This case illustrates the potential for delayed pacemaker lead perforation after an uneventful implantation of an active fixation lead I. Pacing electrode stimulation of the chest wall musculature and absence of a pericardial effusion are unusual features of this presentation.

72 Primary Lymphoma of the Heart

Jeffrey Kuvin, MD; Nisha Parikh, MD; Robert Salomon, MD; Arthur Tischler, MD; Philip Daoust, MD; Yevgeniy Arshanskiy, MD; Karl Coyner, MD; Philip Carpino, PA; Natesa G. Pandian; Carey Kimmelstiel, MD; Caroline Foote, MD; John Erban, MD; Hassan Rastegar, MD

From the Departments of Medicine (J.K., N.P., C.K., N.G.P., C.F., J.E.), Pathology (R.S., A.T., P.D.), Radiology (Y.A.), and Surgery (P.C., H.R.), Tufts-New England Medical Center, Tufts University School of Medicine, Boston, Mass; and the Department of Radiology (K.C.), Brigham and Women's Hospital, Harvard Medical School, Boston, Mass.

(*Circulation*. 2005;112:e5–e6.)

DOI: 10.1161.CIRCULATIONAHA.104.495135

A previously healthy 65-year-old woman presented with palpitations and positional chest discomfort 3 weeks after she sustained chest wall trauma in a motor vehicle accident. Physical examination revealed occasional premature ventricular beats and low-grade fever. Her erythrocyte sedimentation rate was elevated (66 mm/hour). Transthoracic and transesophageal echocardiography revealed a 3 × 3 cm, well-demarcated, homogeneous, round mass moving with the heart adjacent to the right atrium (Figs. 1A and 1B). There was invagination of nearby cardiac chambers but no obstruction to right heart filling. Magnetic resonance imaging (MRI) showed a circumscribed mass with dense tissue characterization (isointense to myocardium) not consistent with blood or fat (Fig. 2A). There was

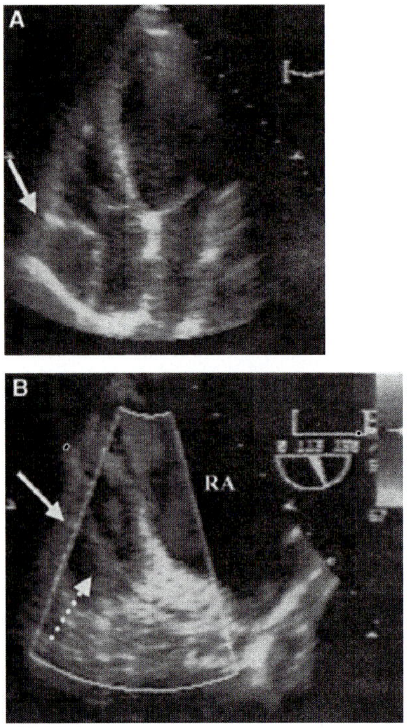

Figure 1. A, Transthoracic echocardiogram, apical four-chamber view. Round mass adjacent to right heart (arrow) with invagination of right atrial wall and right ventricular inflow. **B,** Transesophageal echocardiogram: Well-demarcated mass (arrow) adjacent to the right atrium (RA). A linear structure with color Doppler flow (dashed arrow) is noted within the mass.

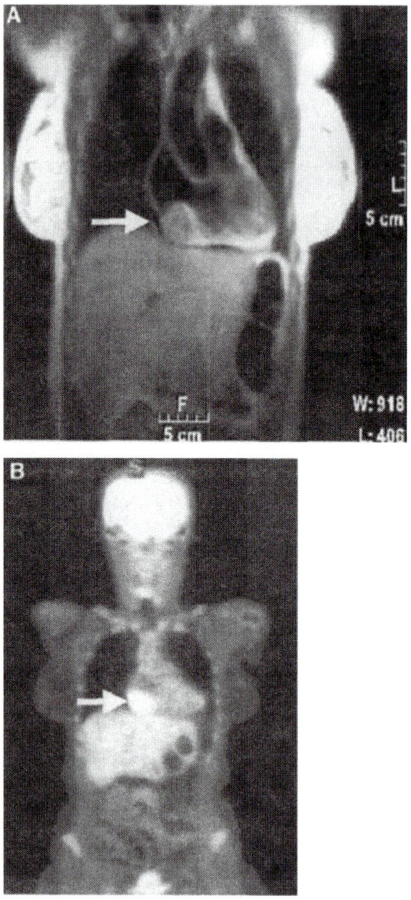

Figure 2. A, MRI, coronal multislice single shot. Round mass in the region of the right atrioventricular groove (arrow), isointense to the myocardium. **B,** F-18 FDG PET imaging, coronal view. Intense focal FDG activity (arrow) adjacent to the right atrium correlates with the round mass shown on the accompanying MRI image.

minimal enhancement of the mass after gadolinium injection. Coronary angiography was normal. Two weeks later, the patient's symptoms improved. Repeat transthoracic echocardiogram showed no change in size or consistency of the mass. A combined positron emission tomography (PET) and computed tomography (CT) scan after administration of F-18 fluorodeoxyglucose (FDG) revealed focal intense activity adjacent to the right heart (Fig. 2B), which correlated with a cardiac wall mass on the CT images. The distribution of F-18 FDG in whole-body imaging was otherwise unremarkable, and no additional abnormal masses were identified.

The patient underwent surgery. The pericardium was thin, with a small amount of cloudy pericardial fluid. A round, firm mass was detected, originating from the atrioventricular groove, attaching to the right atrium and free wall of the right ventricle, and encasing the right coronary artery (Fig. 3A). The mass was excised without removing any portion of right atrium or ventricle. The right coronary artery was preserved by peeling the tumor from the vessel after the mass was divided into two halves (Fig. 3B). Immunophenotyping by flow cytometry and tissue staining demonstrated that the malignant cells were positive for CD45, CD19, and CD20, and were negative for surface immunoglobulin. These findings were diagnostic of a diffuse large B-cell lymphoma (Fig. 4). The pericardial fluid also showed evidence of lymphoma. A bone marrow biopsy obtained from the sternum at time of resection revealed benign lymphoid nodules and a mediastinal node adjacent to the pericardium was negative for lymphoma. The patient made an uneventful recovery from surgery, received systemic chemotherapy, and 1 year later remains in complete remission.

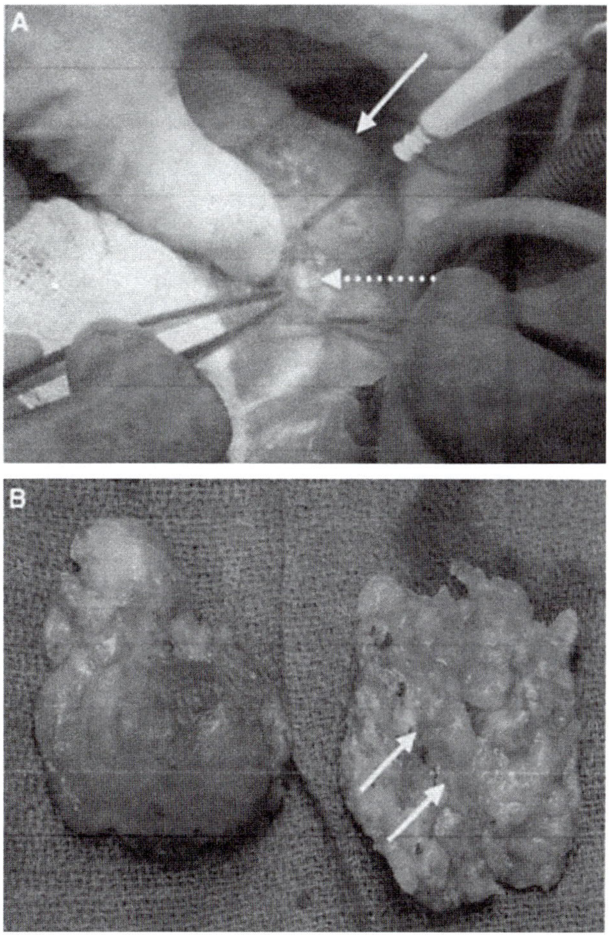

Figure 3. A, Intraoperative photograph of the well-circumscribed epicardial mass adherent to the right heart (arrow), enveloping the right coronary artery (dashed arrow). This vessel corresponds to the color Doppler signal noted on echocardiography in Figure 1B. **B,** Excised lesion (cut into halves) shows a smooth outer surface; the inner surface is indented (arrows) from passage of the right coronary artery.

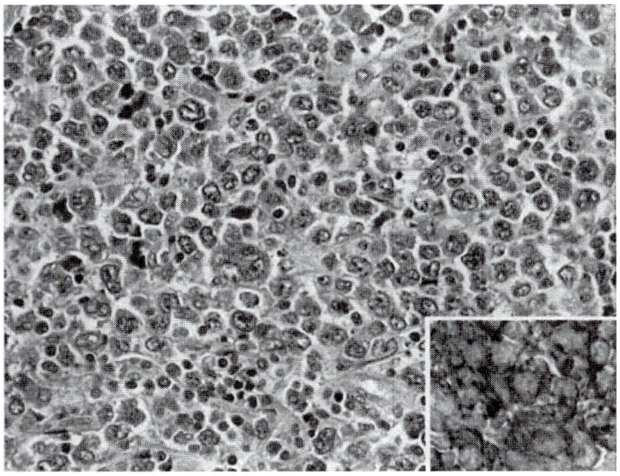

Figure 4. Microscopic pathology (hematoxylin and eosin stain, original magnification ×300) reveals packed sheets of large cells with round, lobulated nuclear contours, fine punctate chromatin, and distinct nucleoli. Frequent apoptotic cells, moderate number of mitoses, and areas of coagulation necrosis were present (not all represented in this image). Immunostaining for CD20 (insert) demonstrates a large B-cell lymphoma.

Section IV

Endocardium and Valves

73

Aortic Valves: Shamrock, Bileaflet, and Lucky?

Warren J. Manning, MD; Craig S. Keighley, MB, BS

From the Cardiovascular Division, Beth Israel Hospital, Boston, Mass.

(*Circulation*. 1995;92:2352.)

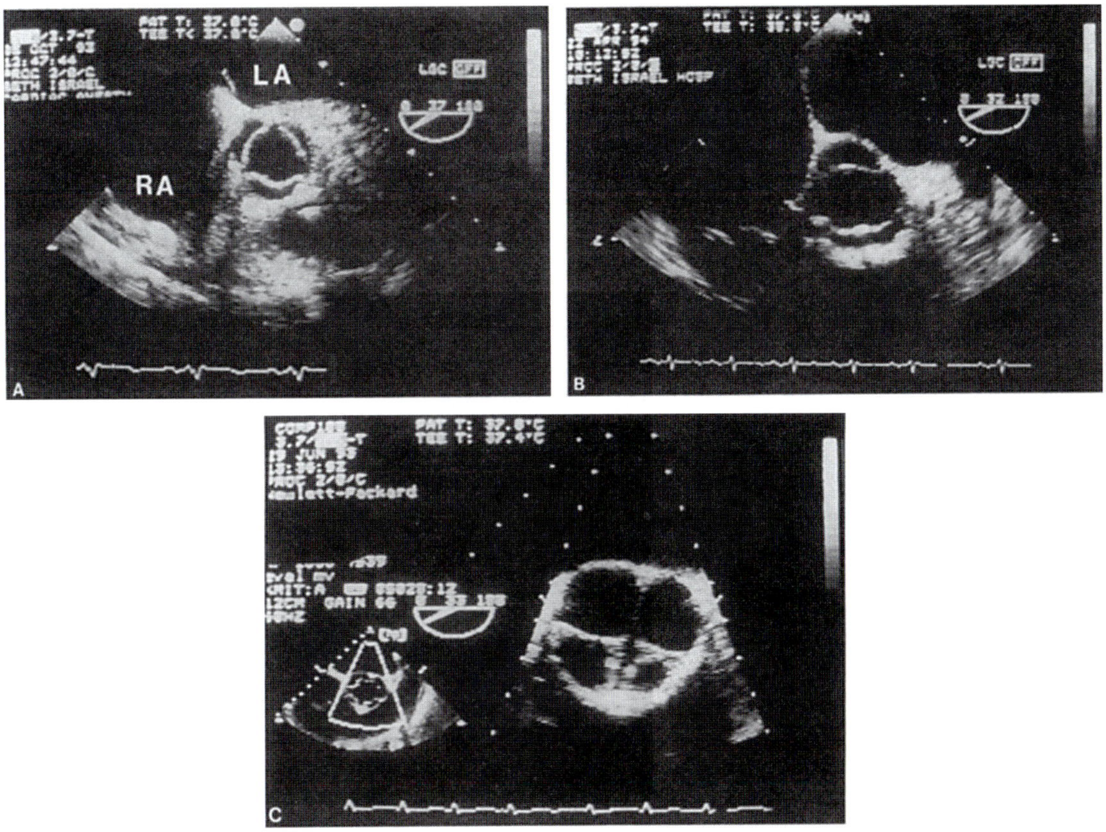

Figure 1. Multiplane transesophageal echocardiography short axis view of the aortic valve with the angle of crystal orientation approximately 35°. **A,** Normal trileaflet aortic valve with commissures at 12-, 5-, and 8-o'clock positions. **B,** Congenital bicuspid aortic valve with commissures at 3- and 9-o'clock positions. **C,** Four-leaflet aortic valve with commissures at 12-, 3-, 6-, and 9-o'clock positions. The bileaflet and four-leaflet aortic valves demonstrated no evidence of aortic stenosis or insufficiency. LA indicates left atrium; RA, right atrium.

74 Fungal Mass on the Tricuspid Valve

James Mathew, MD; Robert Gasior, MD; Natarajan Thannoli, MD

From the Divisions of Adult Cardiology and Cardiothoracic Surgery and the Departments of Medicine and Surgery, Cook County Hospital, Chicago, Ill.

(*Circulation*. 1996;94:2040.)

A 33-year-old man with a history of intravenous drug use was admitted to the hospital with fever, cough, and shortness of breath lasting for about 4 weeks. Physical examination was remarkable for evidence of tricuspid valve (TV) regurgitation. A transthoracic echocardiogram revealed a mass on the TV and an enlarged right atrium. Blood cultures grew *Candida albicans*. The cauliflower-like mass was better visualized on the transesophageal echocardiogram (Fig. 1). The patient was treated with amphotericin B and TV resection. At surgery, the mass attached to the TV filled about 80% of the enlarged right atrium and measured 6.5 × 4.5 cm (Fig. 2). The patient died of multisystem failure from sepsis 8 weeks after surgery.

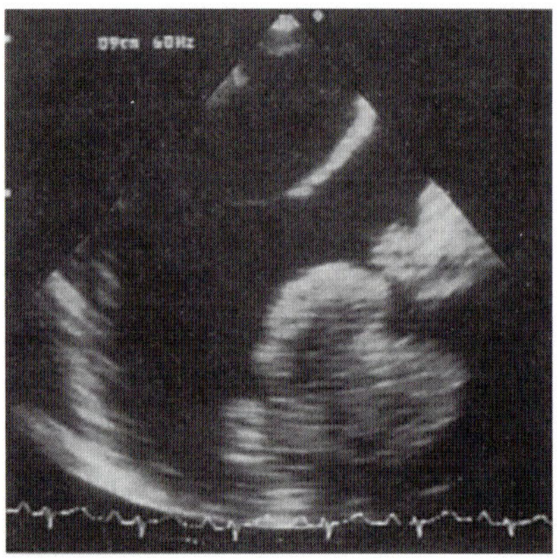

Figure 1. Transesophageal echocardiographic image in a patient with infective endocarditis due to *Candida albicans*.

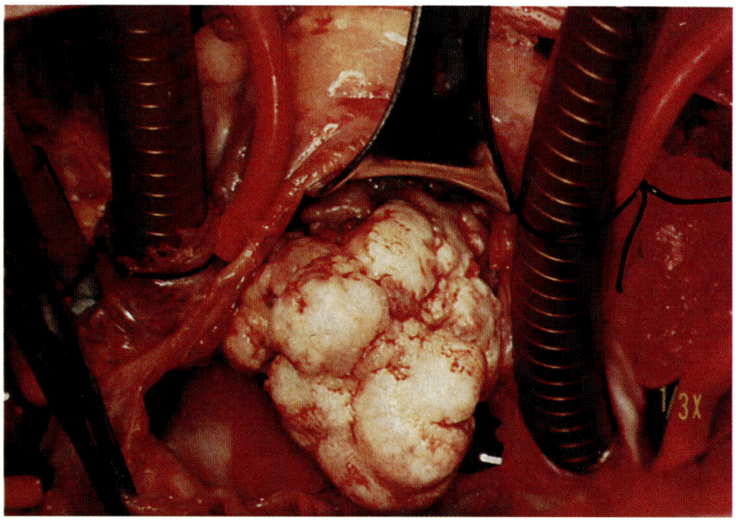

Figure 2. Intraoperative photograph of fungal mass on the tricuspid valve in a patient with infective endocarditis due to *Candida albicans*.

75 Carcinoid Heart Disease

Carlos M. Gaos, MD; Maher M. Nasser, MD; Susan Wilansky, MD

From the Department of Adult Cardiology, St Luke's Episcopal Hospital and the Texas Heart Institute, Houston.

(*Circulation*. 1997;95:1346.)

A 37-year-old Black woman presented with watery diarrhea, facial flushing, and progressive right heart failure. Computed tomography (CT)-guided biopsy of a liver mass revealed a neuroendocrine tumor. Elevated levels of 5-hydroxyindoleacetic acid confirmed the diagnosis of metastatic carcinoid syndrome. A two-dimensional (2-D) Doppler echocardiogram shows the typical findings of carcinoid heart disease.

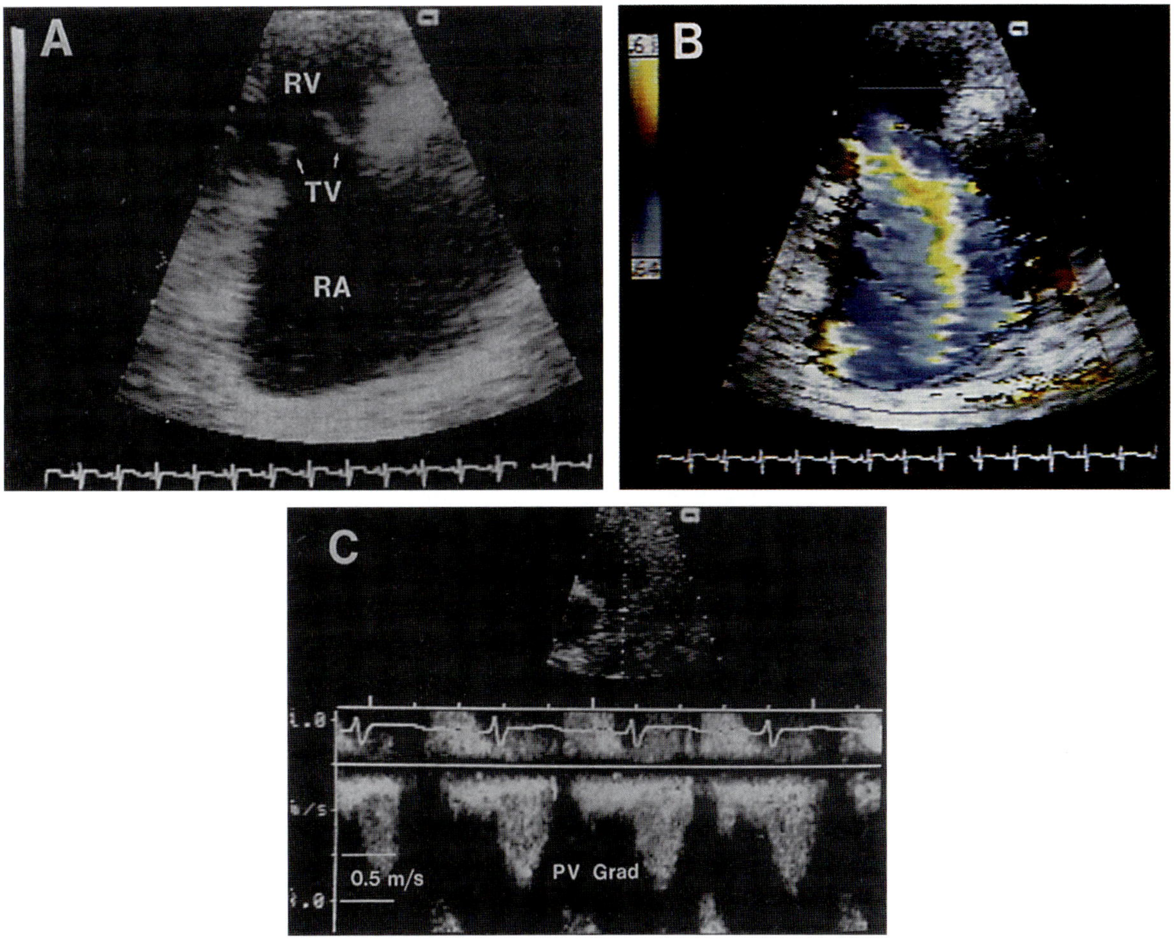

Figure 1. A, 2-D echocardiogram of right ventricular inflow tract view. Tricuspid valve leaflets (TV) are thickened, rigid, and immobile during the entire cardiac cycle. RA indicates right atrium; RV, right ventricle. **B,** Same view as A, with color flow Doppler showing severe tricuspid regurgitation. **C,** Mild pulmonary stenosis, with a peak gradient (PV Grad) by continuous-wave Doppler of 9 mm Hg and mean gradient of 5 mm Hg.

76 Cardiovascular Disease in Ankylosing (Marie-Strümpell) Spondylitis

Azam Ansari, MD; Barry J. Maron, MD

From the Department of Medicine (Cardiovascular Section), Fairview Southdale Hospital, Edina, Minn, and the Cardiovascular Research Division, Minneapolis Heart Institute Foundation, Minneapolis, Minn.

(*Circulation*. 1997;95:2585–2586.)

An 85-year-old man presented for cardiac evaluation before urological surgery with a long history of intermittent stiffness and discomfort in the dorsal spine. An early diastolic murmur (grade 2/6) was heard along the left parasternal border. The sedimentation rate was 91 mm in the first hour.

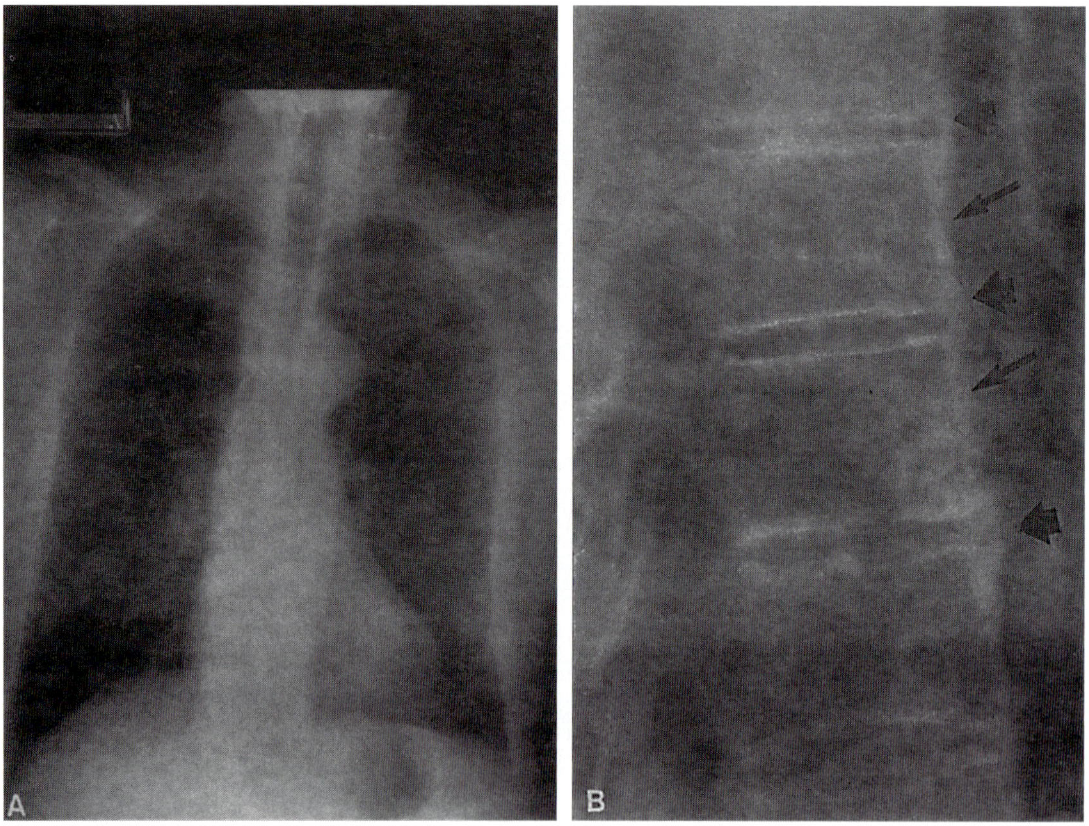

Figure 1. A, Posteroanterior chest x-ray shows mild cardiac enlargement with prominence of aortic knob and left ventricle. **B,** Lateral chest x-ray (focused) shows ossification and calcification of the anterior longitudinal ligament (long arrows); when bridging the adjacent vertebrae, the ligament imparted to the spine the classic "bamboo" appearance (short arrows). Squaring of the vertebral bodies and osteoporosis are also evident.

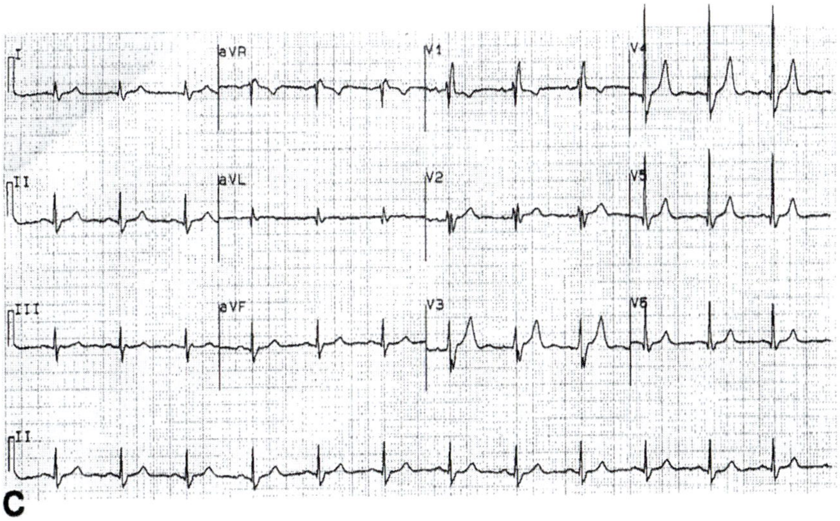

C, Electrocardiogram (ECG) shows complete right bundle-branch block.

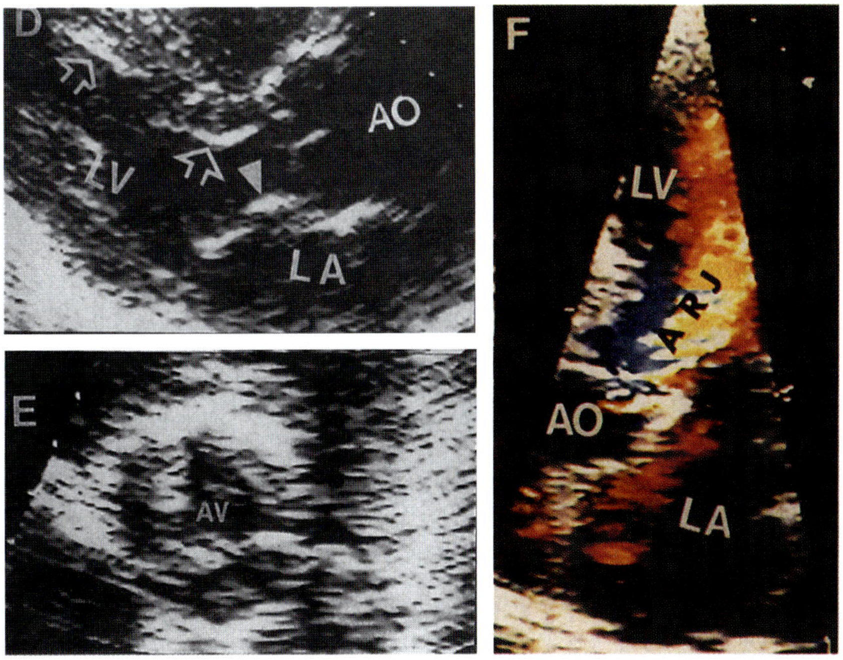

D, Parasternal long-axis echocardiogram: "subaortic bump" represents fibrosis at the mitral-aortic junction (arrowhead); also evident is thickening of the walls of the aortic root and left septal endocardium (arrows). **E,** Parasternal short-axis echocardiogram shows thickened aortic root and valve cusps (AV). **F,** Color-flow Doppler demonstrates aortic regurgitation jet (ARJ) and disturbed blood flow in diastole (mosaic color) below aortic valve orifice (AO) extending into left ventricular cavity (LV). LA indicates left atrium.

77 Quadricuspid Aortic Valve

Efrain Feliciano, MD; Eric Steinberg, MD; Itzhak Kronzon, MD

From the Department of Medicine, Manhattan Veterans Affairs Medical Center (E.F., E.S.), and New York University Medical Center (I.K.), New York, NY.

(*Circulation*. 1998;97:113.)

After a transient ischemic attack, this 68-year-old patient was referred for transesophageal echocardiography to look for a possible cardiac source of embolization. There were no heart murmurs. Transesophageal echocardiography was unremarkable except for the incidental finding of a quadricuspid aortic valve (Fig. 1). Doppler studies demonstrated minimal aortic regurgitation and no stenosis. There was no evidence of any other congenital anomaly. The pulmonary artery and valve were normal (no truncus arteriosus).

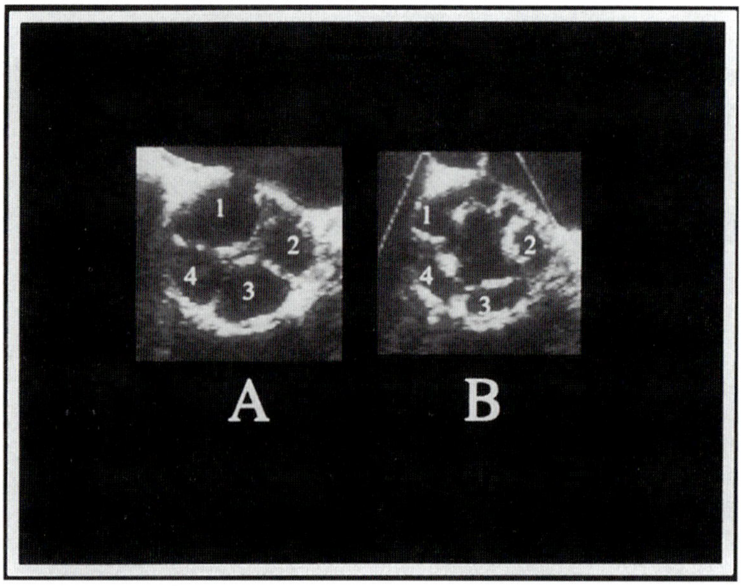

Figure 1. Transesophageal echocardiography of aortic valve shows four cusps (1 through 4). **A,** Diastolic frame; **B,** Systolic frame.

78 Sinus of Valsalva Pseudoaneurysm

Tsung-Ming Lee, MD; Chiau-Suong Liau, MD; Yuan-Teh Lee, MD; Shu-Hsun Chu, MD

From the Departments of Internal Medicine and Surgery (S.-H.C.), College of Medicine, National Taiwan University Hospital.

(*Circulation*. 1998;97:607–608.)

A 59-year-old woman presented with exertional dyspnea this past year. She gave no history of cardiac disease or trauma. On examination, a soft systolic ejection murmur was noted at the left sternal border. Her blood pressure was 110/74 mm Hg, and her pulse rate was 84 bpm. The electrocardiogram (ECG) showed a normal sinus rhythm with T-wave inversion in leads II, III, and aVF. Roentgenography of the heart revealed mild cardiomegaly. Two-dimensional (2-D) transthoracic echocardiography demonstrated a huge cystic mass (9.4 × 8.3 cm) with a ball-like thrombus next to the aortic root extending into the right ventricular outflow tract (Fig. 1). Doppler color flow mapping showed a turbulent flow in this cystic mass (Figs. 2 and 3). Rupture of the sinus of Valsalva with pseudoaneurysm formation was diagnosed. During right heart catheterization, the mean right atrial pressure was 11 mm Hg, the right ventricular pressure was 24/5 mm Hg, the main pulmonary artery pressure was 15/6 mm Hg, and the right pulmonary artery wedge pressure was 7 mm Hg. During left heart catheterization, her aortic pressure dropped from 110/70 to 55/35 mm Hg, and the patient became drowsy. For fear of sudden rupture of the aortic pseudoaneurysm, the patient was immediately transferred to the operating room for open-heart surgery. During surgery, a huge, pulsating mass was noted over the right ventricular free wall extending into the aortic root and causing compression of the right ventricular outflow tract. It was an aneurysm originating from the right coronary sinus, and the aneurysm ruptured into the right ventricular free wall between the epicardium and myocardium. A 5 × 4 × 4 cm thrombus was noted within the aneurysm. No ventricular septal defect was found. The aneurysm was resected, and the rupture site was repaired with a pericardial patch. Microscopic examination of the resected tissue showed an atherosclerotic aorta with a false aneurysm formation in the adventitial area. After the operation, the patient did well.

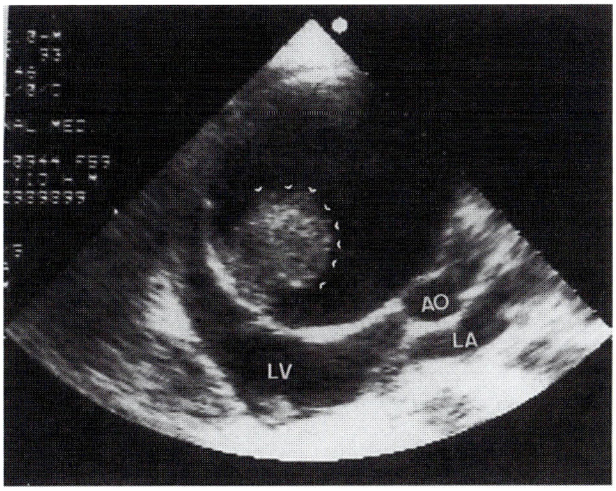

Figure 1. A huge cystic mass with a ball thrombus (arrowheads) in the parasternal long-axis view. Wall motion of this mass was parallel to interventricular septal motion. AO indicates aortic root; LA, left atrium; and LV, left ventricle.

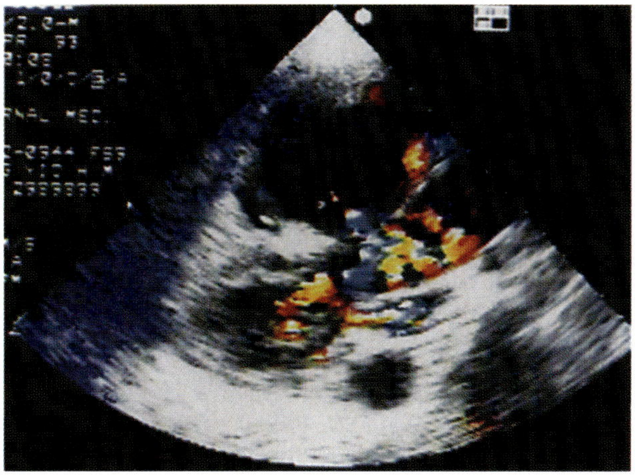

Figure 2. Color flow mapping shows mosaic images at junction of aortic root and neck of pseudoaneurysm.

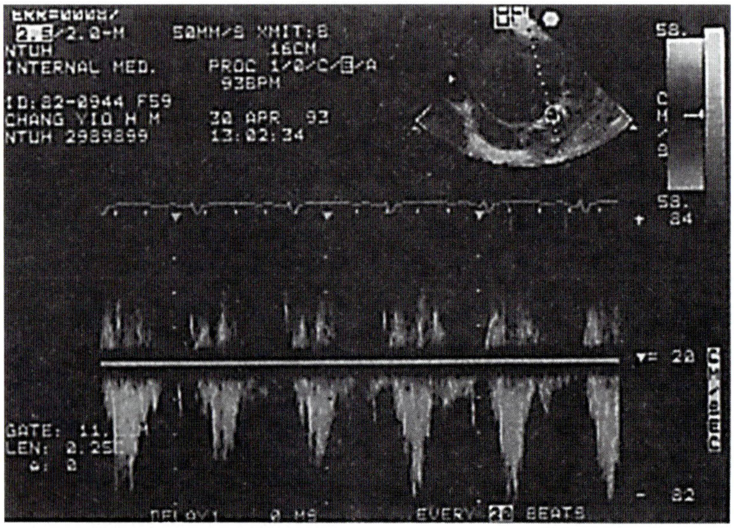

Figure 3. Doppler flow shows systolic flow toward aortic root during systolic phase.

79 Löffler Endocarditis

Friedrich M. Fruhwald, MD; Ferdinand Aglas, MD; Martin Schumacher, MD; Robert Zweiker, MD; Bernd Eber, MD; Werner Klein, MD

From the Department of Internal Medicine, Division of Cardiology, Karl-Franzens University, Graz, Austria.

(*Circulation*. 1998;97:1025.)

Figure 1 shows a case of a rare syndrome, Löffler endocarditis, in vivo by echocardiography in an apical four-chamber view with biventricular apical thrombi.

The patient, a 50-year-old White man, revealed biventricular thrombi despite oral anticoagulation, an eosinophilia of up to 49%, loss of weight (18 kg), and pleural effusion. Echocardiography showed a mass in both ventricles and a restrictive filling pattern that was confirmed by magnetic resonance (MR) imaging of the heart. After initiation of treatment with prednisolone and hydroxyurea, the patient's condition improved markedly, the biventricular mass decreased, and pleural effusion disappeared.

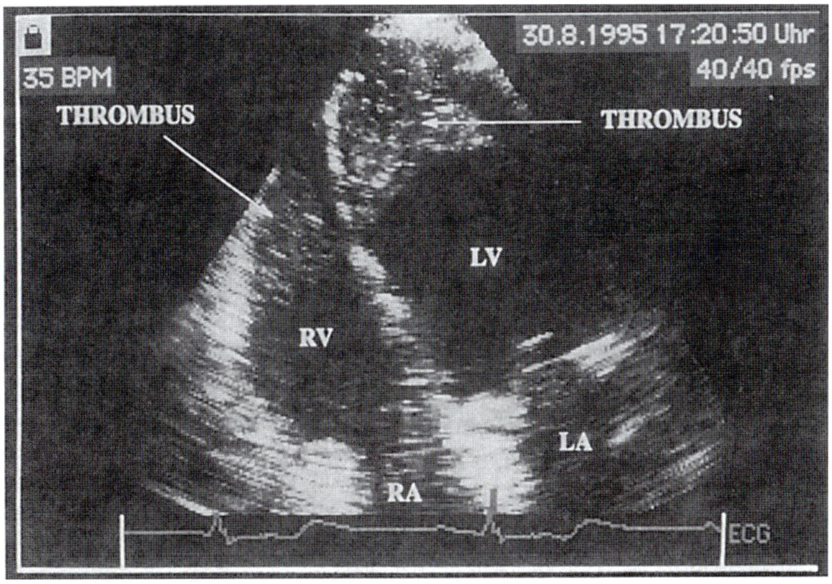

Figure 1.

80

Aortic Valve Stenosis in Alkaptonuria

Misako Hangaishi, MD; Junichi Taguchi, MD; Yuji Ikari, MD; Minoru Ohno, MD; Kiyoshi Kurokawa, MD; Yutaka Kotsuka, MD; Akira Furuse, MD

From the First Department of Internal Medicine, Faculty of Medicine (M.H., J.T., Y.I., M.O.) and the Department of Thoracic Surgery (Y.K., A.F.), University of Tokyo; and the Department of Internal Medicine, Faculty of Medicine, Tokai University, Isehara (K.K.), Japan.

(*Circulation*. 1998;98:1148–1149.)

A 63-year-old man who had previously been diagnosed with alkaptonuria was admitted to our department with severe anemia (hemoglobin, 4.9 g/dL) due to gastrointestinal bleeding and congestive heart failure with severe aortic valve stenosis (AS) and moderate left ventricular hypertrophy.

Alkaptonuria was evidenced by homogentisic acid in the urine (Fig. 1: left, fresh urine; right, urine left to stand for 24 hours) and ochronotic arthropathy in vertebrae, hip, and knee joints. The patient had undergone joint replacement surgery for the right hip and knee 9 months before admission; at that time, preoperative echocardiography revealed moderate AS (pressure gradient of 65 mm Hg). After surgery, he regularly took nonsteroidal anti-inflammatory drugs (NSAIDs) for arthralgia, and these were considered to be the cause of the gastrointestinal bleeding.

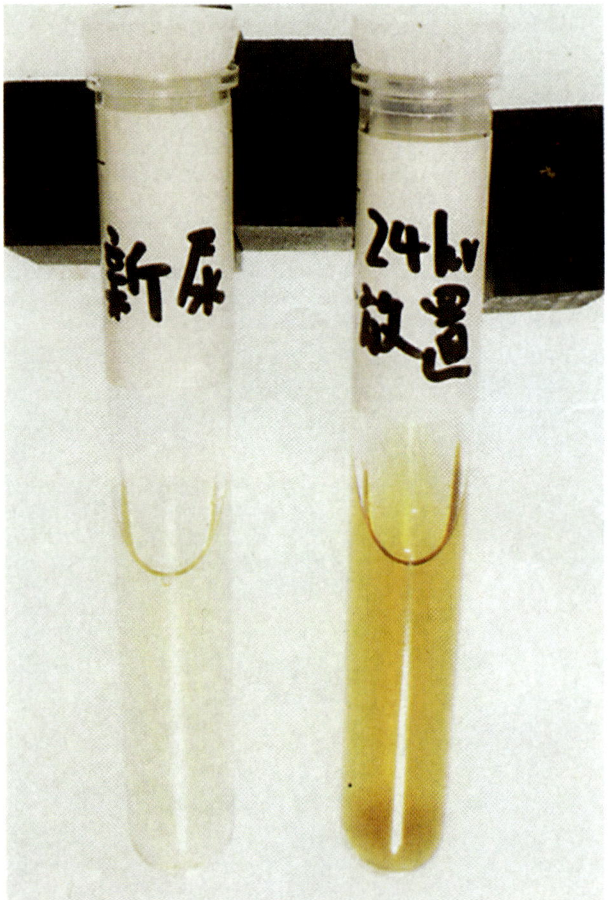

Figure 1.

After anemia and heart failure had been treated, cardiac catheterization was performed. The left ventricular–aortic pressure gradient was 90 mm Hg, with a normal ejection fraction. He had successful aortic valve replacement (Carpentier-Edwards valve). The native valve had massive ochronotic deposition with calcification, although the edge of each cusp was relatively free of degenerative change (Fig. 2). Ochronotic pigmentation was also observed in the aortic lumen (Fig 3, arrow) during the operation.

Alkaptonuria is a rare hereditary disorder (autosomal recessive trait) of tyrosine catabolism. Deficiency of homogentisic acid oxidase leads to

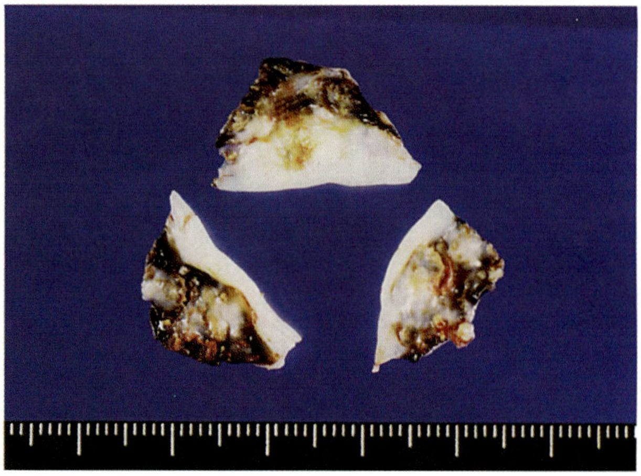

Figure 2.

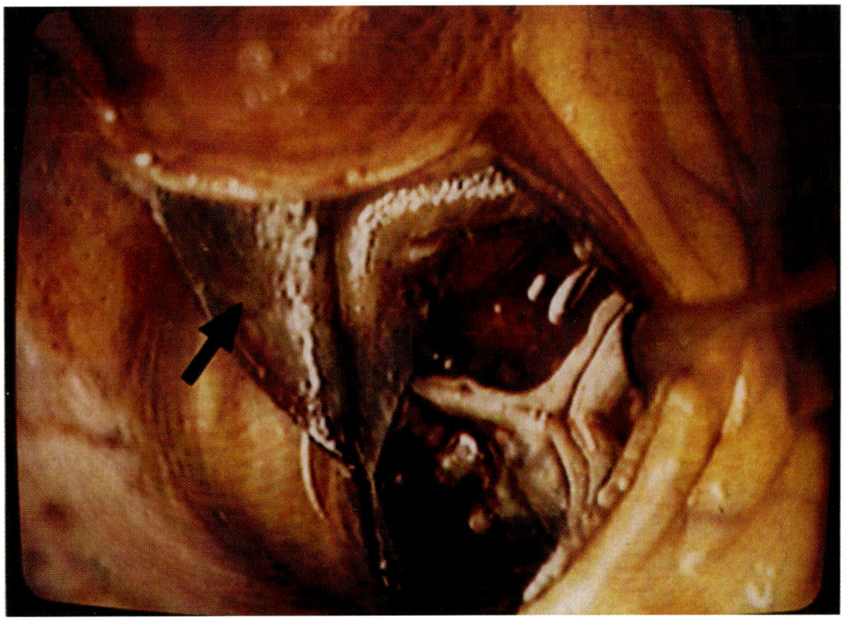

Figure 3.

excretion of large amounts of homogentisic acid in the urine, which darkens on standing, and to accumulation of oxidized homogentisic acid pigment in connective tissue (ochronosis). Patients usually present with degenerative arthritis in middle life. Degenerative cardiovascular disease, especially AS as in this case, has been reported and may be one of the important clinical problems in older patients.

81

Effect of Balloon Dilatation on Aortic Stenosis Assessed by Three-Dimensional Echocardiographic Reconstruction

Philippe Acar, MD; Yacine Aggoun, MD; Zakhia Saliba, MD; Daniel Sidi, MD; Jean Kachaner, MD

From Service de Cardiologie Pédiatrique, Hôpital Necker/Enfants-malades, Paris, France.

(*Circulation*. 1999;99:2598–2599.)

A 10-year-old boy with aortic valve stenosis treated by surgical valvotomy when he was 6 months old underwent balloon dilatation of recurrent aortic stenosis. The procedure was performed through the right femoral artery under general anesthesia with mechanical ventilation. The aortic valve was dilated with a balloon 20 mm in diameter. The peak systolic gradient dropped from 120 to 30 mm Hg after the procedure. Postprocedural aortography showed mild aortic regurgitation.

Multiplane transesophageal echocardiographic images of the aortic valve were acquired with a rotational scan before and after balloon dilatation. Three-dimensional (3-D) views from the aorta were reconstructed (TomTec). The anatomy of the aortic valve and effects of the balloon dilatation are shown on the 3-D views (Figs. 1 through 3).

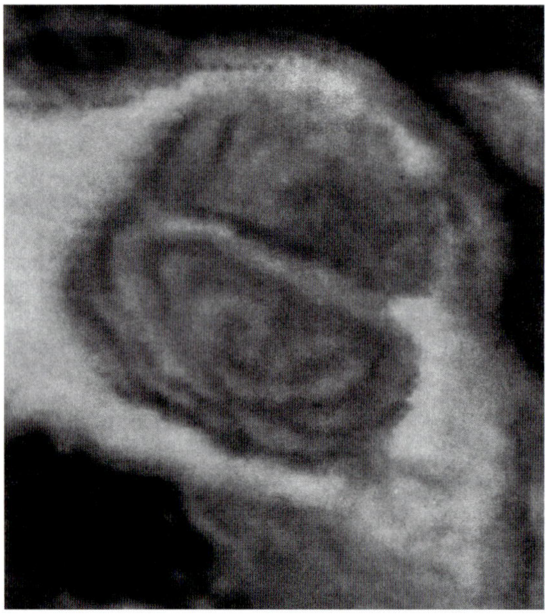

Figure 1. 3-D view from aorta in diastole before balloon dilatation. Aortic valve is bicuspid. Two leaflets have equal areas. Edges of leaflets appear thickened, and waves on their surfaces express flexibility of valve.

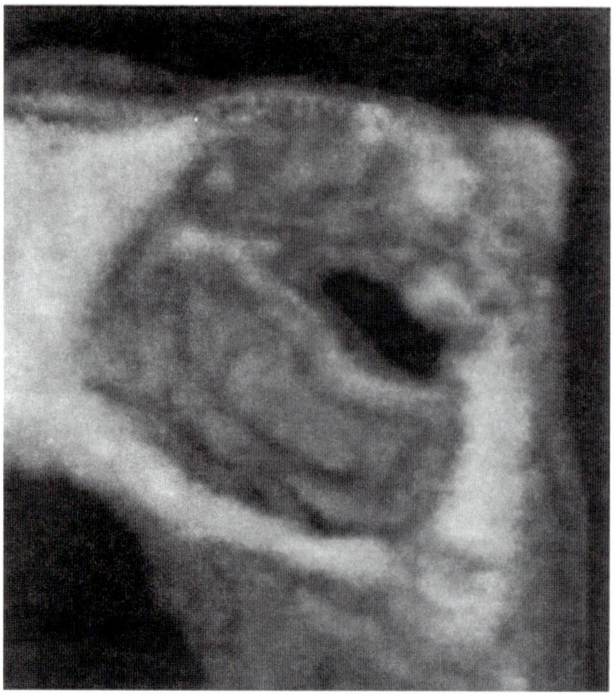

Figure 2. 3-D view from aorta in systole before balloon dilatation. Fusion of anterior commissure associated with thickness of leaflet edges makes valve stenotic. Posterior commissure is free. Opening surface of valve is 0.7 cm^2.

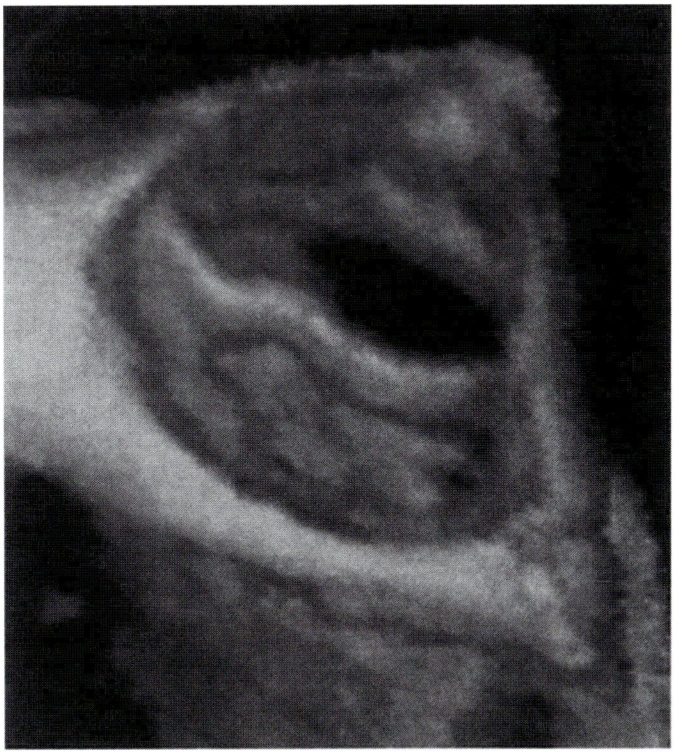

Figure 3. 3-D view from aorta in systole after balloon dilatation. Anterior commissure is clearly opened after balloon inflation. Mild aortic regurgitation assessed by 2-D color Doppler emanates from this commissure. Opening surface of valve is now 1.2 cm^2.

82 Sudden Death of a Woman with Fibroelastoma of the Aortic Valve Chronically Occluding the Right Coronary Ostium

Rossana Bussani, MD; Furio Silvestri, MD
From the Institute of Pathological Anatomy of the University of Trieste, Italy.

(*Circulation*. 1999;100:2204.)

An 89-year-old woman was hospitalized for ischemic cardiopathy and anemia. Her initial ECG showed sinus tachycardia, incomplete right bundle-branch block, and nonspecific ST- and T-wave changes. On day 19 after admission, during a gastroscopy, the patient suddenly collapsed. Cardiopulmonary resuscitation was unsuccessful.

At autopsy, the heart weighed 460 g, and the left ventricular chamber was significantly dilated. The closure line of the free edge of the right aortic cusp presented a pedunculated fibroelastoma whose distal end completely occluded the right coronary ostium (Fig. 1). The posteroinferior wall of the left ventricle, the posteromedial papillary muscle, and the posterior third of the interventricular septum were replaced by fibrous tissue. The aortic valve cusps were slightly sclerotic, with focal fusion of their free edges. The lesion was probably related to healed valvulitis. The postinflammatory endocardial cell damage and the subsequent irregularity of the closure line with exposure of the underlying collagen of the valve probably played a role in the formation of the fibroelastoma.

Systemic embolization is a frequent complication of any cardiac tumor. Occasionally, these lesions may cause obstructive symptoms interacting with the transvalvular blood flow. In the case reported here, the fibroelastoma did not present embolic potential or transvalvular blood flow disorders.

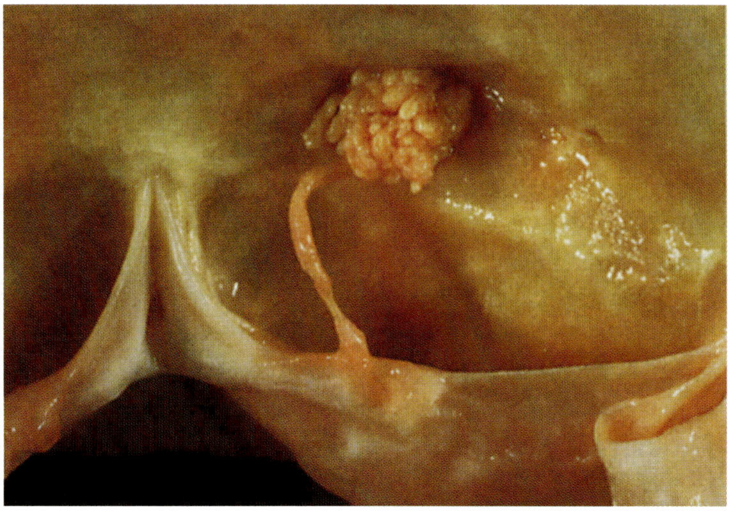

Figure 1.

83

Hemolysis after Mitral Valve Repair

R. Parker Ward, MD; Lissa Sugeng, MD; Lynn Weinert, BS; Claudia Korcarz, DVM; Ralph J. Verdino, MD; Kirk T. Spencer, MD; Roberto M. Lang, MD

From the University of Chicago Medical Center, Department of Medicine, Section of Cardiology, Chicago, Ill.

(*Circulation*. 2000;101:695–696.)

A 54-year-old woman, status post–mitral valve repair for severe mitral regurgitation secondary to mitral valve prolapse, was admitted 7 weeks after surgery with shortness of breath and fatigue. Hematological studies revealed a Coombs-negative hemolytic anemia with a hematocrit of 17.1%, haptoglobin of <7.9 mg/dL (normal 51 to 192 mg/dL), lactate dehydrogenase (LDH) of 3165 U/L, total bilirubin of 6.8 mg/dL (indirect of 6.1 mg/dL), and a peripheral blood smear demonstrating mechanical hemolysis with schistocytosis and red cell fragmentation (arrows, Fig. 1A). A transesophageal echocardiogram revealed partial dehiscence of the mitral valve annuloplasty ring (No. 28 Baxter Physio ring) from the native mitral valve annulus (arrow, Fig. 1B). Color Doppler images demonstrate severe regurgitation with fragmentation of the mitral regurgitation (arrow, Fig. 1C) into a valvular jet and a high-velocity para-ring regurgitant jet. Three-dimensional (3-D) echocardiographic images reveal a paravalvular communication (white arrow, Fig. 1D) created by the dehiscence of the annuloplasty ring from the native mitral valve annulus. 3-D color Doppler images (with color suppression of the lower-velocity valvular regurgitation) demonstrates the high-velocity para-ring regurgitant jet (white arrow, Fig. 1E).

Hemolytic anemia is a reported, although uncommon, complication of mitral valve repair. Mechanisms of hemolysis that have been suggested include collision of the regurgitant jet into the prosthetic ring, fragmentation of the regurgitant jet by a dehisced annuloplasty ring, and rapid acceleration of a jet through a small para-ring channel. The probable mechanism in the present case is fragmentation of the regurgitant jet, with rapid acceleration through the para-ring dehiscence. The patient returned to the operating room for mitral valve replacement, after which the hemolytic anemia resolved.

(Figures follow on next page.)

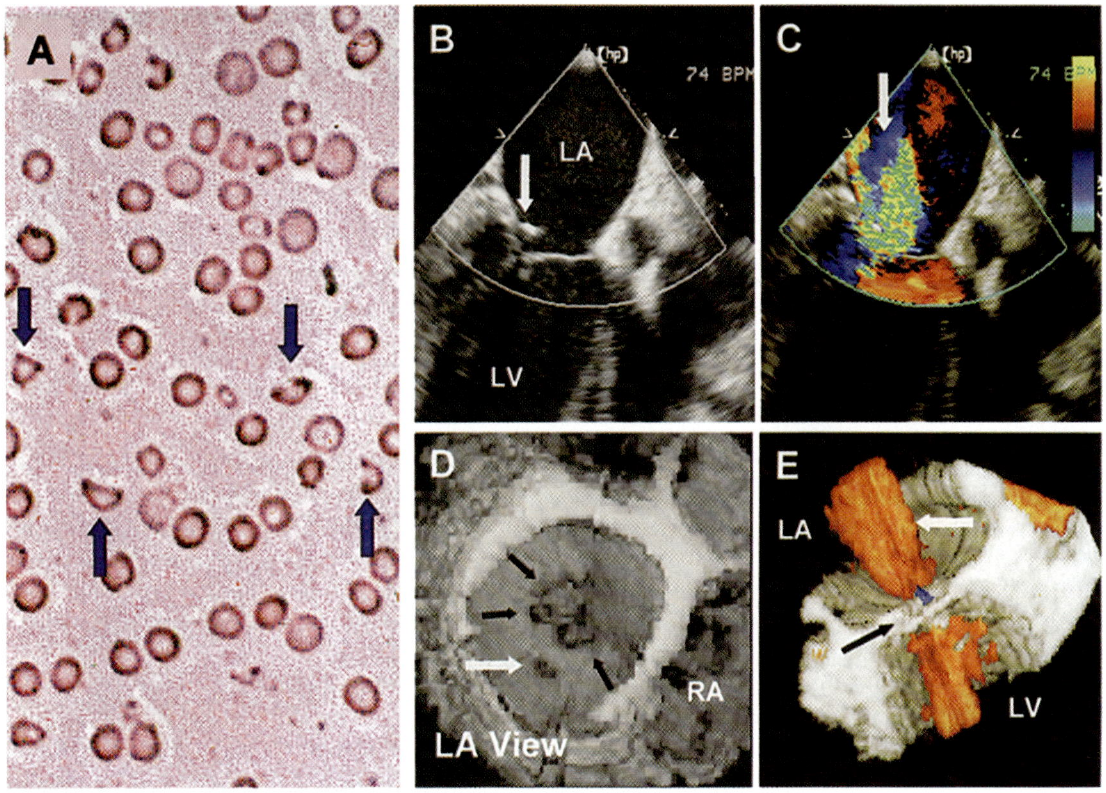

Figure 1. A, Peripheral blood smear revealing schistocytes and red cell fragmentation due to mechanical shearing of red blood cells. B and C, Transverse-plane transesophageal images of mitral valve. **B,** Partial dehiscence (arrow, B) of annuloplasty ring from native mitral valve annulus. **C,** Color Doppler imaging reveals fragmentation of regurgitant flow into a valvular and a para-ring regurgitant jet. **D,** 3-D echocardiographic images of mitral valve from LA view demonstrating an area of dehiscence (white arrow) of annuloplasty ring from native mitral valve annulus (black arrows outline medial border of annuloplasty ring). **E,** Long-axis 3-D color Doppler images of mitral valve and posterior LA wall demonstrate a high-velocity regurgitant jet (white arrow) outside annuloplasty ring. Lower-velocity valvular regurgitant jet has been suppressed (black arrow identifies posterior aspect of annuloplasty ring).

84 Coronary Artery Angiography Using Multislice Computed Tomography Images

Harvey Cline, PhD; Curtis Coulam, MD; Mehmet Yavuz, PhD; Geoffrey D. Rubin, MD; Peter Edic, PhD; TinSu Pan, PhD; Yun Shen, MS; Ricardo Avila, MS; Matthew Turek, MS; Maria Iatrou, PhD; Ann Loree, BS; Nadeem Ishaque, PhD; Robert Senzig, MS

From the Department of Radiology, Stanford University Medical School, Palo Alto, Calif (C.C., G.D.R.); General Electric Corporate Research and Development, Schenectady, NY (H.C., M.Y., P.E., R.A., M.T., M.I., N.I.); General Electric Medical Systems, Milwaukee, Wis (T.P., A.L., R.S.); and Yokogawa Medical Systems, Tokyo, Japan (Y.S.).

(*Circulation.* 2000;102:1589–1590.)

Multislice computed tomography (CT) scanners are the newest class of CT scanners and they have not one but many detectors. These scanners can acquire up to four slices of data from the body in the same time it takes a single-slice CT scanner to acquire one. Multislice CT allows for rapid cardiac imaging during a single breath-hold. A multislice scanner operated in helical mode provides information that can be used to reconstruct three-dimensional (3-D) cardiac images in arbitrary phases of the cardiac cycle.

A 71-year-old man with hypertension, hypercholesterolemia, and known aortic and peripheral vascular disease was imaged with a LightSpeed four-slice, multislice CT scanner (GE Medical Systems). Ten minutes before the cardiac scan, the patient received intravenous contrast material (150 mL of 300 mgI/mL) for a CT study of his abdomen. The cardiac scan was acquired during a 35-s breath-hold, and simultaneous acquisition of the ECG enabled reconstruction using retrospective gating (Fig. 1). The helical pitch was 0.85 (relative to the detector elements), with a 2.5 mm nominal slice thickness (interpolated to 0.625 mm). The interpolated volume elements (voxels) were 0.39 × 0.39 × 0.625 mm in a 512 × 512 × 130 data matrix covering a 200 × 200 × 81 mm volume. The effective temporal acquisition window was 160 ms. Postprocessing tools were used to separate the coronary arteries from the cardiac chamber blood pool. 3-D images can be displayed as projections similar to those obtained at catheter angiography (Fig. 2).

These first results of electrocardiogram (ECG)-gated multislice CT cardiac imaging are encouraging. At present, the quality of these scans is dependent on heart rate, rhythm, and patient ability to suspend respiration. Current developments will make this technique more robust. Increasing the number of detector rows will result in improved temporal and spatial resolution and fewer motion artifacts. Faster and variable gantry rotation speeds will improve temporal resolution and image quality over a greater range of heart rates and rhythms. A cardiac gated-pulse x-ray tube could be used to decrease patient dose if diastolic imaging is sufficient. Imaging of the coronary arteries, for example, can be limited to diastole without a diagnostic penalty. A clinical study comparing multislice CT coronary angiography with conventional x-ray angiography is required for validation of this new method.

Acknowledgments

The authors thank Erdogan Cesmeli, PhD, Siegwalt Ludke, BS, Christopher Hardy, PhD, James Miller, PhD, William Lorensen, MS, Nagesh Mallugari, and Tony Pan for their contributions.

(Figures follow on next page.)

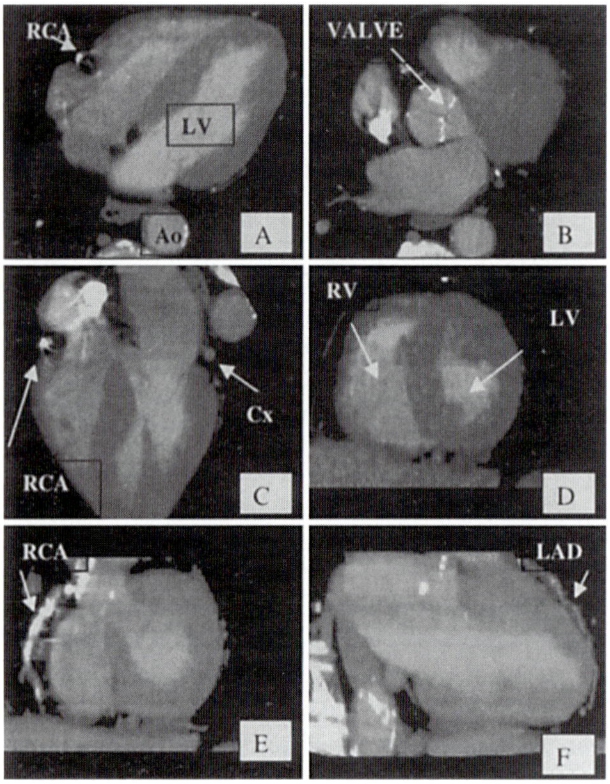

Figure 1. A, Transverse CT section shows calcification in right coronary artery (RCA). **B,** Calcification also exists at edge of 2 aortic valve leaflets. **C,** Images were reformatted to give a longitudinal view that shows both the cross-section of the calcified right coronary artery and the circumflex branch of the left coronary artery (Cx). **D,** Short-axis view was reformatted to show left and right ventricles (LV and RV) at end-diastole. **E,** A 3-mm-thick maximum intensity projection shows right coronary artery calcification. **F,** A 15-mm-thick projection clearly shows left anterior descending coronary artery (LAD). Ao indicates aorta.

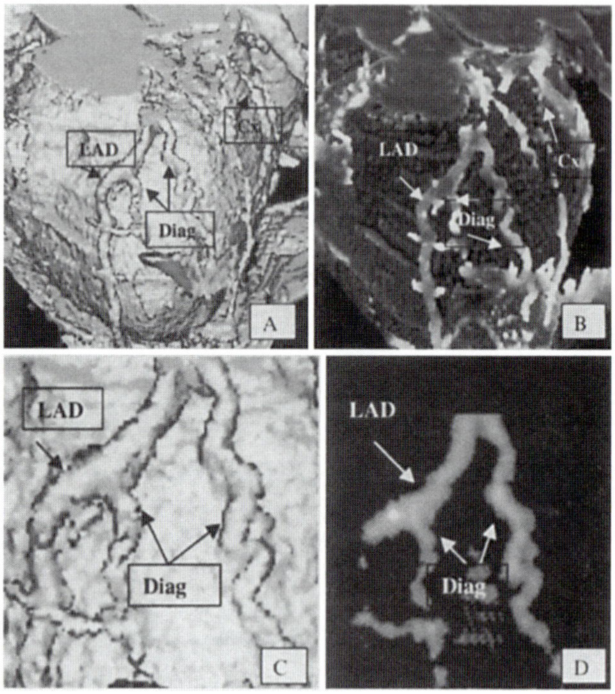

Figure 2. A, Left anterior oblique view surface rendering shows LAD, two diagonal branches (Diag), and the circumflex artery (Cx). **B,** The 3-D multislice CT images were processed with a computer workstation to both remove the blood pool and create a projection through the coronary arteries. **C,** The 3-D surface image is magnified to examine the coronary arteries. **D,** A 5-mm-thick projection through this region is made in an oblique plane tangent to the 3-D surface model.

85 Resolution of Nonbacterial Endocarditis after Surgical Resection of a Malignant Liver Tumor

M. Cockburn, MD; J. Swafford, MD; W. Mazur, MD; G. L. Walsh, MD; J. N. Vauthey, MD

From the Department of Medicine, Cardiology Section (W.M.), Baylor College of Medicine, and the Departments of Cardiology (J.S.), Thoracic and Cardiovascular Surgery (G.L.W.), and Surgical Oncology (M.C., J.N.V.), The University of Texas M.D. Anderson Cancer Center, Houston, Tex.

(*Circulation*. 2000;102:2671–2672.)

A 51-year-old woman presented with significant weight loss and right upper quadrant abdominal pain. A computed tomography scan of the abdomen showed a large mass in the right lobe of the liver, with involvement of the right hemidiaphragm and right lower lobe of the lung (Fig. 1A). A biopsy revealed poorly differentiated adenocarcinoma. The patient was referred to M.D. Anderson Cancer Center for treatment.

During the hospital stay, the patient had intermittent high-grade fever, thrombocytopenia, prolonged prothrombin time and partial thromboplastin time, and elevated D-dimer and fibrinogen levels; all these symptoms are consistent with paraneoplastic chronic disseminated intravascular coagulation. Antibiotics were administered empirically after various cultures, including 3 blood cultures, were obtained. A transesophageal echocardiogram revealed extensive vegetations involving both leaflets of the mitral valve (Fig. 2A). Because all cultures were negative, antibiotics were discontinued and a diagnosis of nonbacterial endocarditis (NBTE) was made. The patient underwent complete surgical resection of the tumor (hepatectomy), including en-bloc resection of the right hemidiaphragm and wedge resection of the lower lobe of the right lung (Fig. 1B). The fever and hematological abnormalities resolved promptly after surgery. The postoperative course was uncomplicated, with hospital discharge on the seventh postoperative day. A transesophageal echocardiogram performed 4 weeks later revealed complete resolution of the vegetations (Fig. 2B).

In a prospective study of 200 patients with solid tumors, the echocardiographic prevalence of NBTE

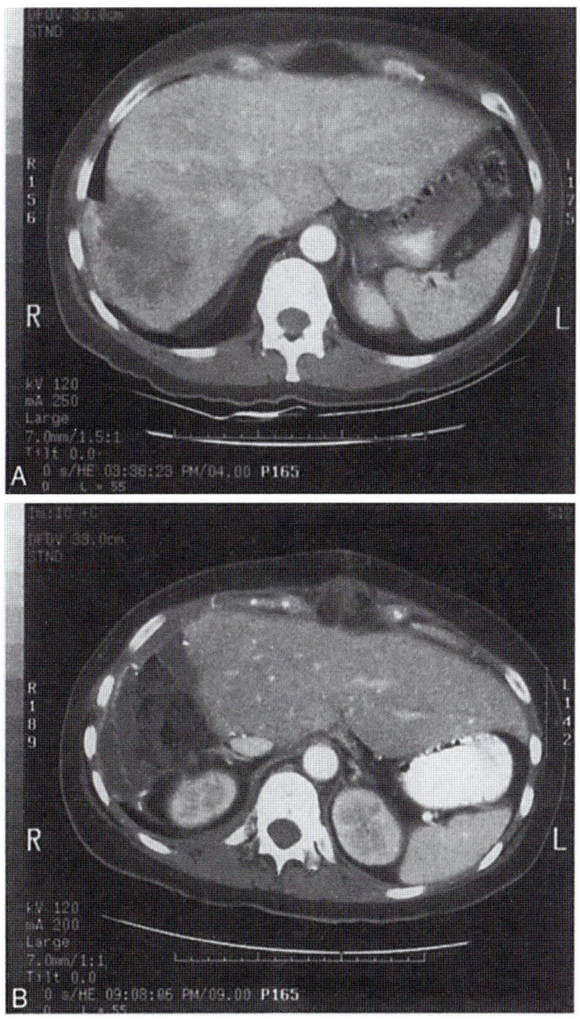

Figure 1. Computed tomography scans of right hepatic lobe tumor involving diaphragm before **(A)** and after **(B)** resection.

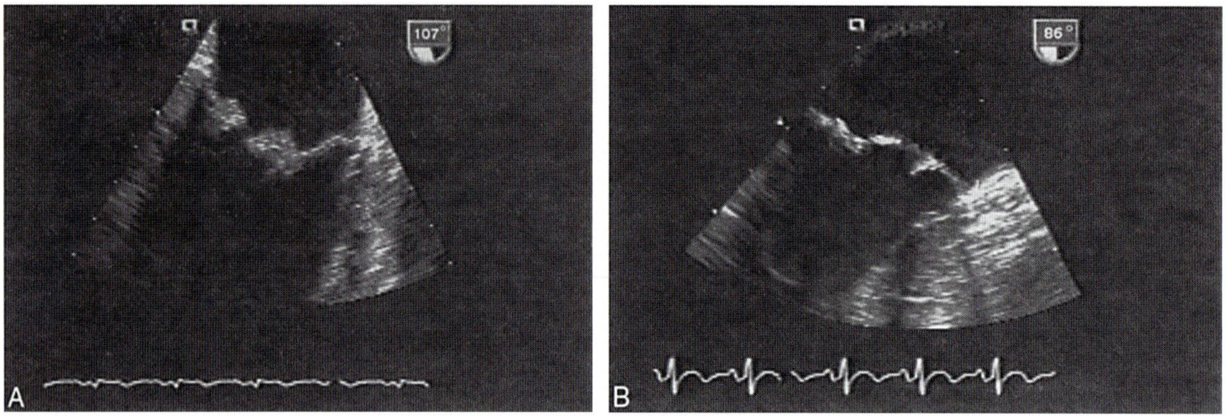

Figure 2. Two-dimensional transesophageal echocardiographs showing mitral valve with vegetations before hepatic resection **(A)** and resolution of vegetations after surgery **(B)**.

was 19%, with predominant mitral valve involvement. NBTE is typically seen in patients with advanced and incurable malignancy. To our knowledge, this is the first documented case of echocardiographic resolution of NBTE.

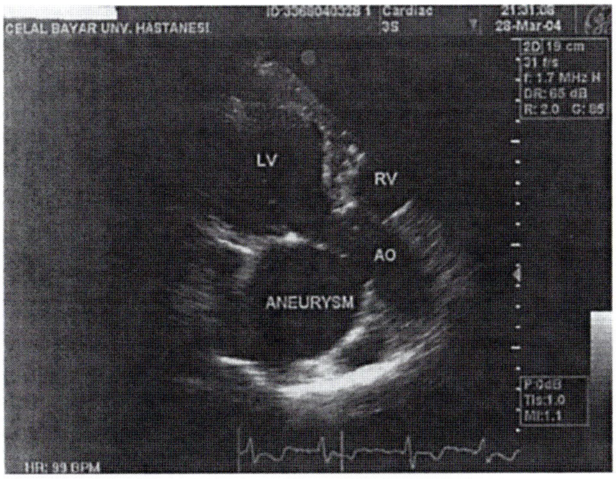

Figure 3. Parasternal short-axis view revealing the origin of cystic mass from the noncoronary sinus of Valsalva. RCC indicates right coronary cusp; LCC, left coronary cusp; RVOT, right ventricle outflow tract; and PA, pulmonary artery.

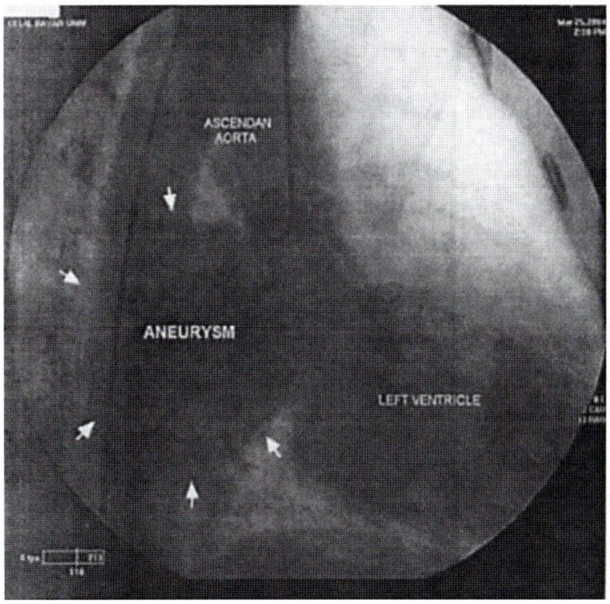

Figure 4. Angiography of the aortic root confirming the giant aneurysm of the sinus of Valsalva and serious aortic regurgitation.

Section V

Pericardium and Myocardium

89 Epitome of Cardiac Tamponade

David H. Spodick, MD, DSc
From the Cardiology Division, St Vincent Hospital, Worcester, Mass.

(*Circulation*. 1993;88:1943–1944.)

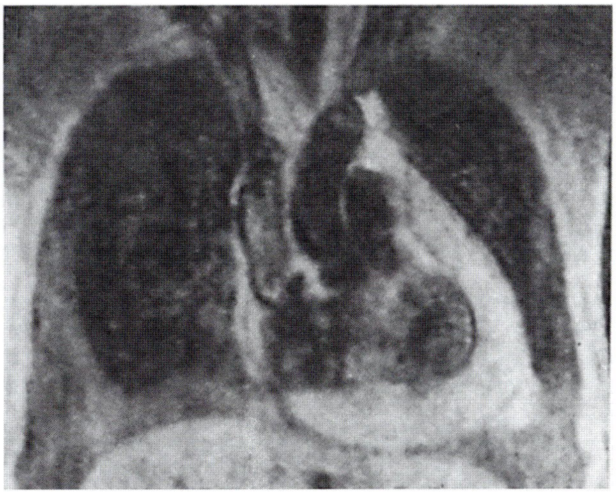

Figure 1. Magnetic resonance image: Large pericardial effusion (pale zone overlying thin dark layer of epicardial fat).

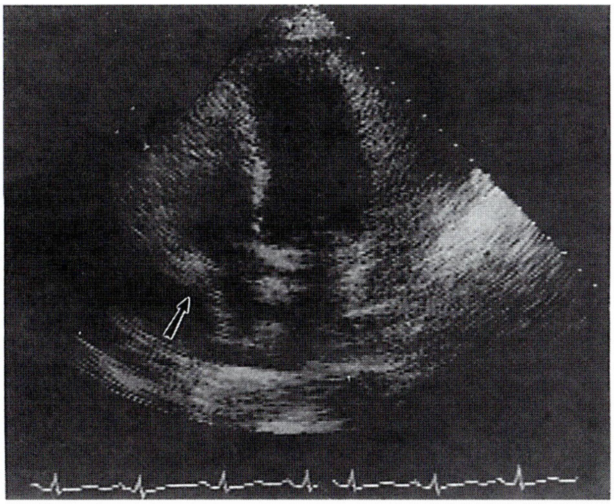

Figure 2. Two-dimensional (2-D) echocardiogram (apical four-chamber scan plane): Circumcardiac pericardial effusion with prominent right atrial collapse (arrow).

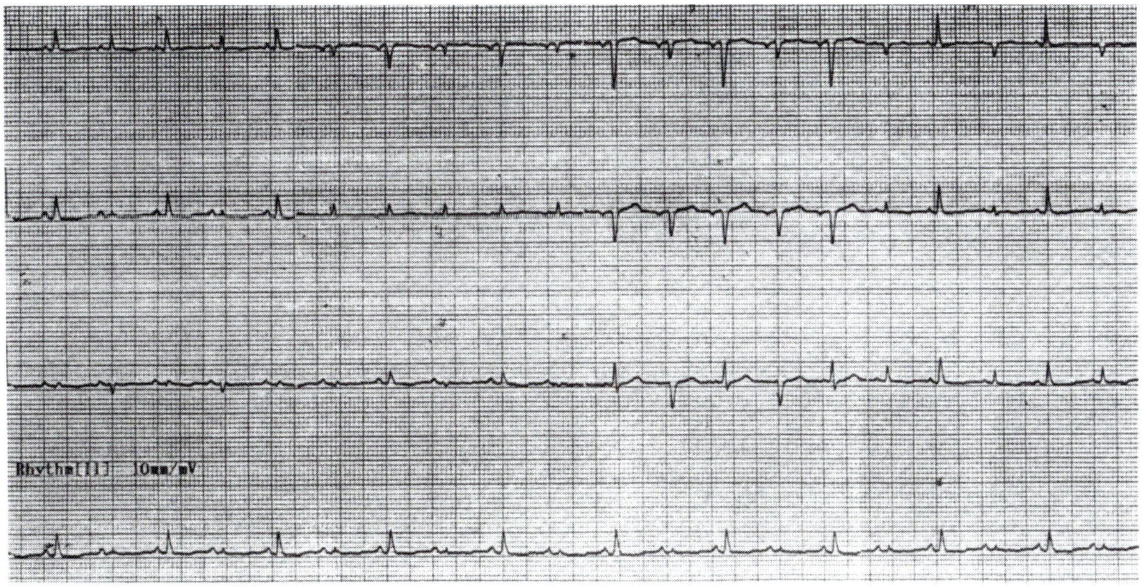

Figure 3. 12-Lead electrocardiogram: Marked electric alternation.

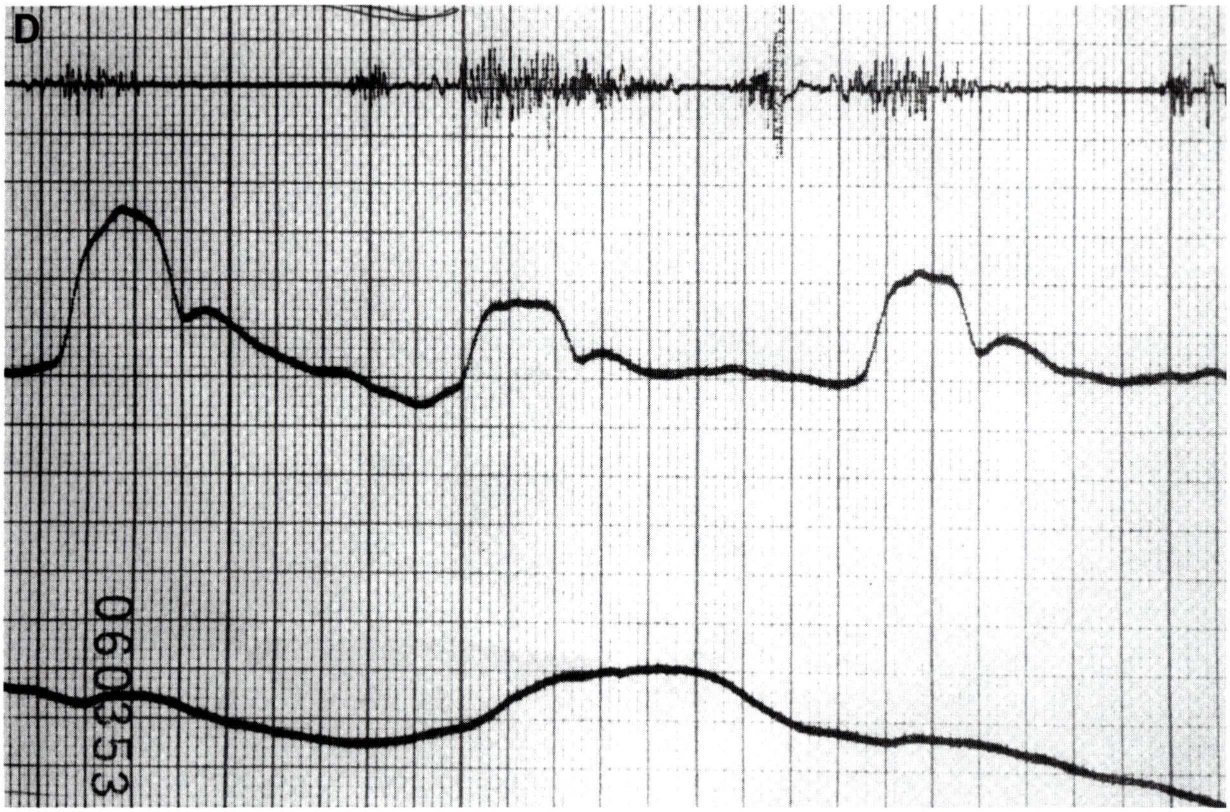

Figure 4. Noninvasive graphics: **Top,** Phonocardiogram showing pericardial rub and diminished first heart sound. **Middle,** Carotid displacement pulse. **Bottom,** Respiratory thermistor (Upward = inspiration). During inspiration the systolic pulse level falls and the rub is accentuated.

90 Calcified Pericardium Causing Cardiac Constriction

Herbert L. Fred, MD; Edie E. Shulman, MD; Andrew C. Nelson, MD; Karen Kerr Botsoe, MD; B. Tharaknath Rao, MD

From the Department of Internal Medicine, Lyndon B. Johnson General Hospital, and The University of Texas Health Science Center at Houston.

(*Circulation*. 1994;90:2546.)

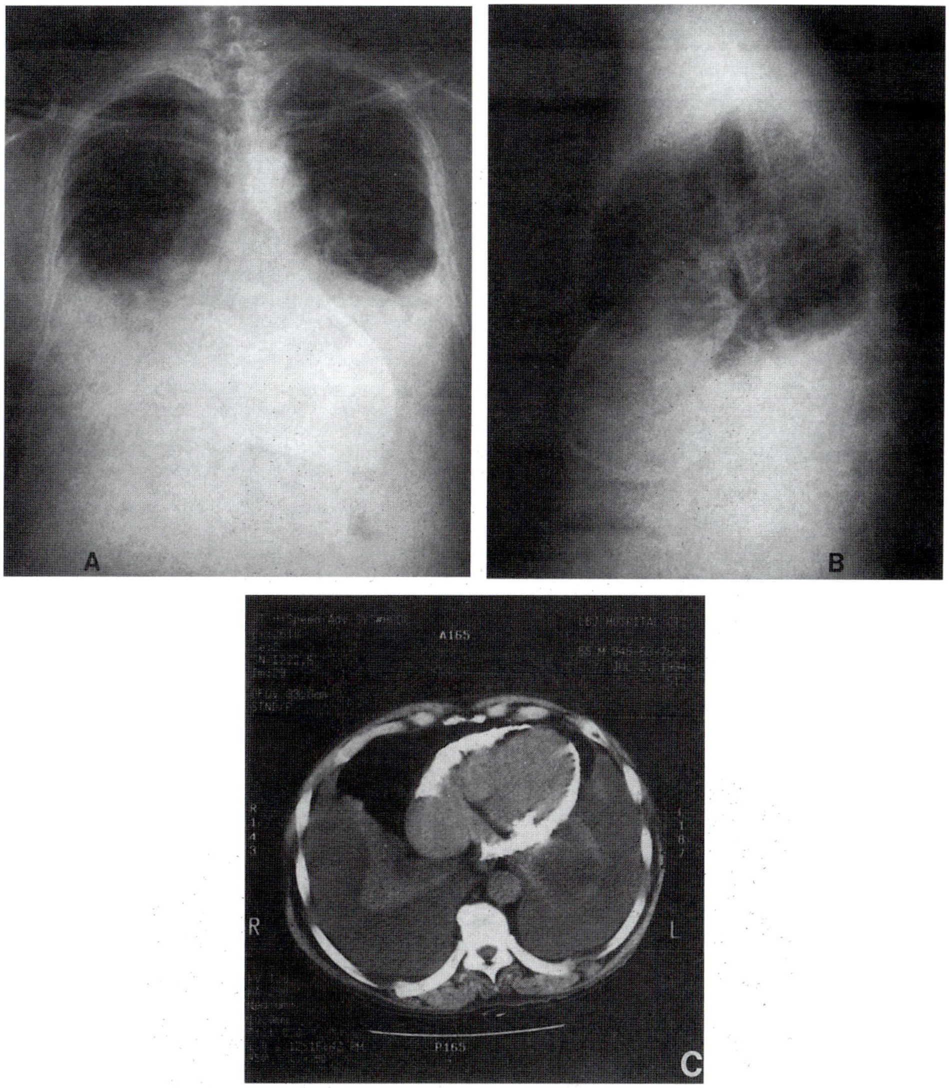

Figure 1. A 55-year-old Mexican man complained of dyspnea, increasing abdominal girth, and swollen legs of 4 months' duration. Pertinent physical abnormalities included distended neck veins, distant heart sounds, hepatomegaly, ascites, and edema of the legs. The electrocardiogram (ECG) showed atrial fibrillation and low QRS voltage. A transthoracic echocardiogram demonstrated biatrial dilatation, normal left ventricular size and function, and thickened pericardium. Radiographs of the chest (Figs. **A** and **B**) showed bilateral pleural effusions, pulmonary vascular prominence, and striking pericardial calcification. Computed axial tomography scan of the chest (Fig. **C**) further delineated the distribution and character of the calcification. Four days after admission, the patient left the hospital against advice and was lost to follow-up. The cause of his calcified pericardium is unknown.

91

Amiodarone Phototoxic Reaction

Manfred Zehender, MD

From the Klinikum der Albert-Ludwigs Universität, Freiburg, Germany.

(*Circulation*. 1995;92:1665.)

Amiodarone (200 mg/d) was used over a 5-year period in a 64-year-old farmer with dilative cardiomyopathy to prevent recurrent sudden cardiac death. During this time, the patient developed the characteristic photosensitivity and blue-gray discoloration of the sun-exposed areas in his face, which typically excluded the area just around the eyes.

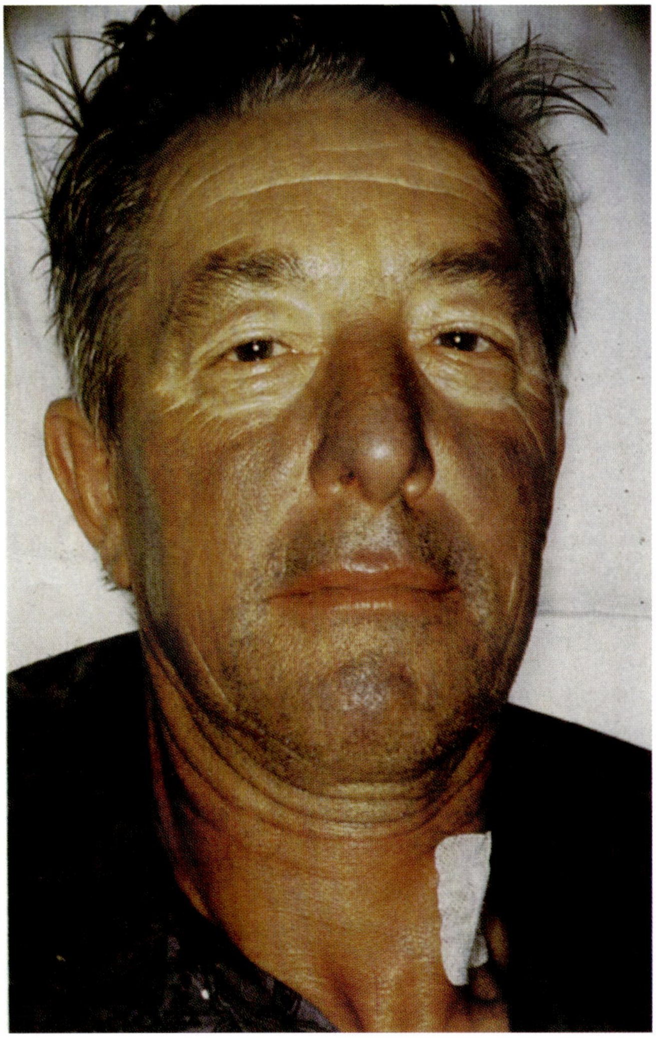

Figure 1.

92 Extreme Left Ventricular Hypertrophy

Barry J. Maron, MD; Brian W. Gross, MD; Stephen I. Stark, MD

From the Minneapolis Heart Institute Foundation, Minneapolis, Minn, and Mercy General Hospital, Sacramento, Calif.

(*Circulation*. 1995;92:2748.)

Hypertrophic cardiomyopathy (HCM), a common cause of sudden death in the young, is characterized by unexplained left ventricular wall thickening in the presence of a nondilated cavity. Although the morphological spectrum is broad, patients with HCM may show the greatest magnitude of wall thickening of any known cardiac disease. The young patient illustrated here shows the most extreme example of hypertrophy yet observed, defining the probable outer limits of ventricular septal thickness in cardiac disease (up to 6 cm).

This young boy (147 lb), a talented athlete, was first identified by echocardiography as having nonobstructive HCM at age 14 after a syncopal spell associated with blood drawing, which was regarded as a vasovagal event. He remained asymptomatic for 2 years until he experienced a cardiac arrest (with documented ventricular fibrillation) while sleeping, from which he was promptly and successfully resuscitated. An automatic cardioverter/defibrillator was implanted, and the patient has survived to date without the device discharging.

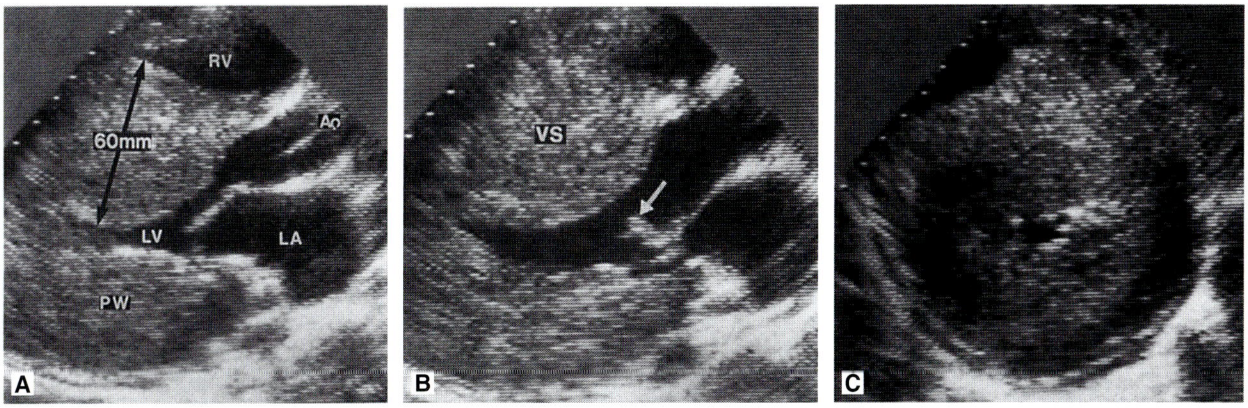

Figure 1. Massive left ventricular hypertrophy in hypertrophic cardiomyopathy. **A,** Parasternal long-axis view in diastole showing ventricular septum (VS in B) bulging into left (LV) and right (RV) ventricular cavities with maximal wall thickness of 60 mm in the midseptal region. Asymmetry between septal and posterior free wall (PW) thickness is evident. The posterior free wall, usually the thinnest portion of the left ventricle in hypertrophic cardiomyopathy, is itself as much as 50 mm in thickness. Calibration dots are 10 mm apart. Ao indicates aorta; LA, left atrium. **B,** Long-axis view in systole showing mild anterior motion of the anterior mitral leaflet (arrow). Doppler-derived left ventricular velocities were normal (1.2 m/s), substantiating absence of outflow obstruction under basal conditions. **C,** Parasternal short-axis view at end systole in the distal portion of the left ventricle showing extraordinary massive wall thickening diffusely involving the wall, in the presence of a diminutive cavity. Calibration dots are 10 mm apart.

93 Detection of Normal Pericardium and of Pericardial Effusion in the Lateral Chest Radiograph

Kyuhyun Wang, MD; Morrison Hodges, MD

From Hennepin County Medical Center, Minneapolis, Minn.

(*Circulation.* 1996;93:1254.)

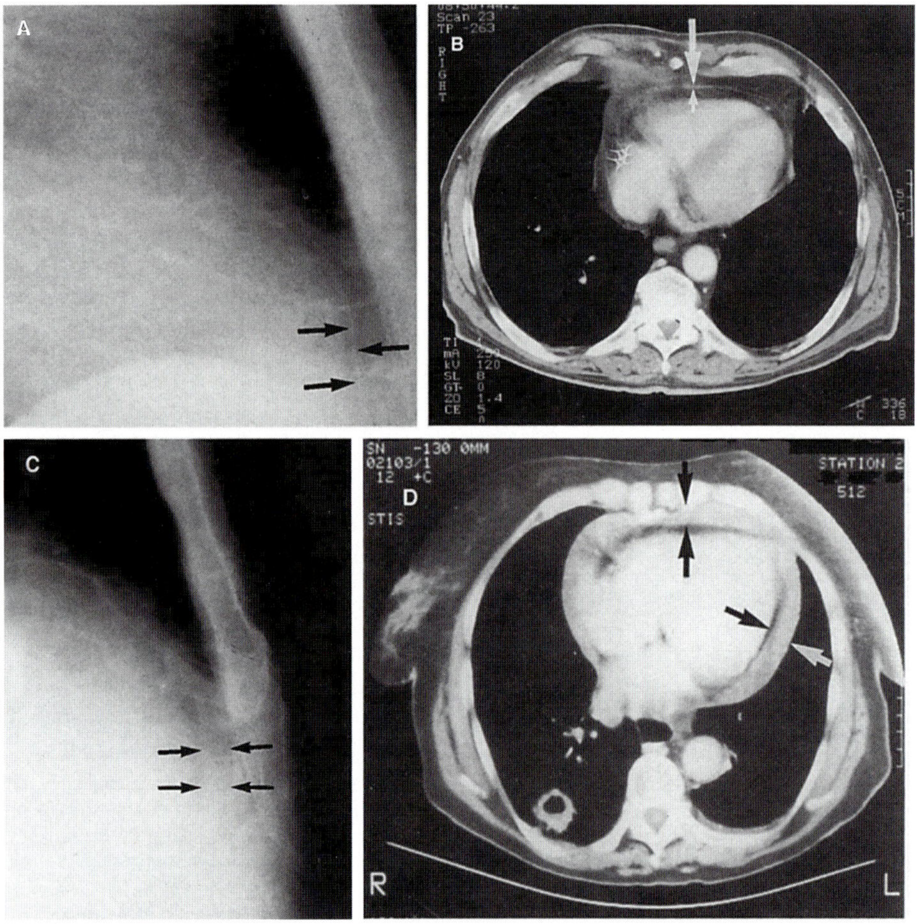

Figure 1. A, Thin linear density in front of the cardiac silhouette and behind the sternum is shown by arrows in a lateral chest radiograph. This density is due to the apposition of the normal visceral and parietal pericardia and is visible as a distinct line because this patient has significant fat beneath the visceral pericardium (epicardium) and also behind the sternum. **B,** A computed tomography (CT) scan of the chest from a different patient who also has significant subepicardial and substernal fat demonstrates how an x-ray beam going across the chest will pick up the normal epicardium-pericardium (arrows) as a thin linear density on a lateral chest radiograph as in A. **C,** A broad band of density (arrows) is present between subepicardial fat and retrosternal fat. The increased width of this band can be due to thickened epicardium, thickened parietal pericardium, fluid between them, or a combination of the three. (In this patient, it is due to pericardial effusion.) **D,** A CT scan of the chest from a different patient demonstrates how an x-ray beam going across the chest will pick up a pericardial effusion (between the arrows) as a wide band of density on a lateral chest radiograph as in C. Thus, a lateral chest radiograph can reveal either normal pericardium or a pericardial effusion, provided that enough subepicardial and retrosternal fat is present.

94 Heart Injury from Firearm

Gilles Montalescot, MD, PhD; Daniel Thomas, MD
From Pitié-Salpétrière Hospital, Paris, France.

(*Circulation*. 1996;94:1489.)

A 20-year-old man was hospitalized because of firearm injury. Projectiles were identified on the chest radiograph (Figs. 1A and 1B). One projectile was found within the heart, as shown on the computed tomography (CT) scan image (Fig. 1C). The echocardiogram localized the projectile in the middle of the septal wall, with intense reverberations originating from the projectile (Fig. 1D; VG indicates left ventricle; VD, right ventricle; OG, left atrium; and OD, right atrium). On repeated echocardiograms, there were no changes in the location of this projectile and no pericardial effusion. The electrocardiogram (ECG) was normal, with only infrequent premature ventricular beats. The patient performed well and had no cardiac symptoms and no signs of hemorrhage. This young patient was discharged from the hospital after a few days of follow-up without specific medical or surgical treatment.

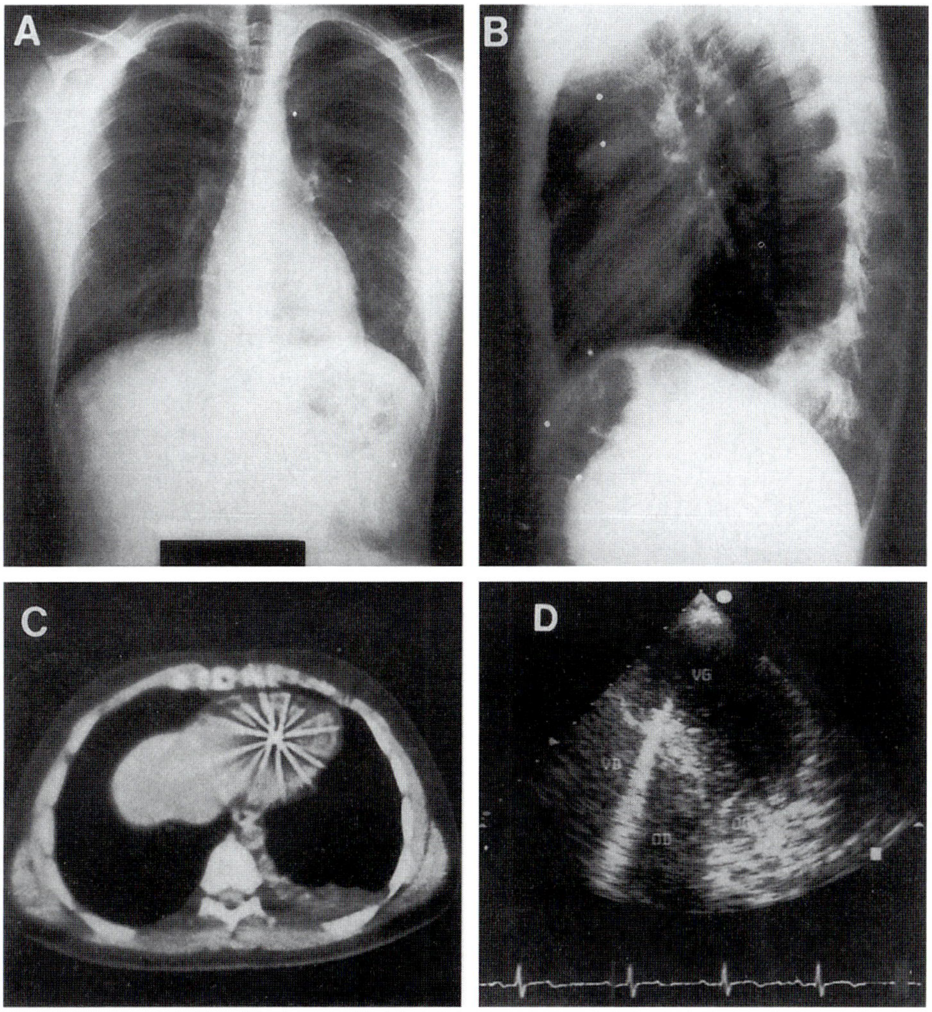

Figure 1.

95

Constrictive Pericarditis with Right Atrial Thrombus

Mitsuru Noma, MD; Tsuyoshi Itoh, MD

From the Department of Internal Medicine, Saga Prefectural Hospital, Koseikan, Saga City (M.N.), and the Department of Thoracic Surgery, Saga Medical School, Saga City (T.I.), Japan.

(*Circulation*. 1996;94:1786.)

Enhanced computed tomography revealed both calcification of the pericardium (white arrows) and a largely right atrial thrombus (dark arrows) in a 53-year-old Japanese man who had had several episodes of systemic and pulmonary embolism (Fig. 1A). At operation, an organized right atrial thrombus (65 g; white arrows in Fig. 1B) and calcified pericardium were successfully removed. There was no left atrial thrombus. Right atrial thrombus formation was considered to be due to hemostasis in the markedly dilated right atrium secondary to decreased diastolic compliance and to atrial fibrillation. After surgery, anticoagulation therapy with warfarin was given to prevent the recurrence of thromboembolism. RA indicates right atrium; RV, right ventricle; LA, left atrium; LV, left ventricle; and SVC, superior vena cava.

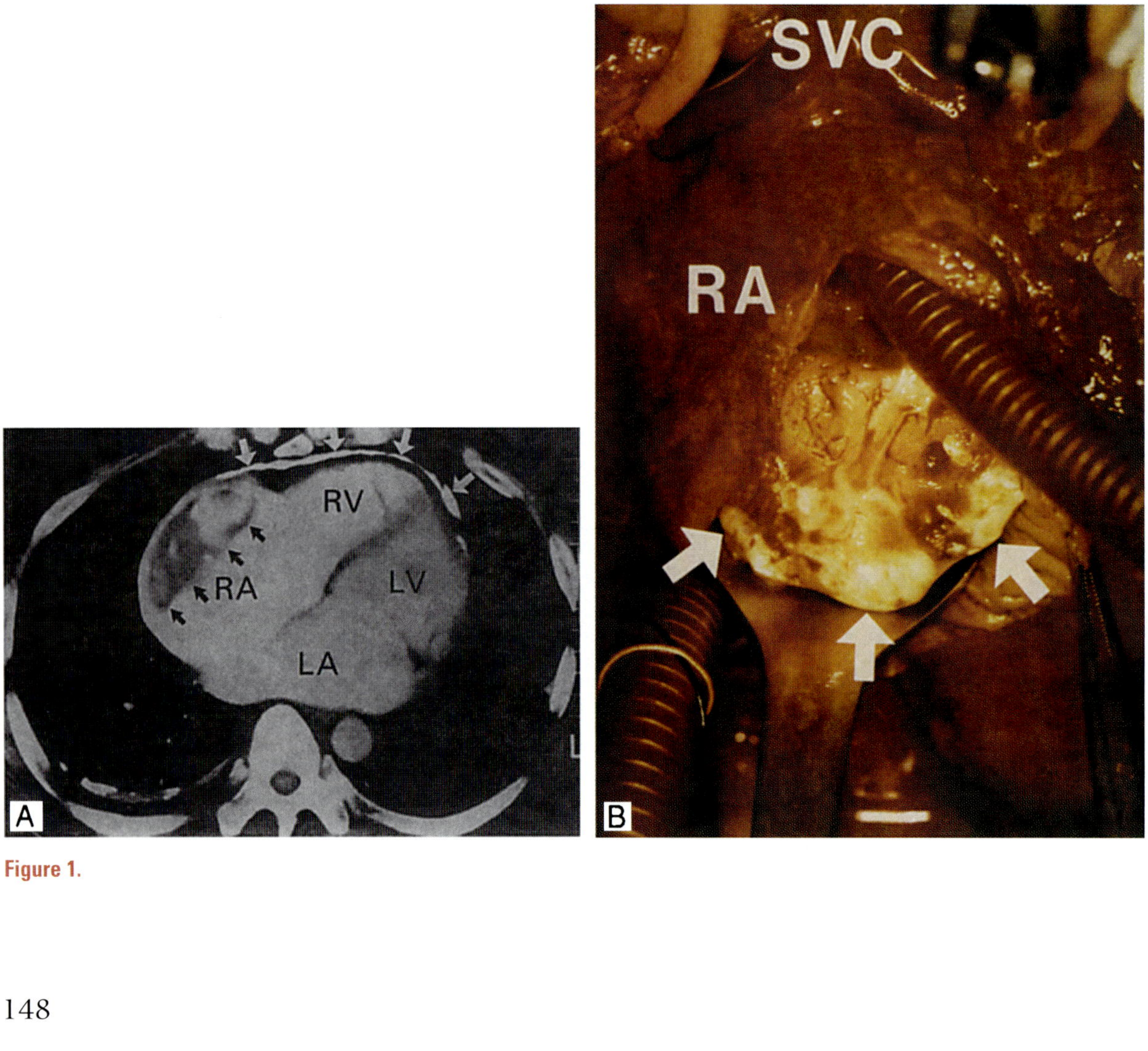

Figure 1.

96 Hydatid Cyst of the Interventricular Septum

Jean F. Aupetit, MD; Bernard Ritz, MD; Marc Ferrini, MD; Michel Coppin, MD; Gérard Champsaur, MD

From the Department of Cardiology, Centre Hospitalier St Joseph–St Luc (J.F.A., B.R., M.F., M.C.) and the Department of Cardiovascular Surgery, Hopital Cardiologique (G.C.), Lyon, France.

(*Circulation*. 1997;95:2325–2326.)

A 22-year-old woman without medical history presented with a grade 3/6 ejectional systolic murmur. She was asymptomatic. An electrocardiogram (ECG) revealed sinus rhythm and nonspecific repolarization changes in the right precordial leads. The chest radiograph was normal. A transthoracic Doppler two-dimensional (2-D) echocardiogram showed a spheroidal, 3-cm-diameter cystic mass in the upper interventricular septum protruding mainly into the left ventricular chamber without creating any significant intraventricular gradient (Figs. 1 and 2). Transesophageal echocardiography demonstrated a liquid mass with a rounded and well-constructed capsule containing an inner sleigh bell (Fig. 3). A computed tomography (CT) scan and nuclear magnetic resonance (NMR) confirmed a round, cystlike structure in the interventricular septum but finally failed to provide much information on the structure and anatomic relationship of the cyst. A blood test showed an erythrocyte sedimentation rate of 60 mm/h and absence of eosinophilia. Serological tests for *Echinococcus granulosus* were positive. Right and left cardiac catheterization showed normal pressures without intraventricular obstruction. Right and left ventricular angiography revealed an intraventricular mass defect in the interventricular septum. Coronary arteriography was normal except for a slightly curved and elongated diagonal branch of the left anterior descending coronary artery but without compression. Abdominal ultrasonographic examination, cranial and abdominal CT scans, and radionuclide bone scan imaging were normal. Surgical ablation was performed through the right ventricle; after the cyst was punctured and its contents were drained, hypertonic glucose solution was instilled, and the cyst capsule was entirely removed. Histopathological analysis of the surgical specimen confirmed a hydatid cyst. Postoperative evolution was uneventful, and the patient remains free of symptoms with normal echocardiography after 4 years of follow-up.

Cardiac hydatid disease is very uncommon. When the cysts are intramyocardial, the most common location is the interventricular septum; the diagnostic value of 2-D transthoracic and especially transesophageal echocardiography is better than that of CT and NMR imaging. Therefore, these methods should be reserved only for the study of extracardiac involvement of echinococcosis.

(Figures follow on next page.)

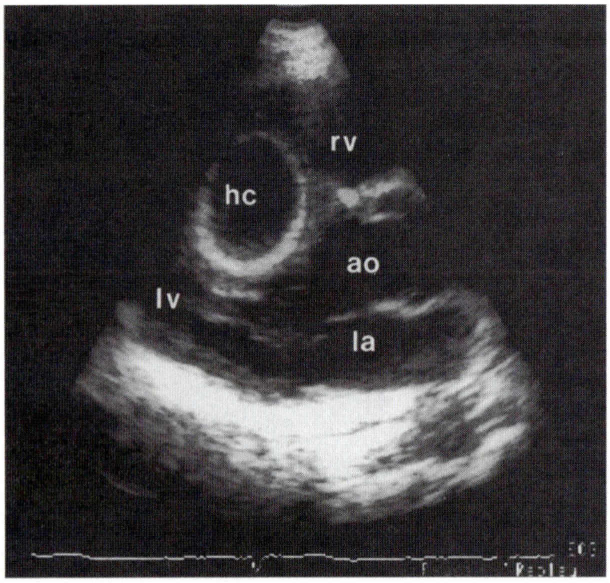

Figure 1. Transthoracic two-dimensional echocardiogram of parasternal long-axis view showing a 3-cm-diameter hydatid cyst (hc) in the upper ventricular septum. la indicates left atrium; lv, left ventricle; rv, right ventricle; and ao, aorta.

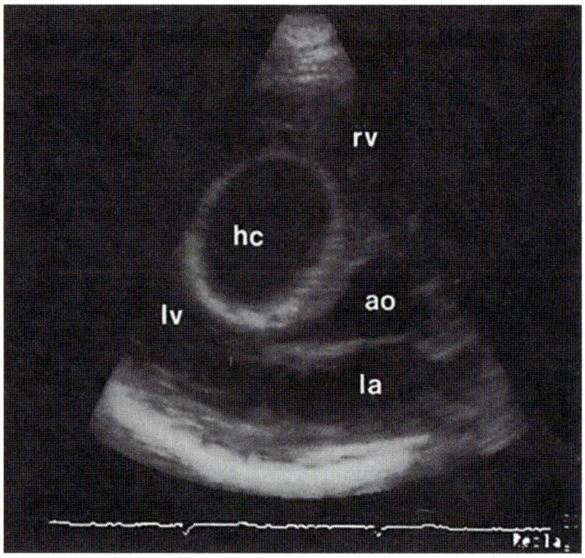

Figure 2. Same as Fig. 1 in another view.

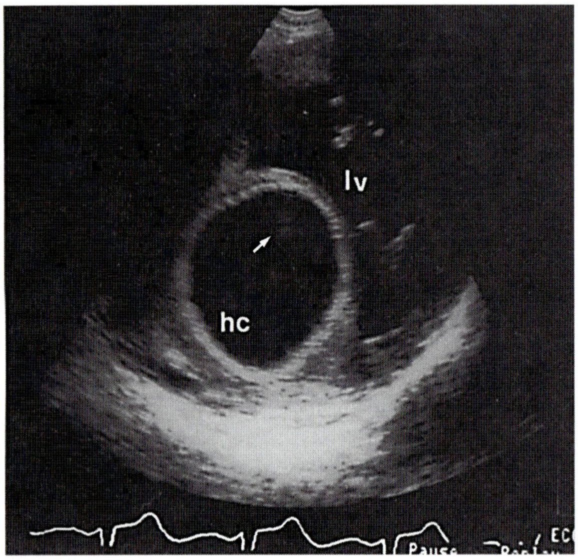

Figure 3. Transesophageal echocardiography showing a hydatid cyst (hc) having a rounded and well-constructed capsule containing an inner sleigh bell (arrow) probably produced by the scolex. lv indicates left ventricle.

97 Ruptured Papillary Muscle

Jason T. Tauke, MD; Susan B. Eysmann, MD
From Northwestern University Medical School, Chicago, Ill.

(*Circulation*. 1997;96:698–699.)

An 82-year-old woman with no significant past medical history presented to the emergency room in cardiogenic shock. After the patient was stabilized with mechanical ventilation and vasoactive medications, an emergency echocardiogram was performed. Figure 1A is a subcostal four-chamber echocardiographic view of the heart, which reveals rupture of the head of the anterolateral papillary muscle. Figure 1B, apical four-chamber echocardiographic view, shows the ruptured papillary muscle; note that the head remains attached to the mitral valve. The ruptured head was noted to prolapse freely into the left atrium, and severe mitral regurgitation was present. After discussion with the patient's family and in accordance with a preexisting living will, further resuscitative efforts were not made, and the patient died shortly thereafter. Postmortem examination revealed a large acute anterolateral myocardial infarction with rupture of the anterolateral papillary muscle (Fig. 1C).

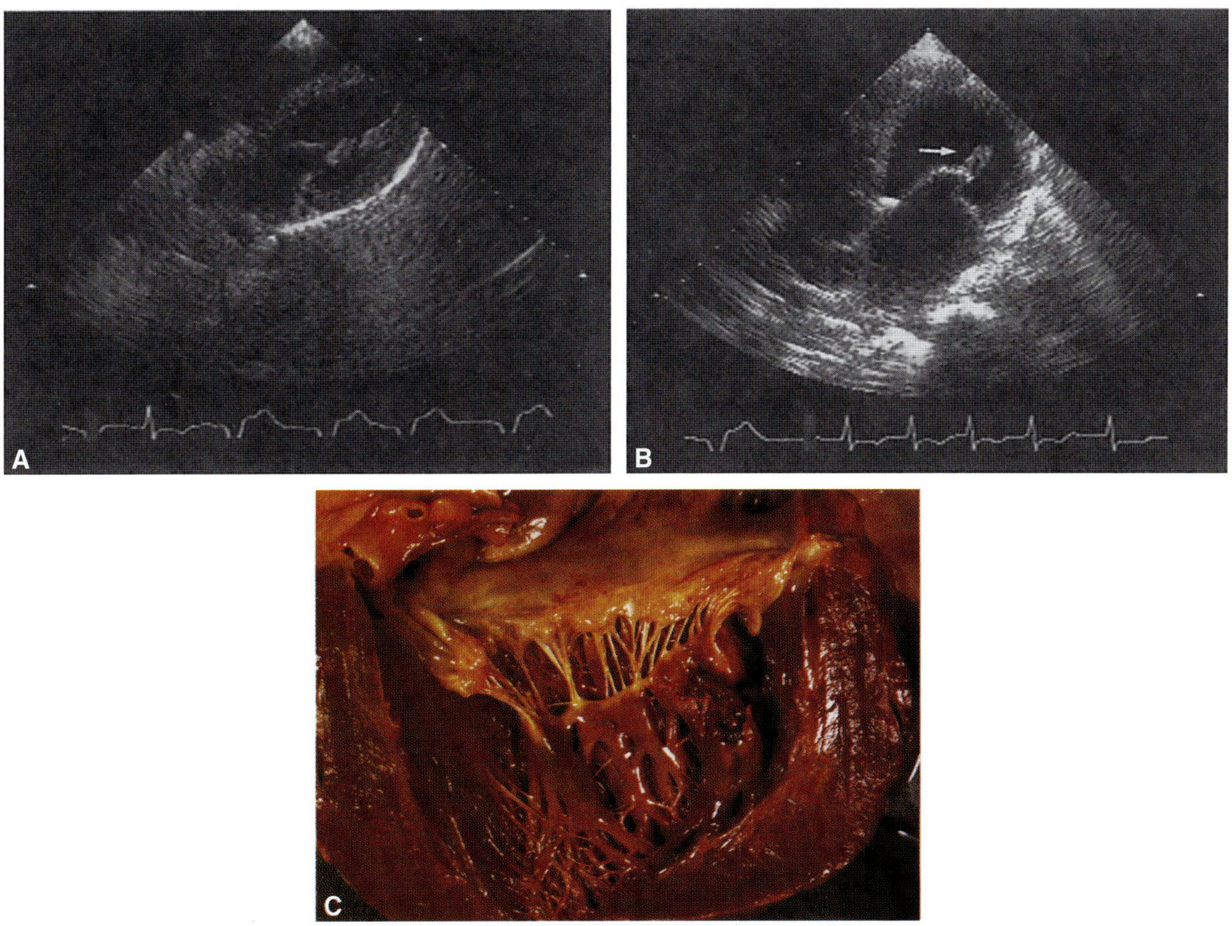

Figure 1.

98 Chagas Disease and Ventricular Aneurysms

Paolo Venegoni, MD; H.S. Bhatia, MD
From the Division of Cardiology, The University of Texas-Houston Medical School.

(*Circulation*. 1997;96:1363.)

A 55-year-old woman presented with shortness of breath and palpitations. She had a history of heart damage with an arrhythmia, which had been detected 16 years previously when she was living in South America. At that time, a diagnosis of Chagas disease was made on the basis of positive blood tests. An electrocardiogram (ECG) showed right bundle-branch block with left anterior hemiblock. Catheterization revealed normal coronary arteries and multiple aneurysmatic dilatations of the left ventricle.

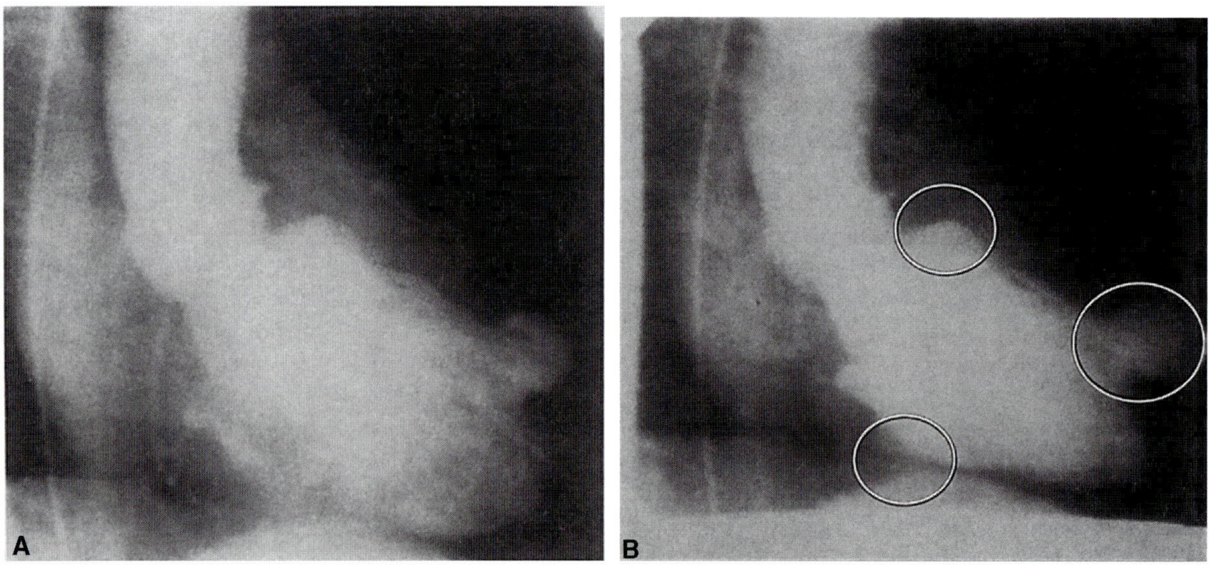

Figure 1. A, Right anterior oblique view of left ventricle. **B,** Multiple left ventricular aneurysms are noted in anterobasal, anterior, and inferior aspects of left ventricle (circled, right).

99

Intrapericardial Teratoma

Maurice Beghetti, MD; Mark Prieditis, MD; Ivan M. Rebeyka, MD, FRCSC;
John Mawson, MBChB, FRACR, FRCPC

From the Divisions of Cardiology (M.B.) and Cardiovascular Surgery (I.M.R.) and the Department of Diagnostic Imaging (M.P., J.M.), The Hospital for Sick Children, University of Toronto, Canada.

(*Circulation*. 1998;97:1523–1524.)

A 1-month-old boy presented with signs of heart failure and tamponade. Two-dimensional echocardiography revealed a complex mass with a large pericardial effusion compressing the heart. Magnetic resonance imaging (Fig. 1) defined the relationship of the mass to the pericardium, myocardium, and great vessels. Complete surgical resection was performed without complication (Fig. 2). Histology of the mass confirmed the presumptive imaging diagnosis of teratoma. The patient remains free of symptoms and tumor 1 year after surgery.

Intrapericardial teratomas are rare primary cardiac tumors usually diagnosed in neonates and infants. They contain endodermic, mesodermic, and neuroectodermic germinal layers. Intrapericardial teratomas are usually benign tumors but may be life threatening because of large pericardial effusion and cardiac compression. Echocardiography generally suggests the diagnosis by showing a heterogeneous intrapericardial mass associated with a pericardial effusion compressing the heart.

Two-dimensional echocardiography is considered to be the best diagnostic imaging modality for primary cardiac tumors, but magnetic resonance imaging may have advantages with large tumors in defining the relationship of the tumor to adjacent structures, in visualizing echocardiographic "blind" spots, and in defining tissue characteristics.

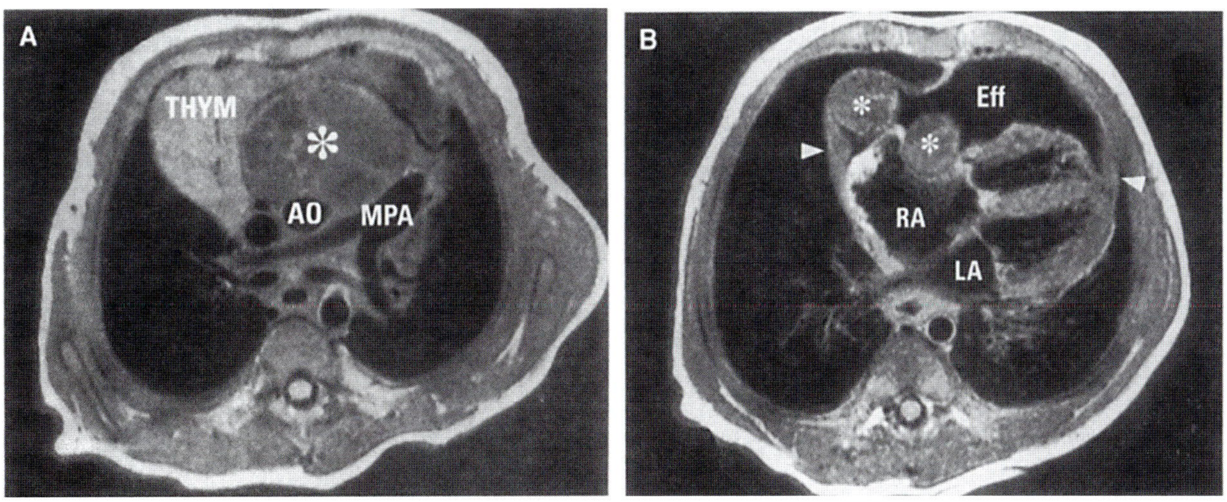

Figure 1. Magnetic resonance imaging. Axial T1-weighted spin-echo images. **A,** Main tumor mass (*) is seen displacing mediastinal structures. Thymus (THYM) is displaced rightward and superiorly (not shown), while aorta (AO) and main pulmonary artery (MPA) are displaced posteriorly and splayed. **B,** Intrapericardial nature of the tumor is demonstrated on a lower image, with tongues of tumor (*) projecting into pericardial space, indenting right atrium (RA). There is an effusion (Eff) and pericardial thickening (arrowheads). LA indicates left atrium.

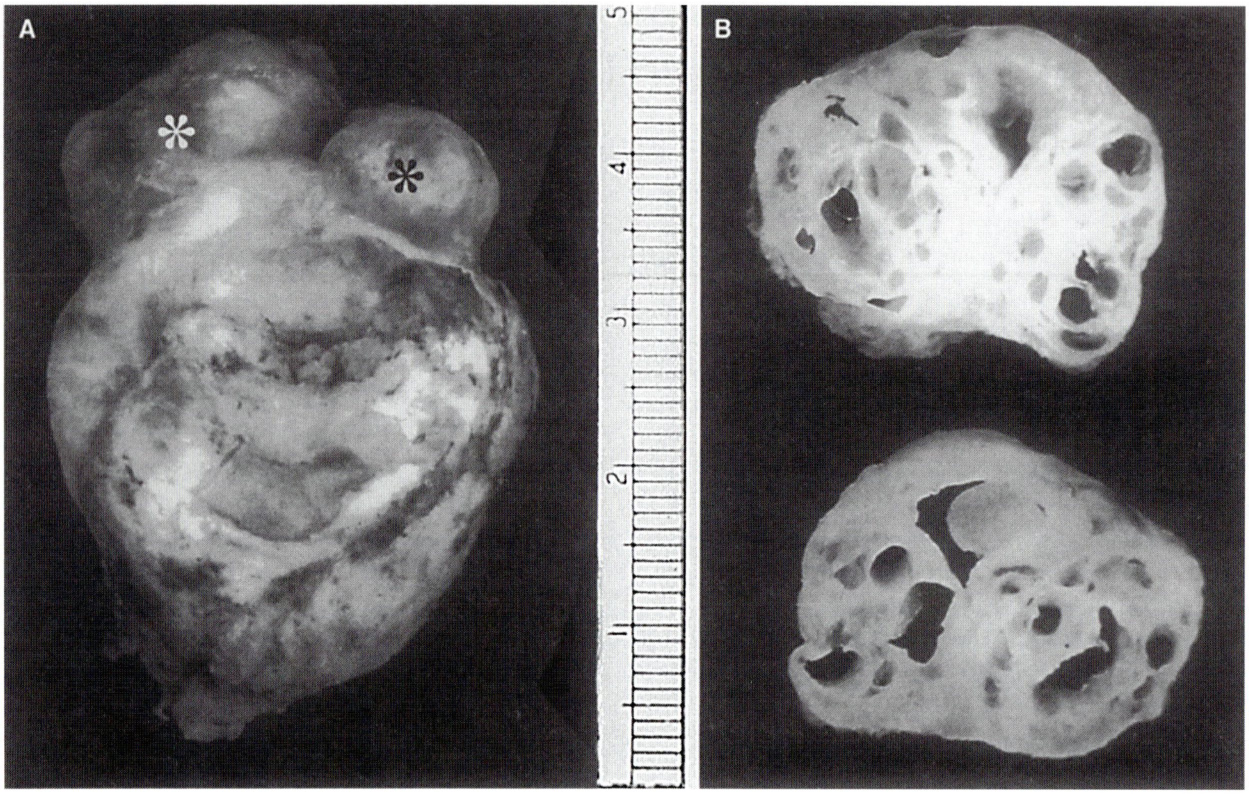

Figure 2. Gross specimens following surgical resection. **A,** Tumor bulk is clearly seen, as are two tumor tongues (*) identified in Figure 1B. **B,** On cut section, cystic and solid nature of lesion is demonstrated, correlating well with variations in signal intensity seen in main tumor mass in Figure 1A.

100 Partial Pericardial Defect

Kean-Wah Lau, MBBS, M Med; Zee-Pin Ding, MBBS, M Med
From Singapore Heart Centre, Singapore General Hospital.

(*Circulation*. 1998;97:1992.)

A 49-year-old healthy-looking man presented with vague chest discomfort in September 1995. Physical examination was unremarkable. Echocardiography revealed mild mitral valve prolapse and an incomplete pericardial echo, arousing suspicion of a partial pericardial defect. A subsequent computed tomography (CT) scan of the thorax clearly demonstrated the incomplete pericardial defect, the rim of which was heavily calcified and constricted the partially herniated right and left ventricles (Fig. 1). Except for a mild focal compression at the junction of the middle and distal third of the left anterior descending coronary artery, there was no significant coronary artery abnormality on contrast angiography. On hemodynamic evaluation, no gradient was detected across the ventricular constriction. The CT findings were confirmed during surgical pericardiotomy (Fig. 2). Since surgery, the patient has remained physically well and asymptomatic.

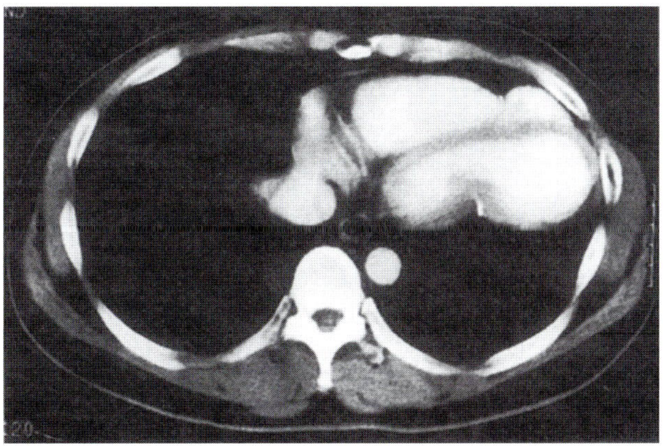

Figure 1. CT scan of thorax, depicting localized partial absence of pericardium with protrusion and compression of both ventricles through defect. Rim of defect was heavily calcified.

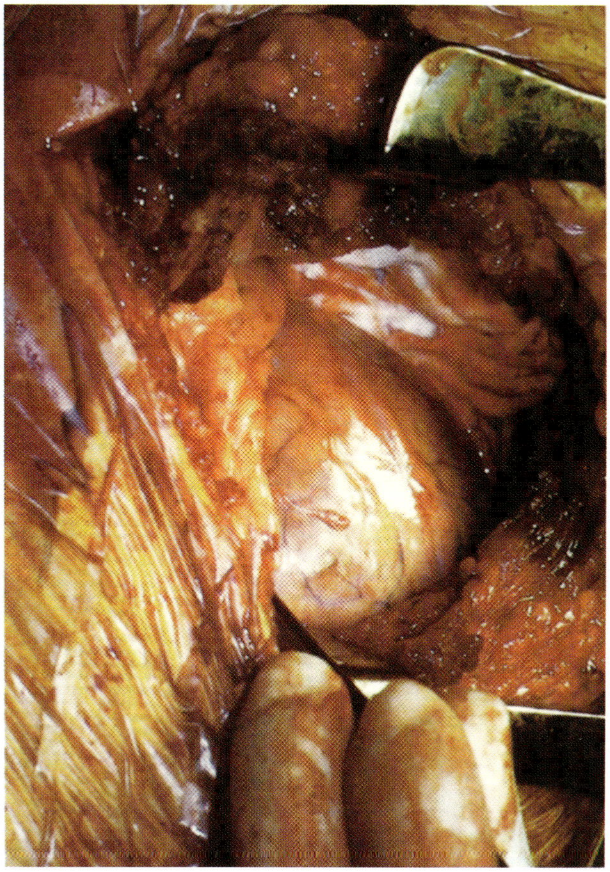

Figure 2. Intraoperative visualization and confirmation of pericardial anomaly. During surgery, a pair of bone cutters was required to cut through heavily calcified pericardial band, which was partially constricting herniated ventricles.

101 Amyloidosis with Cardiac Involvement

Ho-Joong Youn, MD; Jang Seong Chae, MD; Kyo Young Lee, MD; Soon Jo Hong, MD

From the Department of Internal Medicine (H.-J.Y., J.S.C., S.J.H.), and Clinical Pathology (K.Y.L.), The Catholic University of Korea.

(*Circulation*. 1998;97:2093–2094.)

A 59-year-old woman was admitted because of lethargy. She had been treated for heart failure for 5 years before admission, which progressed to include lower-extremity edema as well as orthopnea and nocturnal dyspnea.

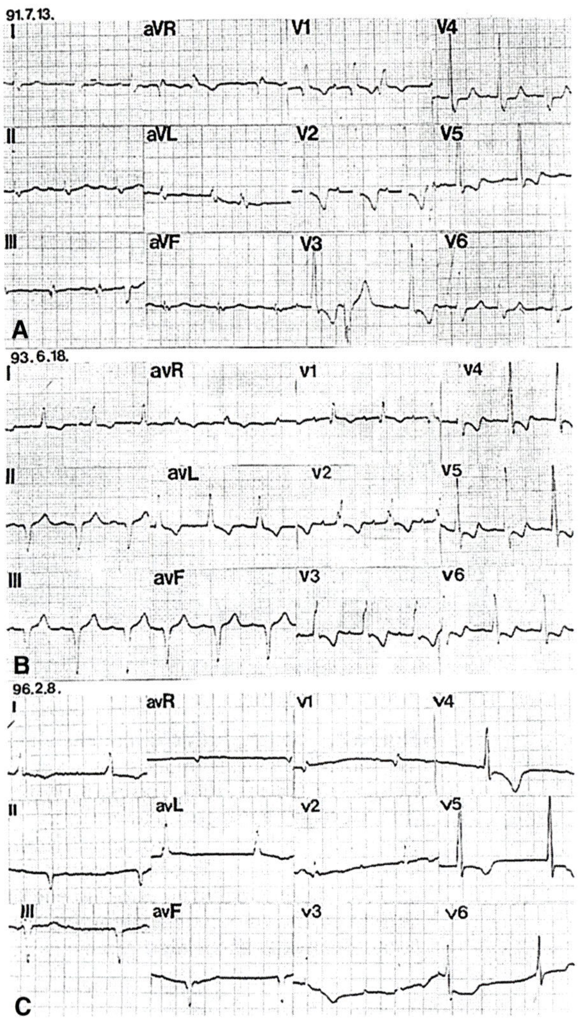

Figure 1. Serial ECG changes. **A,** Sinus rhythm at 80 bpm with first-degree AV block (PR interval, 0.22 second) and right bundle-branch block. **B,** Sinus rhythm at 90 bpm with first-degree AV block (PR interval, 0.24 second), right bundle-branch block, and left axis deviation. **C,** Complete AV block at 48 bpm and low voltage.

The serial ECGs and echocardiographic findings are summarized in Figures 1 and 2. Forearm skin, rectal (Fig. 3), and endomyocardial biopsies (Fig. 4) were performed.

On the basis of our findings (Figs. 1 through 4), the diagnosis of amyloidosis with cardiac involvement was confirmed. Placement of a permanent pacemaker (VVI type) for the treatment of complete atrioventricular block resulted in marked improvement in dyspnea and lethargy.

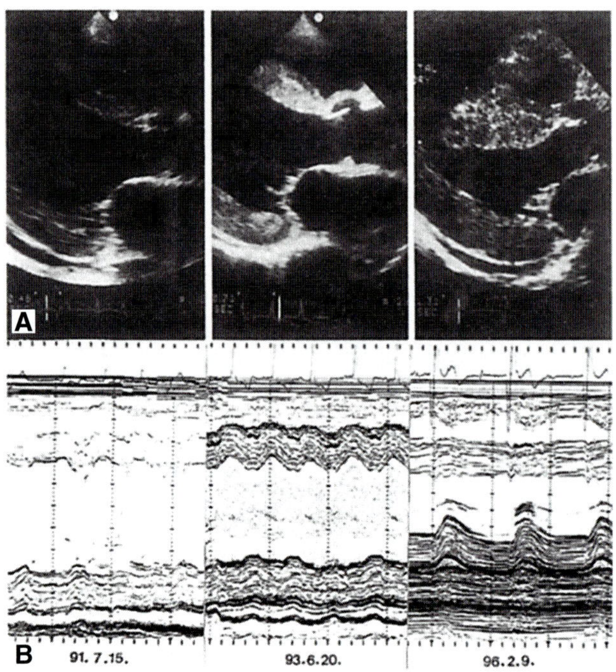

Figure 2. A, Serial two-dimensional echocardiographic findings. Thickening of all myocardial walls and valves; "patch amorphous, high-intensity echoes" in left ventricular myocardium; and a small pericardial effusion were noted (top left). **B,** Serial M-mode echocardiography showed gradual increase of interventricular septal, left ventricular posterior wall, and right ventricular wall thickness.

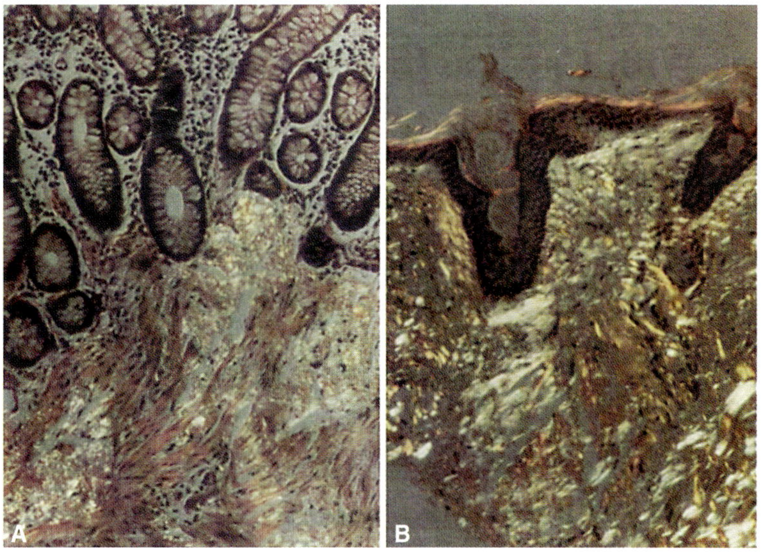

Figure 3. A, Lamina propria and mucosa of rectum. **B,** Dermis of skin showing yellow-green birefringence after Congo red stain under polarizing microscopic examination (×100).

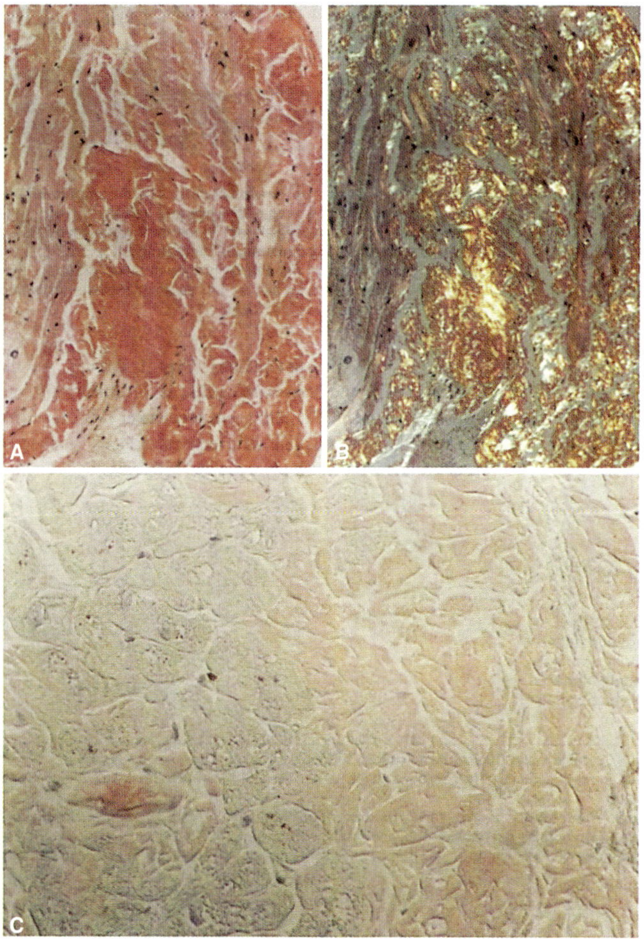

Figure 4. A, Amyloid material stained red within the cardiac muscle cells with Congo red stain (×100). **B,** Typical yellow-green birefringence after Congo red stain under polarizing microscopic examination (×100). **C,** Positive reaction of amyloid material between atrophic cardiac muscle cells with monoclonal murine antibody of amyloid associated protein (×200).

102 Iron Deposition in Myocardium Documented on Standard Computed Tomography in Cardiac Hemochromatosis

Shinichi Niwano, MD; Junji Yokoyama, MD; Hiroe Niwano, MD; Yoshifusa Aizawa, MD

From the First Department of Internal Medicine, Niigata University School of Medicine, Niigata, Japan.

(*Circulation*. 1998;97:2371.)

A 46-year-old woman with pure red-cell aplasia suffered blood transfusion of >200 units, that is, >20 g in iron weight, over 4 years because treatment with a series of immunosuppressants resulted in no effect. Tissue iron deposition caused by iron overload resulted in skin discoloration, hepatic injury, diabetes mellitus, and slight left ventricular dysfunction. Left ventricular end-diastolic and end-systolic dimensions were 45 and 33 mm, respectively, on echocardiogram, and left ventricular ejection fraction was 52%. On standard computed tomography (CT), that is, one scan per 4 seconds, the liver showed a high-density signal before use of contrast medium as a result of iron deposition (Fig. 1). On the same series of CT scans, the left ventricular wall could also be identified as a high-density signal, with neither gated scanning nor cine scanning used (Fig. 2).

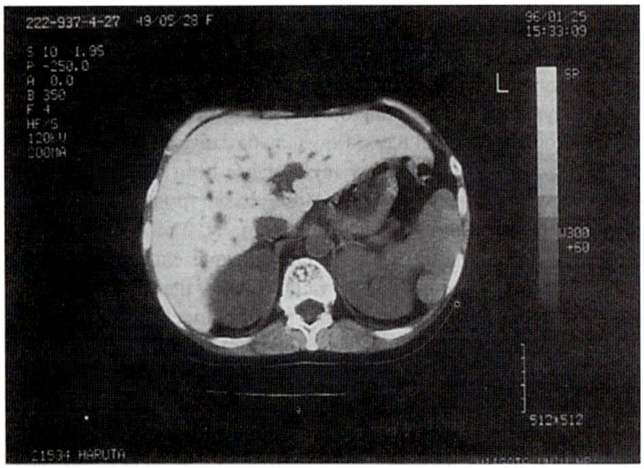

Figure 1. Standard-plane CT scanning of abdomen without contrast enhancement at level of first lumbar vertebra. Whole liver clearly appeared as high-density area because of tissue iron deposition. Bile ducts and hepatic vessels were identified as low-density area, as observed in normal subjects.

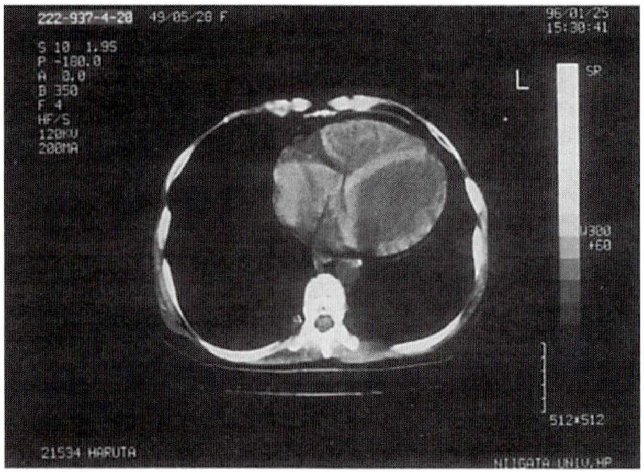

Figure 2. Standard-plane CT scanning of chest without contrast enhancement at level of seventh thoracic vertebra. Gated scanning was not used, and scanning speed was one scan per 4 seconds. Right ventricle (top), left ventricle (bottom), and left atrium were scanned at this level. Left ventricular wall and part of right ventricular wall could be identified as high-density area as a result of iron deposition in myocardium.

103 Cardiac Tuberculosis

Sanjay C. Dhar, MD, MRCP; Sean Hayes, MD; Bojan Cercek, MD; Michael C. Fishbein, MD, MACP

From the Departments of Pathology and Medicine, Cedars-Sinai Medical Center, Los Angeles, Calif.

(*Circulation*. 1998;98:730.)

A 63-year-old man was admitted with a history suggestive of worsening heart failure over a duration of 6 months, recurrent ventricular tachyarrhythmias, poor response to medical treatment, and low-grade fever.

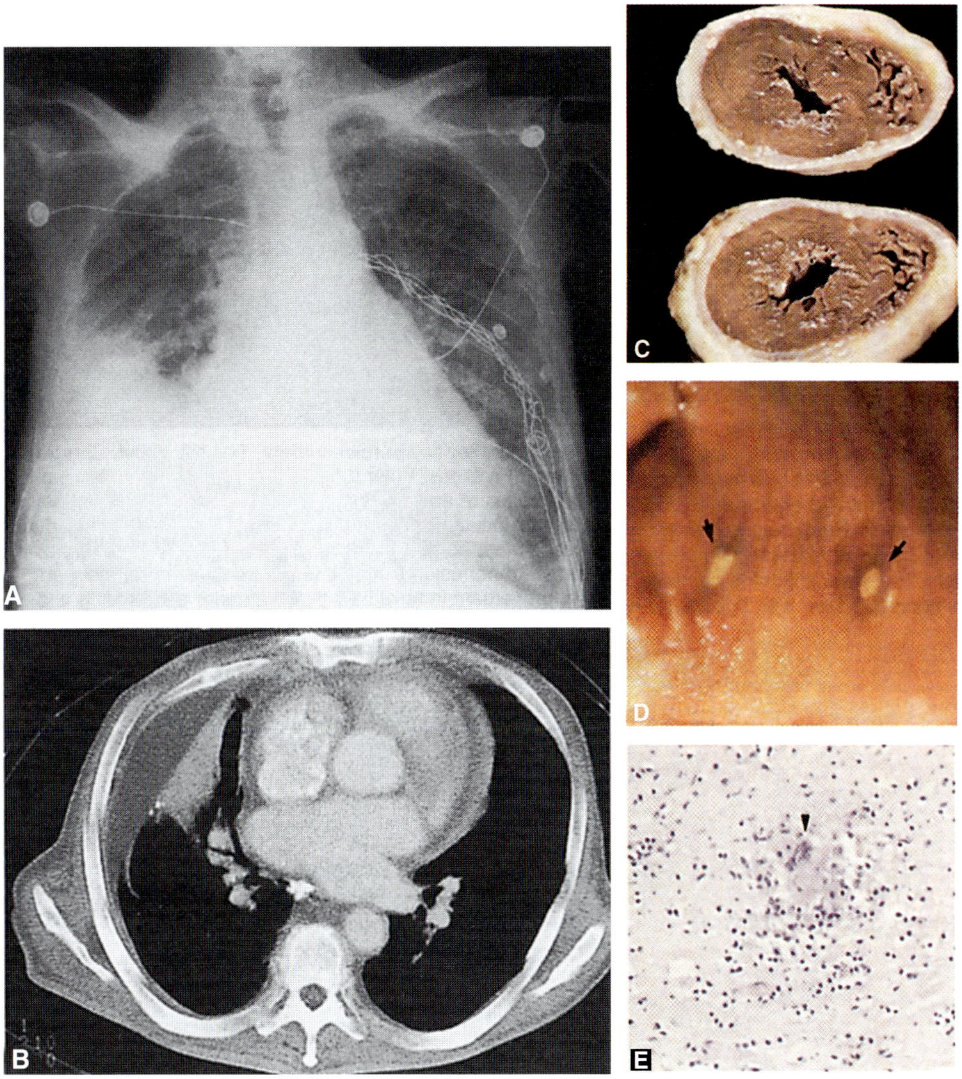

Figure 1. A, Chest radiograph revealed right-sided pleural effusion, cardiomegaly, and borderline perihilar edema. **B,** Computed tomography (CT) scan of chest confirmed right-sided pleural effusion and also revealed pericardial effusion and pericardial thickening. **C,** Cross-section of heart shows thickened pericardium. **D,** Close examination of apical myocardium (arrows) revealed myocardial tubercles. **E,** Higher magnification confirmed presence of granulomas (arrowhead) with giant cells and positive staining for acid-fast bacilli, not seen in this slide.

104 A Broken Heart

Haim Z. Brandspiegel, MD; Roger A. Marinchak, MD; Seth J. Rials, MD, PhD; Peter R. Kowey, MD

From the Division of Cardiovascular Diseases, Lankenau Hospital and Medical Research Center, Wynnewood, Pa, and Department of Medicine, Thomas Jefferson University Hospital, Philadelphia, Pa.

(*Circulation*. 1998;98:1349.)

A 70-year-old woman with no past cardiac history was admitted for near collapse and chest discomfort that occurred when she was informed that her husband of 45 years had died in our hospital of congestive heart failure and refractory ventricular arrhythmias. The electrocardiogram (ECG) revealed minor anterior ST-segment elevations and inferolateral ST-segment depressions, which resolved after intravenous nitroglycerin was administered. Cardiac enzymes were minimally but definitely elevated.

The patient underwent cardiac catheterization, which revealed normal coronary arteries. The left ventriculogram showed anterolateral akinesis and apical hypokinesis, as depicted in Figure 1. The patient was discharged on aspirin and amlodipine. An echocardiogram repeated 3 months later was normal. She has no memory of the entire hospitalization but continues to grieve for her husband.

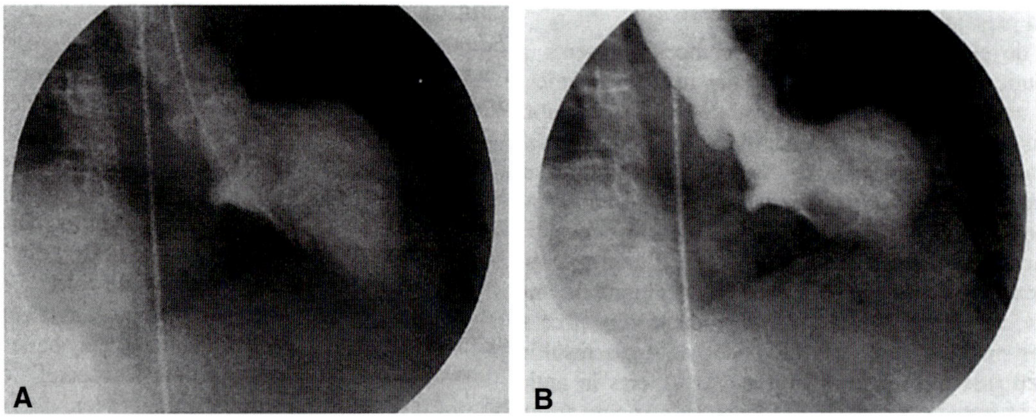

Figure 1. Left ventriculogram during diastole **(A)** and systole **(B)** showing anterolateral akinesis and apical hypokinesis.

105

Restrictive Cardiomyopathy Secondary to Fabry Disease

Warren J. Cantor, MD; Jagdish Butany, MB, BS; Mark Iwanochko, MD, MSC; Peter Liu, MD

From The Toronto Hospital, Toronto, Ontario, Canada.

(*Circulation*. 1998;98:1457–1459.)

A 53-year-old woman presented with progressive dyspnea. Family history was positive for Fabry disease. Cardiac MRI showed marked thickening of the left ventricle (Fig. 1, arrow). Cardiac catheterization revealed a mean right atrial pressure of 16 mm Hg with large *a* waves up to 26 mm Hg (Fig. 2, arrow). A right ventricular endomyocardial biopsy was performed. Light microscopy (Fig. 3) showed myocardial fiber hypertrophy and periodic acid-Schiff (PAS)-positive vacuoles. Electron microscopy (Fig. 4) showed complex concentric lamellar bodies (arrows) characteristic of Fabry's disease. Leukocyte α-galactosidase activity was decreased, confirming the diagnosis. The patient remained severely symptomatic despite medical therapy and was referred for cardiac transplantation. The explanted heart is shown in Figure 5.

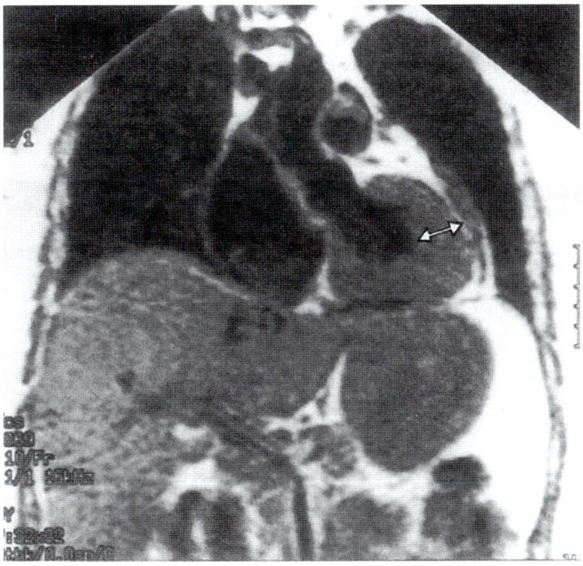

Figure 1. Cardiac magnetic resonance imaging (MRI) (T1-weighted spin echo). Field of view 24 × 24 cm. Slice thickness 5 mm. Coronal view (TE = 12 ms, TR = 869 ms).

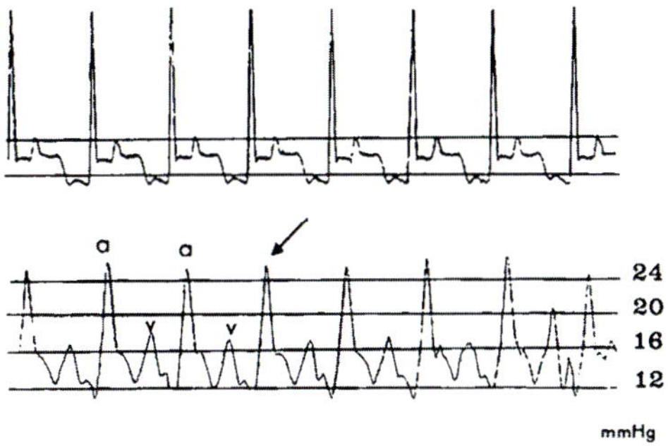

Figure 2. Right atrial pressure tracing with simultaneous electrocardiogram (ECG).

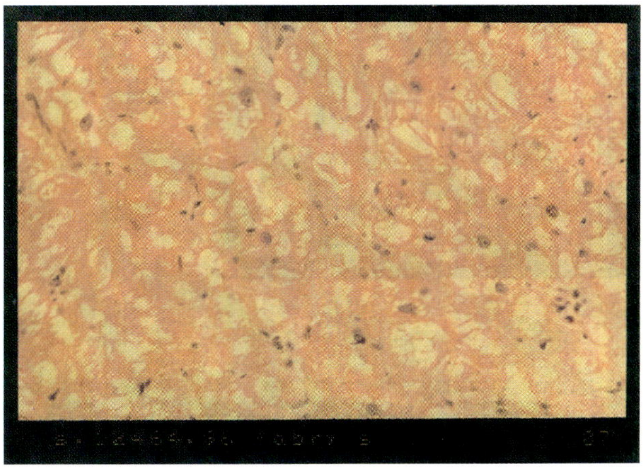

Figure 3. Light microscopy of tissue from cardiac biopsy (Elastic trichrome stain. Original magnification ×200).

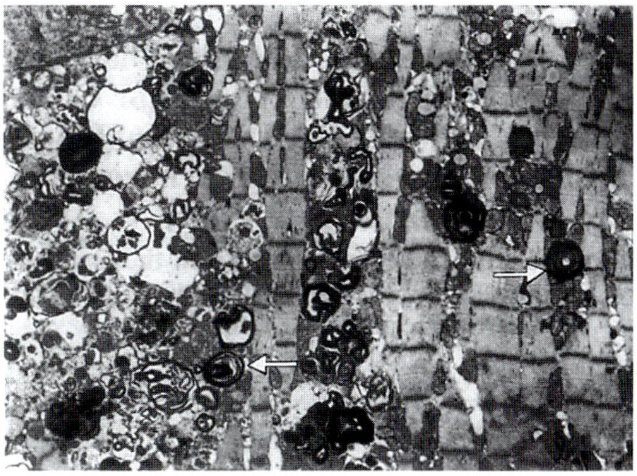

Figure 4. Electron microscopy of cardiac tissue (original magnification ×2000).

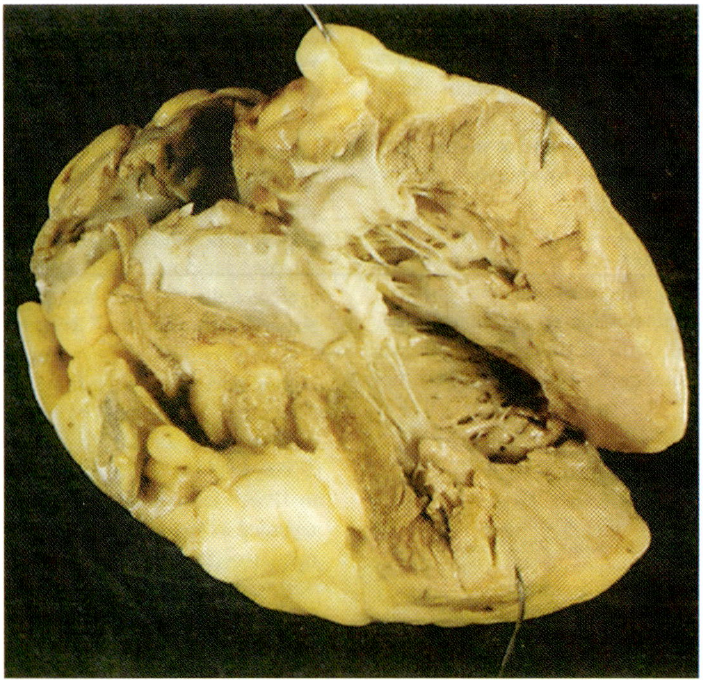

Figure 5. Gross specimen of explanted heart.

106 Right Ventricular Dysplasia with Biventricular Involvement

Bruno Pinamonti, MD; Lorenzo Pagnan, MD; Rossana Bussani, MD; Claudio Ricci, MD; Furio Silvestri, MD; Fulvio Camerini, MD

From the Departments of Cardiology (B.P., F.C.), Radiology (L.P., C.R.), and Pathology (R.B., F.S.), Ospedale Maggiore and University, Trieste, Italy.

(*Circulation*. 1998;98:1943–1945.)

A 23-year-old man was admitted to the hospital with severe heart failure and cachexia. Ventricular arrhythmias and progressive heart failure (predominantly right heart) had been observed in the previous 3 years. Physical examination was unremarkable except for a widely split second heart sound, a systolic left precordial lift, third and fourth heart sounds, and signs of increased venous pressure. Chest radiography showed significant cardiomegaly. The electrocardiogram (ECG) was characterized by right atrial enlargement, low QRS voltages, wide complexes in the right precordial leads (epsilon waves), and negative T waves. Nonsustained ventricular tachycardia with polymorphic configuration was observed at ambulatory ECG monitoring.

The echocardiogram (Fig. 1) disclosed severe right ventricular enlargement, with aneurysm at the level of the outflow, severe depression of systolic pump function, and multiple wall bulges. The left ventricle was not dilated but showed severe diffuse hypokinesis and depression of the ejection fraction (20%).

Considering the severity of clinical symptoms refractory to medical treatment and the echocardiographic findings, a cardiac transplantation was scheduled; unfortunately, the young patient died a few weeks later in low output during an acute febrile illness.

Postmortem examination was compatible with a severe form of biventricular dysplasia, with severe widespread myocardial atrophy and fibrofatty substitution (Fig. 2).

Postmortem magnetic resonance imaging (MRI) examination of the heart (T1-weighted spin-echo technique) showed severe right ventricular enlargement, with wall thinning and increased brightness,

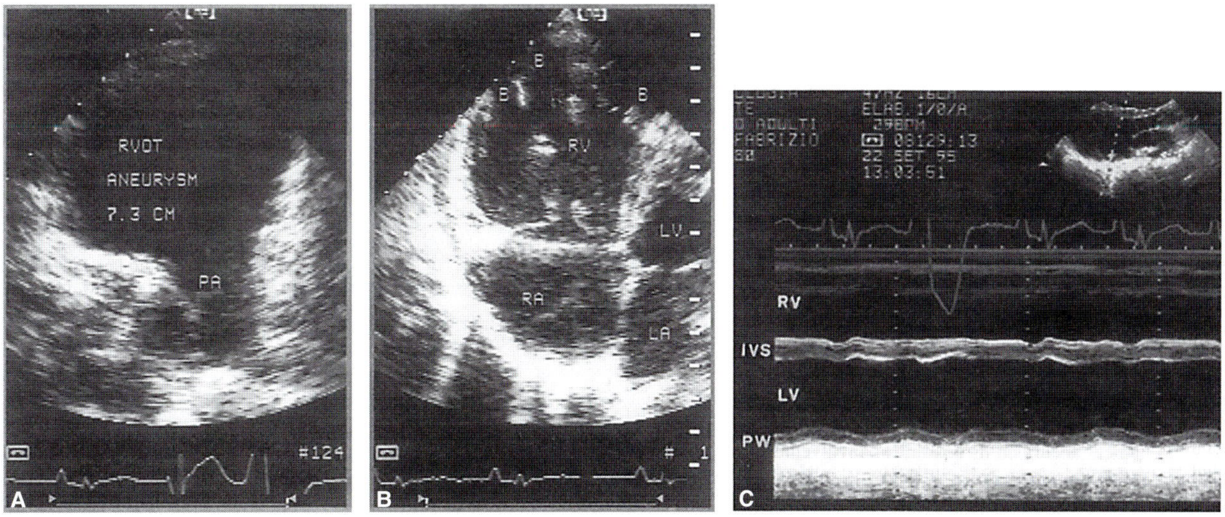

Figure 1. A and B, Two-dimensional echocardiography. **A,** Parasternal short-axis view at basal level. **B,** Modified apical four-chamber view. Both frames in systole. Severe right ventricular (RV) enlargement with aneurysmal dilatation of outflow tract (RVOT) and multiple wall bulges (B) are present. PA indicates pulmonary artery; RA, right atrium; LV, left ventricle; and LA, left atrium. **C,** M-mode echocardiographic tracing at ventricular level. RV is severely enlarged; LV is not enlarged, but severe hypokinesis of both septum (IVS) and posterior wall (PW) is evident.

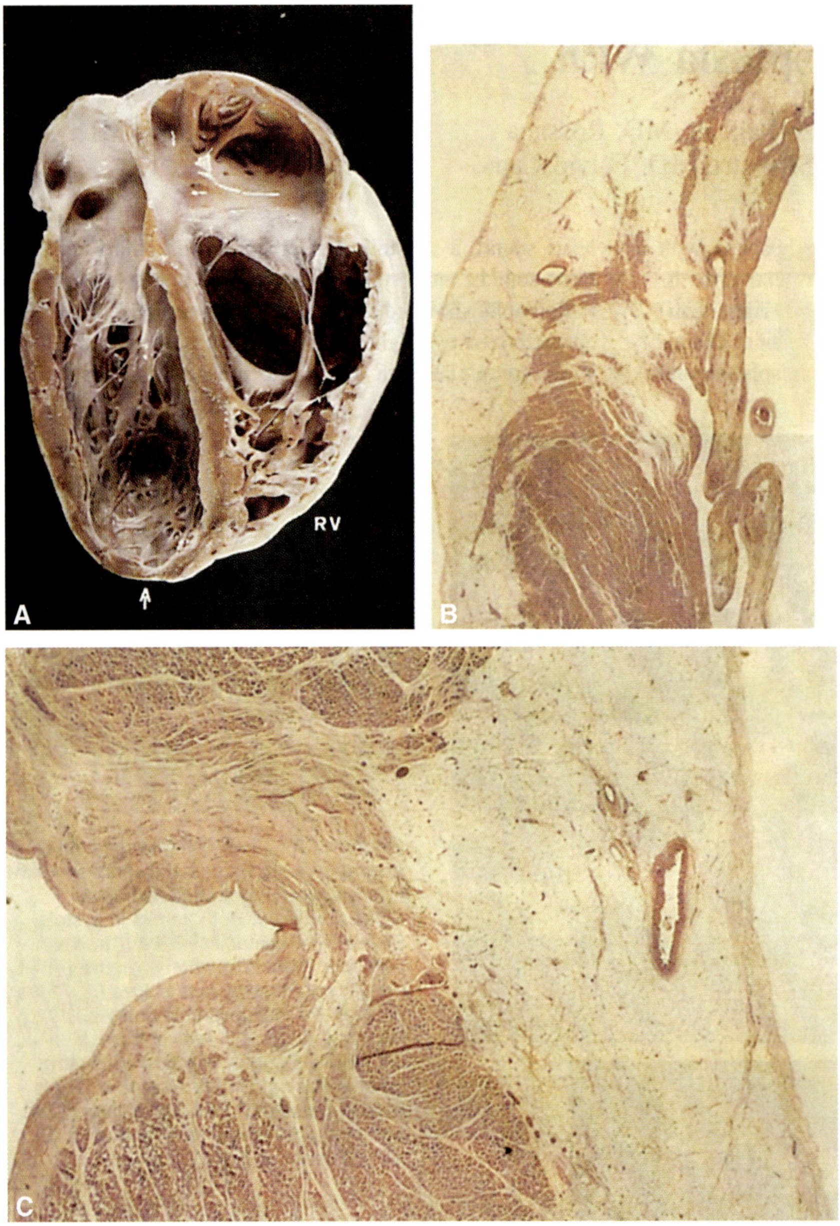

Figure 2. A, Postmortem pathological section of heart (four-chamber): severe widespread fatty infiltration of right ventricular (RV) wall is present; an apical aneurysm is present at left ventricular level (arrow). **B,** Histological section at level of RV inflow (hematoxylin-eosin, ×2.5): severe transmural fibrofatty infiltration of RV wall is present, compatible with RV dysplasia. **C,** Histological section at level of left ventricle (outflow) (hematoxylin and eosin, ×2.5) shows focal severe fibrofatty infiltration with myocellular atrophy, compatible with left ventricular involvement by pathological process.

compatible with fatty infiltration (Fig. 3); focal hyperintensity was also present at the level of the left ventricular apical aneurysm as a result of involvement by the pathological process.

Arrhythmogenic right ventricular dysplasia is a recently described cardiomyopathy characterized by predominant right ventricular involvement with myocardial atrophy and fatty or fibrofatty substitution, clinical signs of ventricular arrhythmias, and rarely, heart failure. Biventricular involvement was observed in several cases. MRI has the unique capability to identify noninvasively the structural abnormalities that characterize this disease, particularly the fatty infiltration.

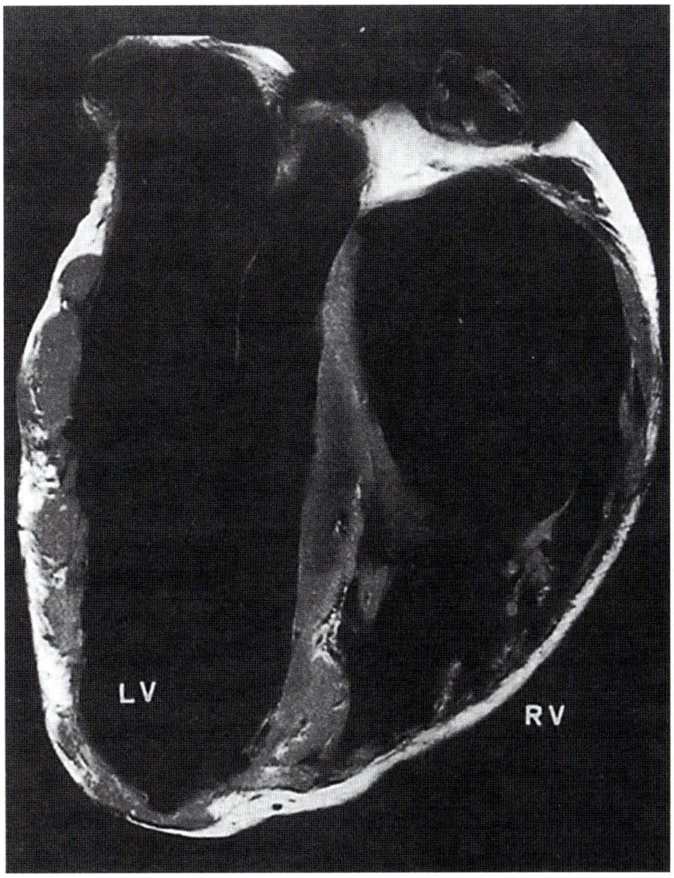

Figure 3. Postmortem MRI (four-chamber view, similar to pathological section, Fig. 2A) shows extensive hyperintense signal at level of right ventricular (RV) wall, compatible with fat; hyperintense areas are also evident at left ventricular level (LV). Note close relationship between presence of fat at pathology and hyperintense areas at MRI.

107 Sewing Needle Transfixing the Posterior Wall of the Left Ventricle Causes Death

Marcos A. Rossi, MD, PhD; Daniel G. Alvarenga, MD; Rovana S. Agrizzi, MD

From the Departments of Pathology and Internal Medicine, Faculty of Medicine of Ribeirão Preto, University of São Paulo, Ribeirão Preto, SP, Brazil.

(*Circulation*. 1999;99:843–844.)

Self-mutilation with a sewing needle and a fatal outcome due to a penetrating wound of the heart is exceedingly rare. To the best of our knowledge, the present image represents the best-illustrated case of such an occurrence.

A 64-year-old woman, a dressmaker, was admitted to the University Hospital because of intense dyspnea. On physical examination, the patient was pale, cyanotic, afebrile, and sweating profusely. The blood pressure was not obtainable. An ECG revealed ST-segment elevation >2 mV in inferior leads and >1 mV in lateral leads. A QRS pattern suggestive of myocardial necrosis was seen in lead V. The chest film showed an indistinct aortic contour, opacification of the space between the aorta and pulmonary artery, mediastinal widening, and interstitial pulmonary edema. Under the assumption that she had diaphragmatic myocardial infarction, she was medicated accordingly. After transfusion of packed red cells, the blood pressure rose (60 mm Hg systolic, 50 mm Hg diastolic), and the patient presented little clinical improvement. Thereafter, her responsiveness gradually declined, terminating in cardiac arrest and death 15 hours after entry. Five days earlier, the patient had been admitted to a Basic Health Unit complaining of epigastric pain radiating to the precordium. The physical examination revealed pallor and hypotension. Transfusion of fresh whole blood was given, and she was discharged in an improved condition. The patient had a past history of depression.

At autopsy, a sewing needle was found transfixing the posterior wall of the left cardiac ventricle (Fig. 1). The tip of the needle could be seen extruding from the middle of a subepicardial hemorrhage in the upper third of the diaphragmatic surface of the heart, close to the atrioventricular grooves. This was associated with hemopericardium (≈250 mL), a small laceration (3 to 4 mm in diameter) of the posterior parietal pericardium close to the inferior esophagus, and mediastinal hematoma. The radiograph of the heart showed the sagittal position of the needle, with the eye inside the left ventricular cavity. The sagittal sectioning of the heart showed a roughly conical area of myocardial hemorrhagic infiltration with the base outside around the 4-cm-long needle. Microscopically, the needle orifice was surrounded by a collar of myocardial necrosis and degeneration, hemorrhage, fibrin, edema, bacterial colonies, and an acute neutrophilic inflammatory infiltrate. The shape of the myocardial hemorrhagic infiltration clearly indicates that the perforation of the heart occurred from outside inward. It is likely that the patient swallowed the needle, which entered the heart from the lower esophagus.

It is difficult to understand why the patient failed to notice the needle injury, but self-mutilation may occur in depressive syndromes, usually in association with severely depressed sensibility to pain. In addition, it is well-known that needles can easily and rapidly migrate through tissues.

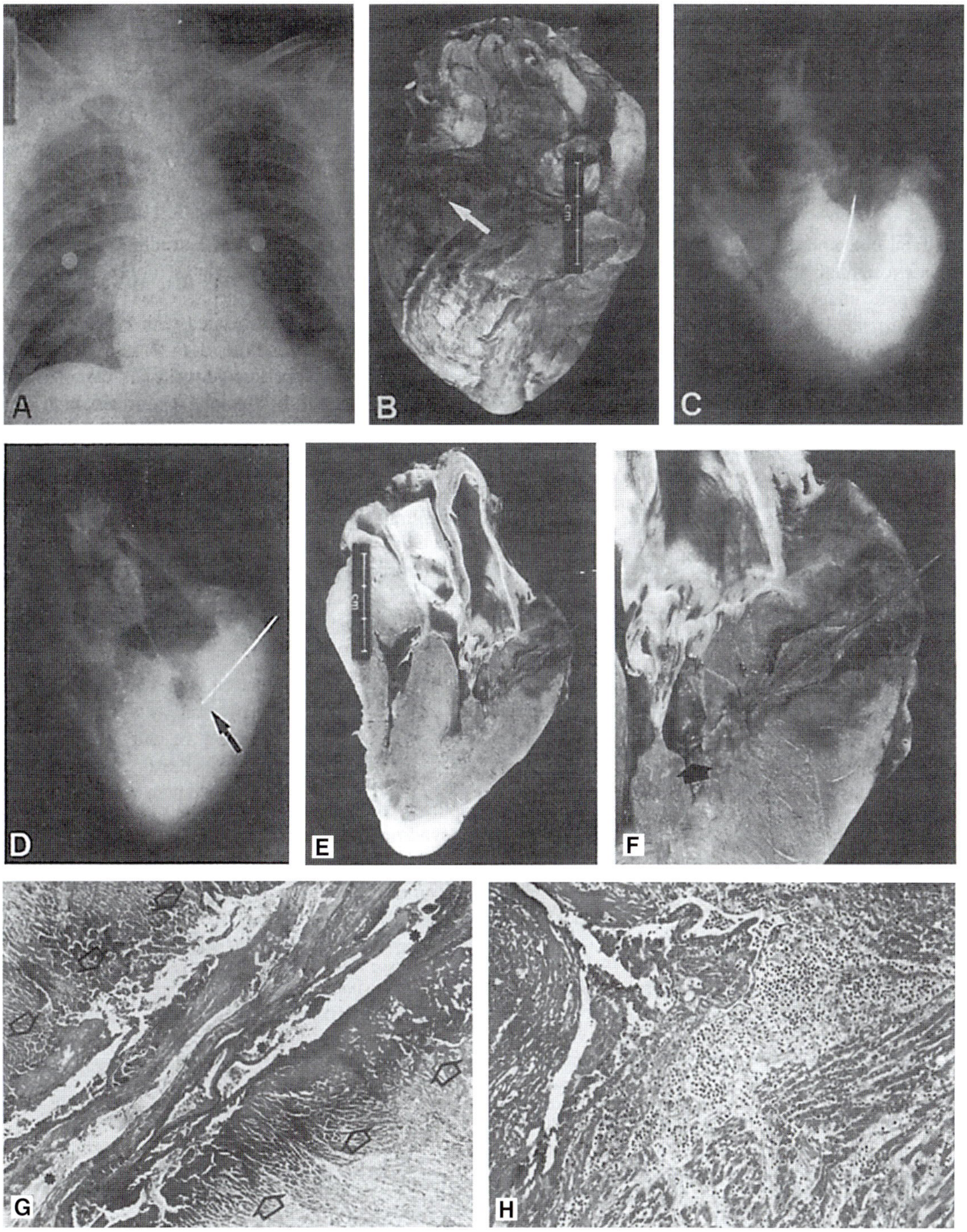

Figure 1. A, Chest film showing indistinct aortic contour, opacification of space between aorta and pulmonary artery, mediastinal widening, and interstitial pulmonary edema. **B,** Sewing needle transfixing left ventricular posterior wall. Four millimeters of tip of needle (arrow) can be seen extruding from middle of subepicardial hemorrhage in upper third of diaphragmatic surface of heart, close to atrioventricular grooves. **C** and **D,** Postmortem radiographs of heart show sagittal position of needle, with eye inside left ventricular cavity (arrow). **E** and **F,** Sagittal sectioning of heart shows a roughly conical area of myocardial hemorrhagic infiltration with base outside around 4-cm-long needle, which has its eye inside left ventricular cavity (arrow). **G,** Microscopically, needle orifice (*) is surrounded by a collar (delimited by open arrows) of myocardial necrosis and degeneration, hemorrhage, fibrin, edema, bacterial colonies, and a neutrophilic inflammatory infiltrate (hematoxylin and eosin stain, ×30). **H,** Higher magnification of border of this collar showing myocyte necrosis and degeneration, bacterial colonies, and marked neutrophilic infiltrate (hematoxylin-eosin stain, ×90).

108 Laser Channels after Percutaneous Transmyocardial Revascularization

Emerson C. Perin, MD; Hans J.F. Dohmann, MD; Hans F.R. Dohmann, MD; Nelson Durval S.G. de Mattos, MD; Luis Antonio Carvalho, MD

From the Department of Adult Cardiology, Texas Heart Institute/St Luke's Episcopal Hospital, and Baylor College of Medicine, Houston, Tex.

(*Circulation*. 1999;99:2218.)

A 62-year-old Brazilian White woman with a history of diabetes mellitus had undergone coronary artery bypass grafting to the left anterior descending coronary artery and right coronary artery in 1991. Four years later, she developed recurrent symptoms of angina; angiography revealed occlusion of both saphenous vein grafts. Her native circumflex system remained patent, but her native left anterior descending and right coronary artery vascular beds were diffusely diseased. The left ventricle was hypertrophic, with preserved function. The patient was not considered to be a suitable candidate for either redo bypass graft surgery or catheter-based therapies. Despite maximum medical therapy, her angina pectoris (Canadian Cardiovascular Society class III) persisted.

On April 26, 1998, she became the first patient in Brazil to undergo a percutaneous transmyocardial revascularization (PTMR) procedure, which was performed with the Eclipse PTMR system (Eclipse Surgical Technologies). The patient was treated successfully, with multiple channels made in the inferior and anterior walls. Her preprocedure and postprocedure left ventricular angiograms are shown in Figures 1 and 2, respectively. The postprocedure angiogram demonstrates the presence of patent channels in the anterior-apical region. The proximal portions of the channels adjacent to the endocardium show defined borders. As the channels come nearer to the subepicardium, the borders become wider and less defined. Although the long-term patency of the channels is questionable, the immediate anatomic results of PTMR are clearly demonstrated.

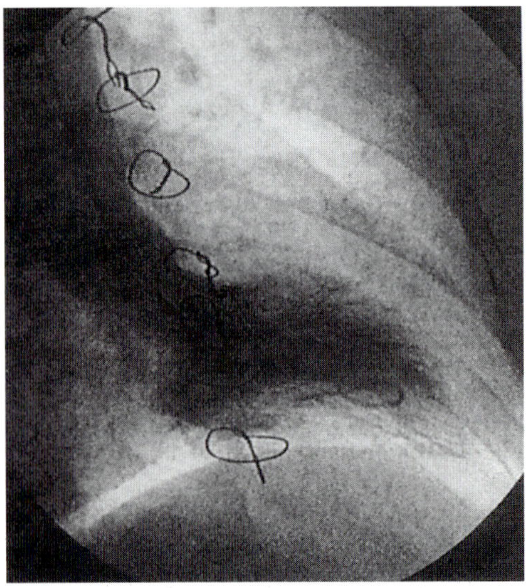

Figure 1.

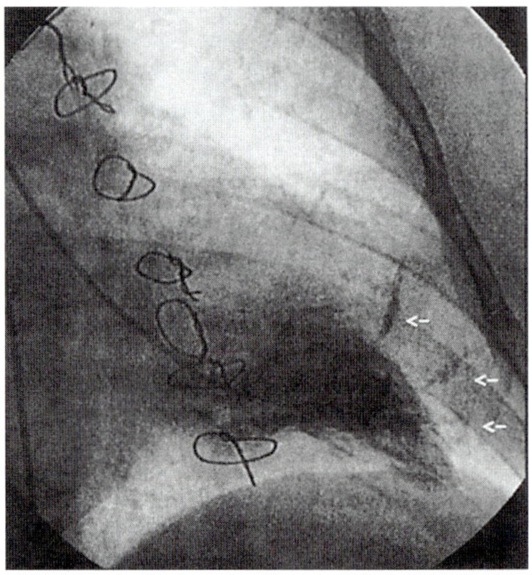

Figure 2.

109 A Bullet in the Heart

Nestor Wainsztein, MD; Branco Mautner, MD

From the Institute of Cardiology and Cardiovascular Surgery, Favaloro Foundation, Buenos Aires, Argentina.

(*Circulation*. 1999;100:1361.)

A bullet located in the interventricular septum is shown in frontal (Fig. 1A) and right lateral (Fig. 1B) chest radiography and in an echocardiogram (Fig. 1C); RA indicates right atrium; RV, right ventricle; LA, left atrium; and LV, left ventricle. Superior white arrow, labeled BULLET, shows the bullet located at the interventricular septum). It is from a 37-year-old policeman who was shot while on duty. The bullet entered the right hemithorax, rupturing the right ventricular free wall and ending in the interventricular septum. A right thoracotomy was performed, a hemopericardium drained, and the right ventricle repaired. The bullet was not removed. Images were made during the patient's recovery.

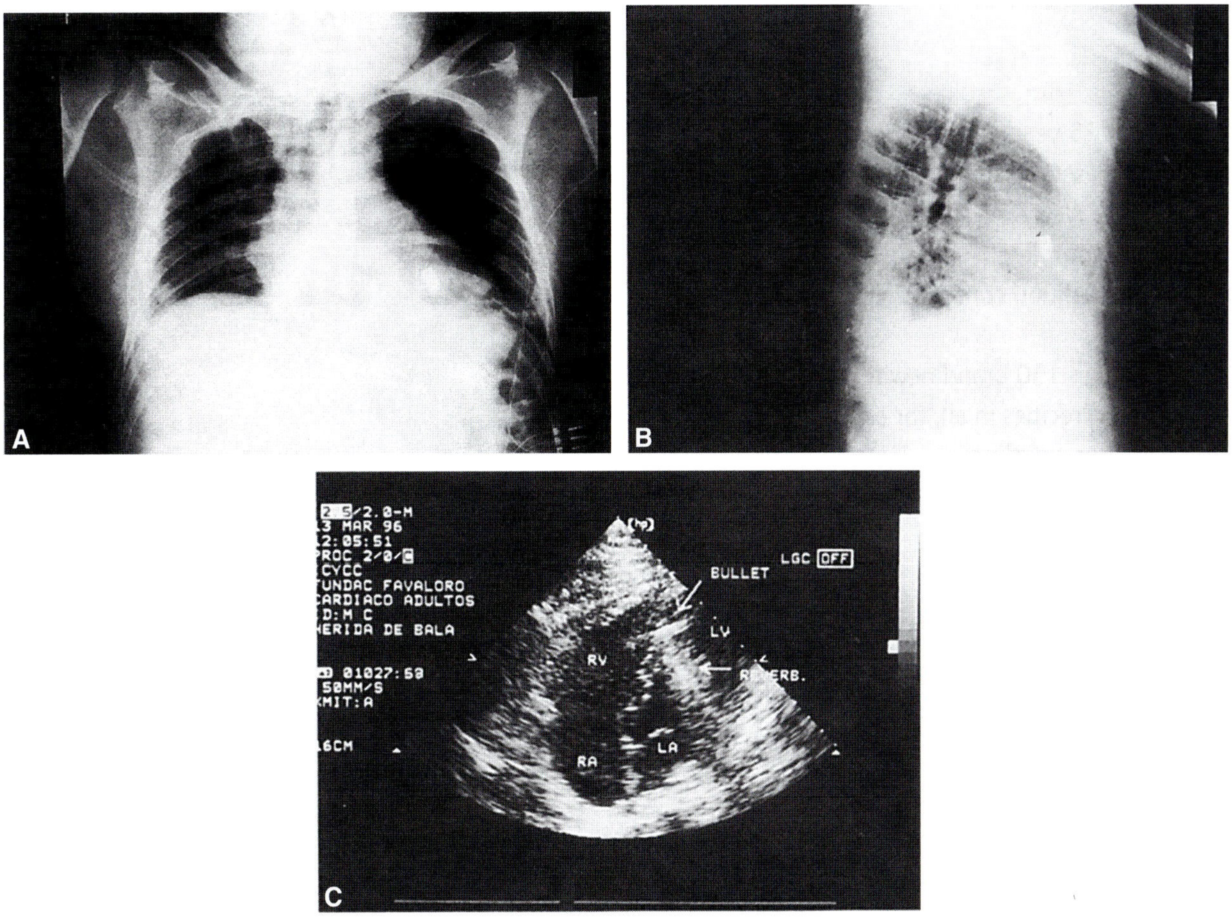

Figure 1.

110 "Switched" Precordial Leads

J. Willis Hurst, MD

From the Department of Medicine, Emory University School of Medicine, Atlanta, Ga.

(*Circulation*. 2000;101:2870–2871.)

Most physicians and technicians have, at one time or another, inadvertently "switched" the extremity leads in preparation for the recording of an electrocardiogram (ECG). This is so common that some modern ECG machines advise the operator that he or she has switched the leads.

Misplacement of the electrode positions is the most common error related to recording the chest leads. The next most common cause of error is probably switching the V_1 and V_2 electrode positions on the chest. This error is easy to make because the wires attached to the lead selector box are adjacent to each other.

During our cardiology morning report, I was shown several ECGs. Two of them were quite unusual. I could not construct the spatial direction of the mean QRS vectors; the frontal plan calculation was easily diagrammed, but the anterior-posterior direction could not be constructed. One of these tracings is shown in Figure 1. There was a tall R wave in lead V_1, a small R wave in lead V_3, and tall R waves in leads V_4 through V_6. The resultantly negative QRS complex at position V_3 was out of place. It appeared that the QRS complex in lead V_3 was more likely recorded from the V_1 position and the QRS complex in lead V_1 was recorded from the V_3 position. If this was true, how did it happen?

I inspected the ECG machine that was used by the new night technician. Inspection of the lead selection box yielded the explanation. The lead wire that was labeled at its end as V_1 was plugged into the V_3 receptacle of the lead selector box and the lead wire labeled V_3 was plugged into the V_1 receptacle of the lead selector box. The new night technician had undoubtedly looked only at the labeling at the end of wires. The corrected ECG is shown in Figure 2.

How could this happen? The wire that connects the lead selector box to the electrode placed on the chest may occasionally break near the clamp used to attach the wire to the electrode. When this happens, the wire must be replaced. In this case, it appears that two wires were replaced. The individual who made the replacement plugged lead V_1 into the V_3 position on the box and plugged V_3 into the V_1 position on the box (Fig. 3).

There are other abnormalities in the tracing. They are not discussed here because the purpose of this communication is to point out what must be an uncommon type of "switched" chest leads. The computer, of course, failed to recognize the error.

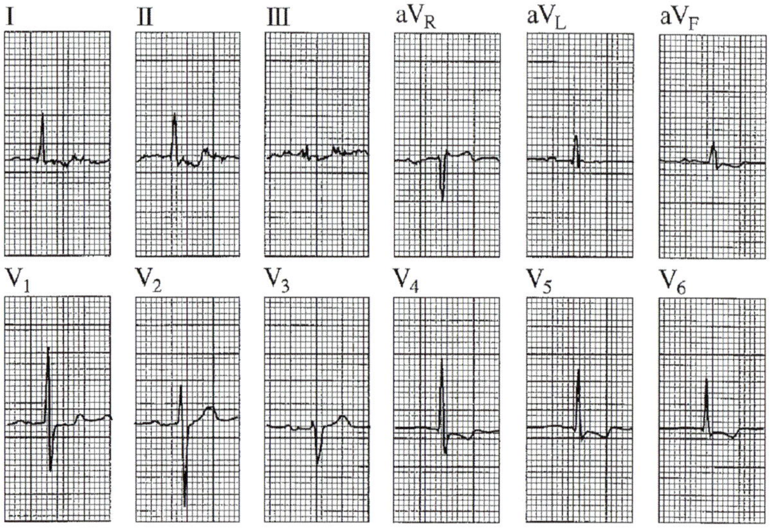

Figure 1. ECG showing switched chest leads V_1 and V_3.

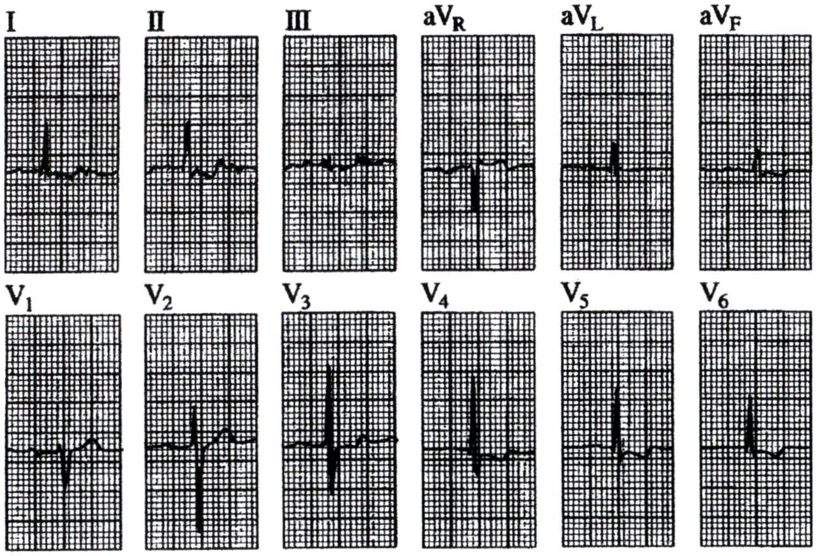

Figure 2. ECG showing corrected chest leads.

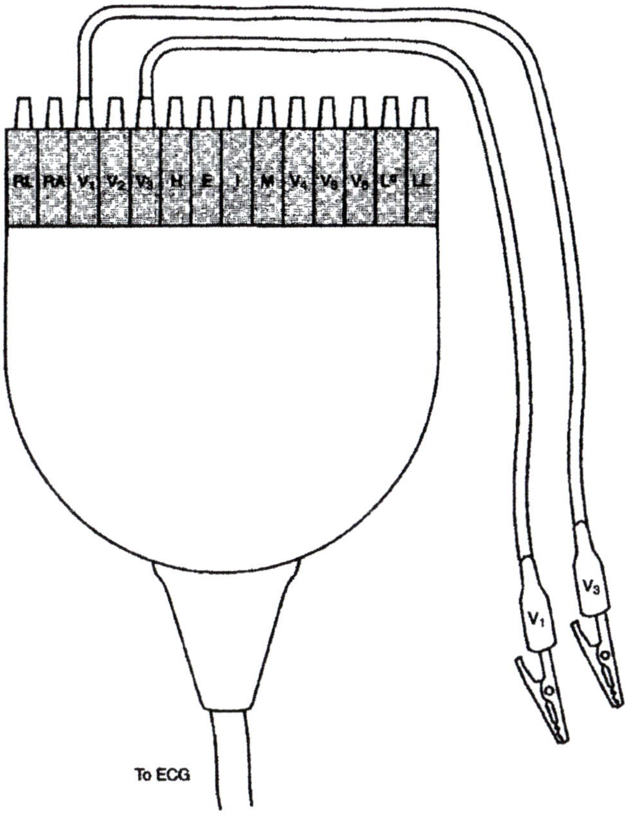

Figure 3. Source of error. Note that lead V_1 is attached to position V_3 on the lead selector box and that lead V_3 is attached to position V_1 on the box.

111 Myocardial Infarction after Dog Bite

Christoph Scharf, MD; Urs Widmer, MD
From the Department of Medicine, University Hospital, CH-8091 Zurich, Switzerland.

(*Circulation*. 2000;102:713–714.)

A 36-year-old man who had undergone splenectomy several years earlier as a result of trauma was admitted with malaise and scattered hemorrhagic lesions on his nose (Fig., 1A). Two days earlier, his dog had bitten him. The next day, he developed chills, watery diarrhea, and vomiting. On admission, the patient complained of chest discomfort. On physical examination, his core temperature was 37.8°C, his blood pressure was 80/60 mm Hg, his heart rate was 90 beats/min, and his respiration was 10 breaths/min, with normal cardiopulmonary auscultation. At the site of the dog bite, a discrete lesion was visible, without any sign of infection (Fig. 1B). The surface ECG showed ST elevation in the inferolateral leads (Fig. 1C). Laboratory examination revealed a white blood cell count of 32,400 cells/μL, a C-reactive protein level of 549 mg/dL, a creatinine level of 268 μmol/L, disseminated intravascular coagulation with thrombocytopenia of 31,000 cells/μL, and D-dimers of 10.2 mg/L. Creatine kinase levels rose from 788 IU/L to 3029 IU/L after 6 hours, and they peaked at 3306 IU/L after 12 hours. The troponin-I concentration rose from 1.2 μg/L to 108 μg/L after 6 hours and declined to 38 μg/L on the second hospital day.

Diagnostic procedures included a thorough examination of the peripheral blood smear (Pappenheim stain). Polymorphonuclear leukocytes showed intracytoplasmic rods, which were gram-negative (Fig., 1D). A presumptive diagnosis of *Capnocytophaga canimorsus* sepsis complicated by acute myocardial infarction was made on the basis of clinical presentation, ECG tracing, and laboratory results. Treatment with meropenem, heparin (10,000 IU per day), and isotonic fluid administration was begun. Coronary angiography was performed the next day, and it demonstrated normal vessels without signs of atherosclerosis. Transthoracic echocardiography showed normal valves, diffuse hypokinesia, and a decreased ejection fraction of 35%. The patient recovered rapidly and was dismissed in good condition after 2 weeks of antibiotic treatment. Blood cultures taken at admission yielded *Capnocytophaga canimorsus* (formerly designated DF-2 by the Centers for Disease Control).

When acute myocardial infarction occurs in patients with bacteremia, it usually results from hypotension or from endocarditis with septic emboli to the coronary arteries. In our patient, however, and in 3 others with *Capnocytophaga canimorsus* bacteremia, acute myocardial infarction developed in the absence of both hypotension and endocarditis.

Acknowledgment

We thank Mrs R. Ruegg, Chief Technician of Hematology, University Hospital, Zurich, for her collaboration.

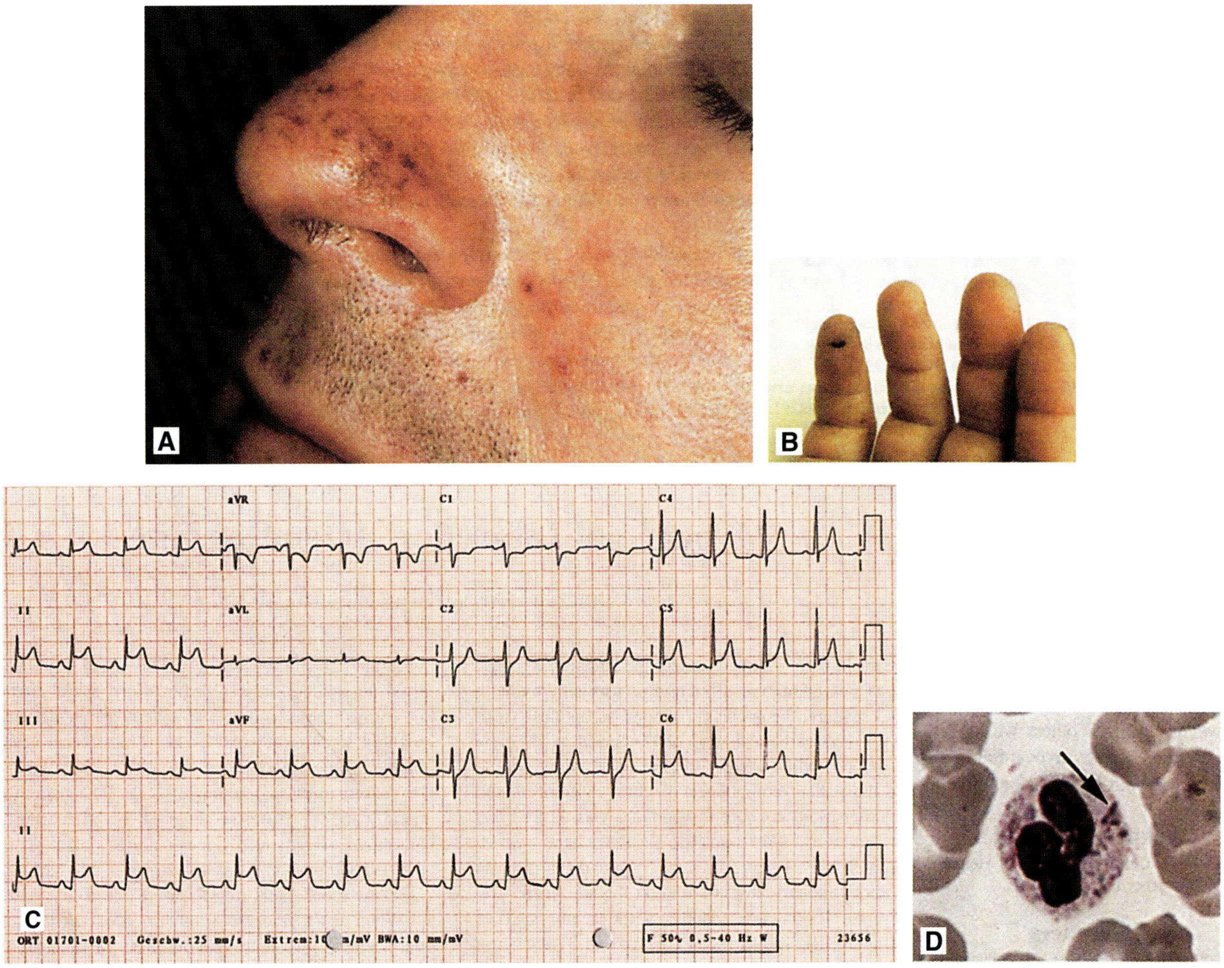

Figure 1. A, Hemorrhagic lesions on the nose made the patient seek medical attention. **B,** Easily overlooked bite wound had no signs of local infection. **C,** ECG demonstrated transmural ischemia in the inferolateral leads. **D,** Polymorphonuclear leukocyte contains intracytoplasmic rods (arrow).

112 Another Broken Heart

Herbert L. Fred, MD

From the Department of Internal Medicine, The University of Texas Health Science Center at Houston, Tex.

(*Circulation*. 2002;105:779.)

DOI: 10.1161/hc0602.101547

A 69-year-old woman underwent a coronary artery bypass procedure (allegedly on Valentine's Day). A portable chest film obtained on the second postoperative day showed a striking radiolucent line bisecting the patient's heart (Fig. 1). On a follow-up film made several hours later, the line had disappeared, proving that it was an artifact and not the result of the surgeon's knife (or Cupid's arrow). The cause of the artifact remains a mystery.

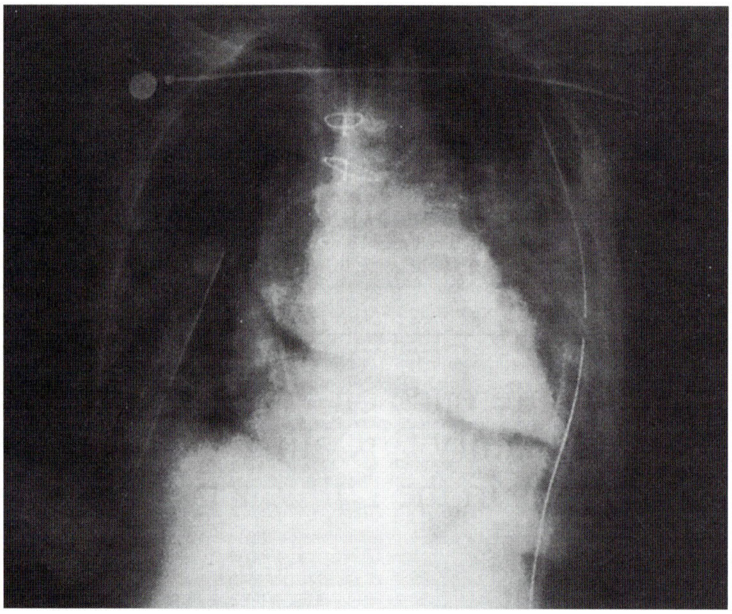

Figure 1. Portable chest film showing mysterious, holiday-appropriate artifact.

113

Left Ventricular Involvement in Arrhythmogenic Right Ventricular Cardiomyopathy

J.A. McCrohon, MD, PhD; A.S. John, MD; C.H. Lorenz, PhD; S.W. Davies, MD; D.J. Pennell, MD

From the Departments of Cardiovascular Magnetic Resonance (J.A.M., A.S.J., C.H.L., D.J.P.) and cardiology (S.W.D.), Royal Brompton Hospital, London, UK.

(*Circulation*. 2002;105:1394.)

DOI: 10.1161/hc1102.104521

A 55-year-old woman presented with an 18-month history of progressive dyspnea, exertional chest tightness, and palpitations associated with light-headedness. Resting electrocardiogram showed sinus rhythm and incomplete right bundle branch block with nonsustained ventricular tachycardia of left bundle branch morphology on 24-hour recording. Thallium scintigraphy reported partial thickness infarction of the inferior wall and reversible ischemia in the anterior wall. Cardiac catheterization showed "disorganized" function of the left ventricle (LV) and severe hypokinesis of the inferior wall and mid-anterior wall. The left coronary system was normal, and the right coronary showed a 50% distal stenosis. Cardiovascular magnetic resonance (CMR) assessment confirmed an enlarged LV with severe hypokinesis of the inferior wall and hypokinesis and focal thinning of the mid anterior wall. The right ventricle (RV) was also abnormal with reduced systolic function, elevated end-systolic volume, dyscoordinate free wall contraction, and an area of prominent dyskinesis in the basal to mid inferolateral RV (Fig. 1). T1-weighted spin-echo images showed fat deposits within the myocardium of the anterior and inferior LV walls and throughout the RV free wall with marked thinning in the areas of dyskinesis (Fig. 2). There was no LV or RV myocardial infarction or macroscopic fibrosis on late enhancement imaging after gadolinium. These features are consistent with arrhythmogenic right ventricular cardiomyopathy with florid LV involvement. Fatty subepicardial deposits of the LV have been documented at autopsy in 64% of arrhythmogenic right ventricular cardiomyopathy cases but are rarely so clearly seen in life. The patient has been referred for electrophysiological testing and investigation of first-degree relatives.

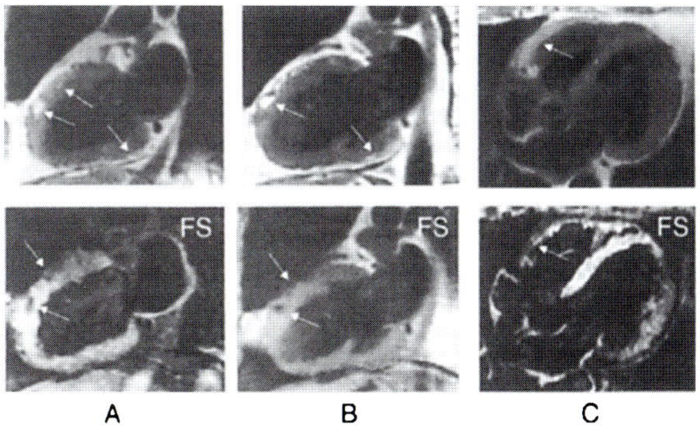

Figure 2. T1-weighted turbo spin-echo images before (upper panel) and after (lower panel) the application of a fat saturation pulse over the region of interest. The arrows (upper panel) point to areas of fatty infiltration of the anterior and inferior myocardium from the epicardial surface. Fatty infiltration is confirmed by the nulling of these areas (black regions) using a fat saturation prepulse in the same plane. The RV free wall shows diffuse high signal consistent with fat (**C**, top), which is nulled using a fat suppression sequence (**C**, bottom) to reveal a remaining thin layer of RV myocardium. FS indicates fat saturation.

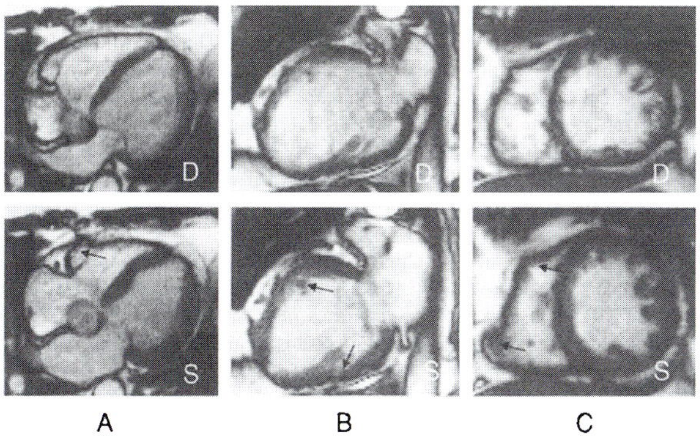

Figure 1. True FISP cine images in the horizontal and vertical long-axis (**A** and **B**) and short-axis planes (**C**) showing a dilated left ventricle with arrows demonstrating mid-anterior and inferior wall hypokinesis and RV free wall dyskinesis and associated wall thinning. S indicates systole; D, diastole.

114 Eosinophilic Pericarditis and Myocarditis

Qiang Li, MD, DSc; Deepali Gupta, MD; George Schroth, MD; Catalin Loghin, MD; George V. Letsou, MD; L. Maximilian Buja, MD

From Department of Medicine/Division of Cardiology (Q.L., G.S., C.L.), Department of Cardiothoracic and Vascular Surgery (G.V.L.), and Department of Pathology and Laboratory Medicine (D.G., L.M.B.), the University of Texas Health Science Center at Houston.

(*Circulation*. 2002;105:3066.)

DOI: 10.1161101.CIR.0000016787.93662.DO

A 58-year-old African-American woman with long-standing asthma presented with a 1 month history of severe dyspnea on exertion, orthopnea, and weight loss. One week before hospitalization, she could only sleep sitting in a chair. She was found to have 50% eosinophils on peripheral blood smear without bone marrow malignancy. Cardiac enzymes were elevated. Electrocardiography revealed low-voltage QRS complexes without ST or T wave changes. Chest radiograph showed bilateral pleural effusions. Echocardiography documented a restrictive filling pattern with normal systolic function and a pericardial effusion. A pericardial window was performed through a left anterior thoracotomy, and 400 mL of bloody pericardial fluid was withdrawn. Pericardial biopsy (Fig. 1) and myocardial biopsy (Fig. 2) confirmed the diagnosis of eosinophilic pericarditis and eosinophilic myocarditis. These are features of Löeffler fibroplastic parietal endocarditis, which can lead to endomyocardial fibrosis and restrictive cardiomyopathy.

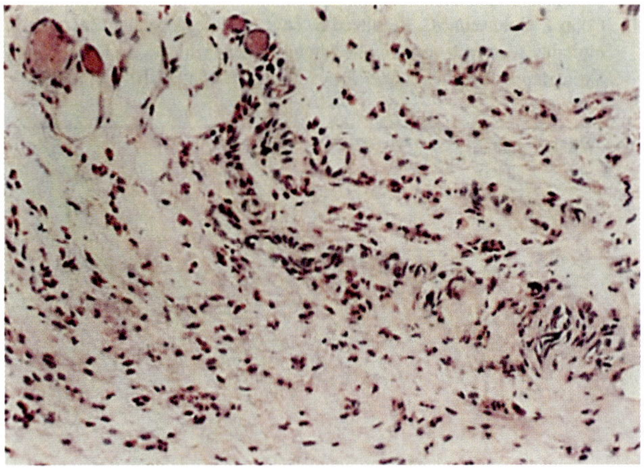

Figure 1. Pericardium: eosinophilic infiltrates and chronic inflammation. (Hematoxylin and eosin stain [HE], ×200).

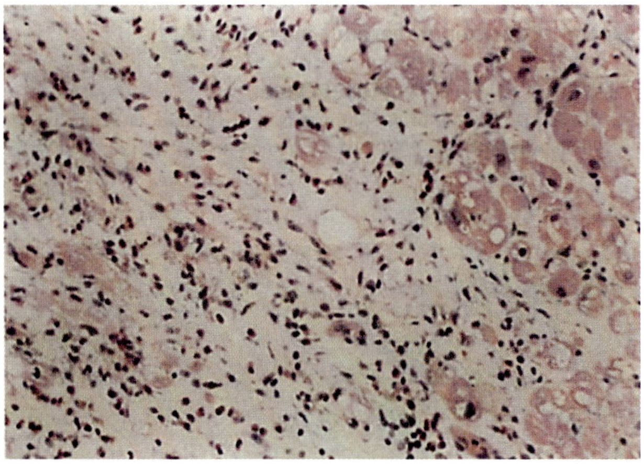

Figure 2. Myocardium: myocardial eosinophilic infiltrates with fibrosis and myocyte degeneration (HE, ×200).

115 Ventricular Fibrillation during Swimming in a Patient with Long-QT Syndrome

Peter Ott, MD; Frank I. Marcus, MD; Arthur J. Moss, MD

From the University of Arizona Health Sciences Center (P.O., F.I.M.), Tucson; and University of Rochester School of Medicine and Dentistry (A.J.M.), Rochester, NY.

(*Circulation*. 2002;106:521–522.)

DOI: 10.1161/01.CIR.0000018643.56813.8C

A 32-year-old woman was diagnosed with long-QT syndrome in 1997. One year later, a single-chamber implantable cardioverter-defibrillator (ICD) was implanted after multiple episodes of syncope. She has had no syncope or ICD discharge during the last 19 months.

She passed out while swimming. She was pulled from the water semiconscious by her 13-year-old daughter and did not remember receiving an ICD shock. A 12-lead ECG showed a QT interval of 600 ms (Fig. 1). The ICD interrogation revealed ventricular fibrillation followed by correct arrhythmia detection and successful termination by defibrillation through the device (Fig. 2). This occurred at the time she was swimming.

Swimming appears to be a specific trigger of arrhythmias in long-QT 1 syndrome. Why swimming has such a specific correlation with the long-QT 1 syndrome is unclear. It is tempting, however, to speculate that this activity may provide particularly intense sympathetic stimulation due to physical exertion, possibly combined with fear.

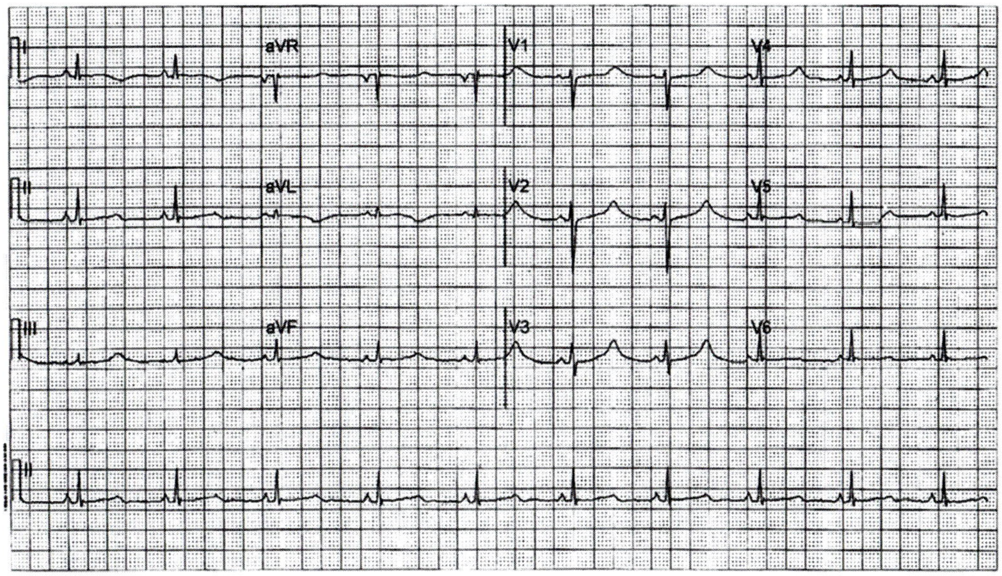

Figure 1. Twelve-lead surface electrocardiogram (ECG) (25 mm/s; 1 mV/cm) showing sinus rhythm at a rate of 60 bpm. There is a markedly prolonged QT interval (600 ms; best seen in leads I and aVL) with a broad-based T wave characteristic of the long QT 1 syndrome.

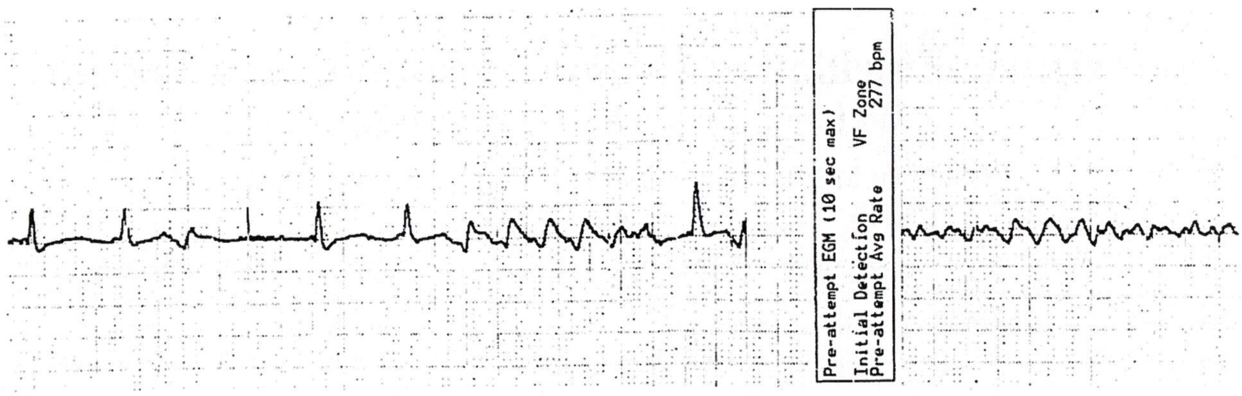

Figure 2. Displayed are the ventricular electrograms (recorded from the shock electrode) from the episode during swimming (25 mm/s). The onset of ventricular fibrillation appears to be preceded by premature ventricular beats and a brief run of ventricular tachycardia.

116 Magnetic Resonance Imaging of Impending Left Ventricular Rupture after Acute Myocardial Infarction

Antonello Zoni, MD; Arianna Arisi, MD; Domenico Corradi, MD; Diego Ardissino, MD

From the Division of Cardiology (A.Z., A.A., D.A.) and Department of Pathology and Laboratory Medicine (D.C.), University Hospital, Parma, Italy.

(*Circulation*. 2003;108:498–499.)

DOI: 10.1161/01.CIR.0000079054.75843.7A

A 63-year-old man with a history of arterial hypertension was admitted to the Cardiology Intensive Care Unit with an inferior acute myocardial infarction. The patient received 10 + 10 units of reteplase. Transthoracic echocardiogram showed an akinetic inferior wall and depressed systolic function (ejection fraction = 40%). Cardiac magnetic resonance imaging (MRI) (Siemens Somaton Vision, 1.5 T) performed 4 days after the infarction for investigative purposes showed an infarct of the left ventricular inferior and posterior walls. The right ventricle was also partially involved. After gadolinium injection, a transmural serpiginous hypoenhancement signal was present in the infarcted area, consistent with myocardial hemorrhage and suggesting impending cardiac rupture (Fig. 1). The patient suddenly died 5 hours after the MRI study. Autopsy showed an inferoposterior infarct involving the right ventricle. A myocardial rupture was present in the middle portion of the posterior wall corresponding to the hemorrhagic area detected by MRI (Fig. 2). Histological examination showed myocardial necrosis and diffuse interstitial hemorrhage (Fig. 3).

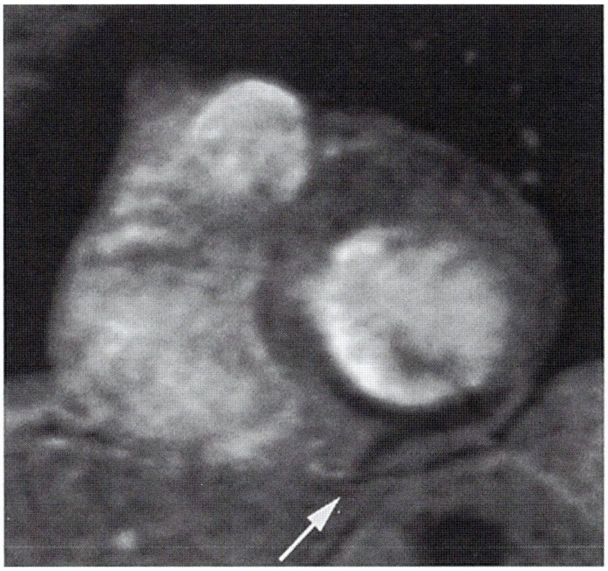

Figure 1. Cardiac MRI of acute myocardial infarction. Gradient-echo fast low-angle shot (2-D-FLASH) sequence after gadolinium injection; note in the infarcted area a systolic hypoenhancement signal proceeding from the endocardium to the epicardium suggesting impending rupture (arrow).

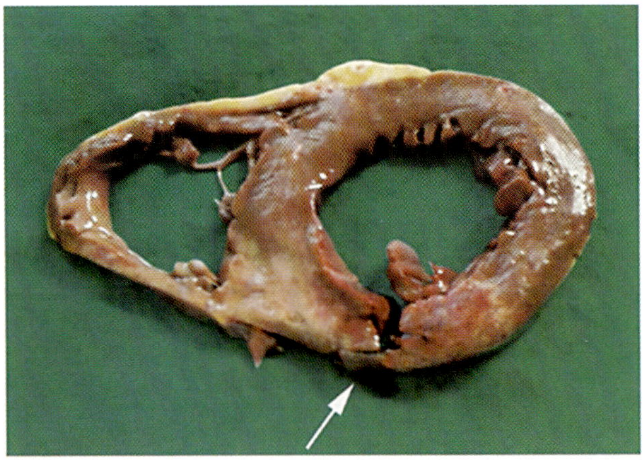

Figure 2. Cardiac rupture in middle portion of infarcted posterior wall (arrow).

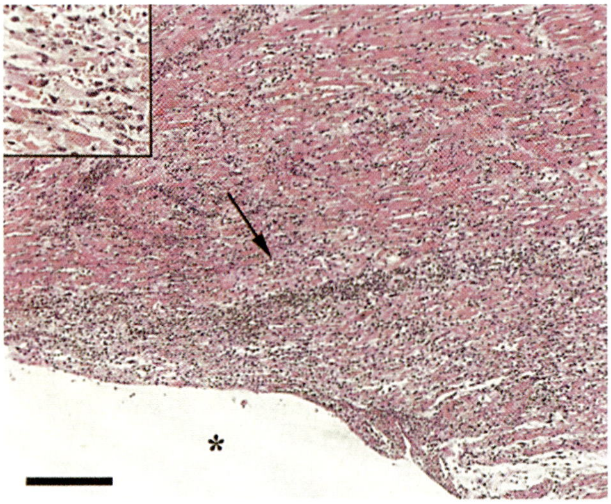

Figure 3. Histological examination. Left ventricular posterior free wall rupture (*) at the site of myocardial infarction. Insert (magnification of area indicated by arrow) shows injured myocytes with destruction of the architecture and diffuse interstitial hemorrhage. Hematoxylin and eosin; magnification in larger portion of figure, ×4. Bar = 300 μm.

117

Traumatic False Aneurysm of the Left Ventricle

Elmar Spuentrup, MD; Henning Schubert, MD

From the Department of Diagnostic Radiology, Technical University of Aachen, Aachen, Germany (E.S., H.S.), and Department of Medicine (Cardiovascular Division), Beth Israel Deaconess Medical Center and Harvard Medical School, Boston, Mass (E.S.).

(*Circulation*. 2004;109:550.)

DOI: 10.1161/01.CIR.0000109526.50291.56

A 34-year-old man was involved in a severe traffic accident 3 years before his current admission and sustained multiple rib and midfacial fractures as well as lung contusion. After 2 months, complete restitution was seen on chest x-ray. Three years later, the patient was scheduled for reconstructive surgery of the midface. Physical examination and laboratory findings at that time were normal. The preoperative chest x-ray, however, demonstrated a large calcified mass adjacent to the anterior wall of the left ventricle (Fig. 1). The mass was confirmed by multislice chest computed tomography (CT) (Fig. 2A) and magnetic resonance imaging (MRI) (Figs. 2B through 2D). It was partly filled with floating blood via a small defect of the anterior wall of the left ventricle (arrows in Figs. 2A through 2D) while major portions were thrombolized as seen by high signal intensity on black-blood MRI (Fig. 2C). Cine MRI (Fig. 2D) demonstrated normal thickening of the myocardium, even adjacent to the defect of the myocardial wall. No evidence of coronary artery disease or history of myocardial ischemia was found. Based on these findings, the diagnosis of a traumatic false aneurysm of the anterior left ventricular wall was established.

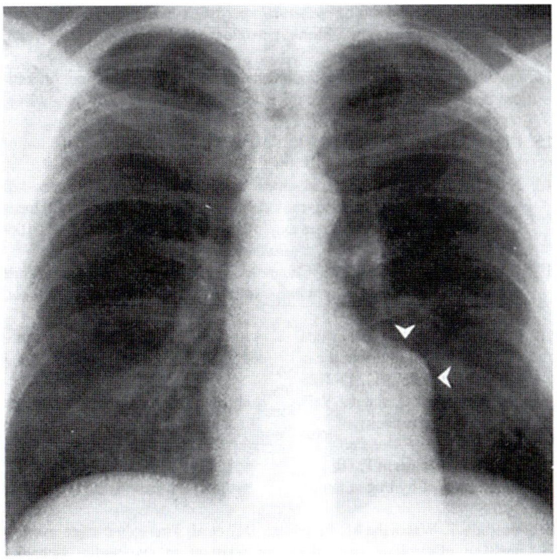

Figure 1. Chest x-ray demonstrating a calcified mass adjacent to the left ventricle (arrowheads).

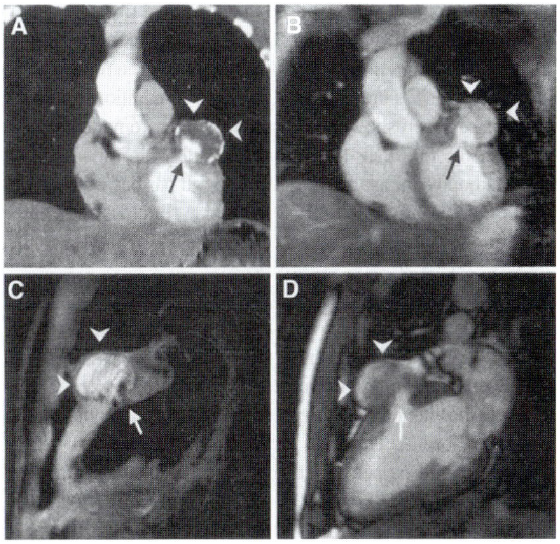

Figure 2. A, Multislice CT of the chest after intravenous contrast medium administration, arterial phase, and coronal reconstruction. The mass (arrowheads) is partly filled with blood via a small defect of the anterior wall of the left ventricle (arrow), whereas the major portion is thrombolized. The wall is partly calcified. B through D, Corresponding MRI. **B,** Navigator-gated T2-prepared and fat-suppressed cardiac-triggered 3-D gradient echo sequence (TR = 7.0 ms, TE = 2.2 ms, 1×0.7 mm in-plane resolution, coronal slice orientation). **C,** Navigator-gated dual-inversion recovery black-blood turbo spin-echo sequence (TR = 2 heartbeats, TE = 26 ms, 2-chamber view). On this sequence, the thrombolized portion is seen with a bright signal. **D,** Cine balanced fast field echo (TR = 3.2 ms, TE = 1.6 ms, 20 heart phases, diastolic frame, two-chamber view).

118 ST-Segment Elevation Resulting from Hyperkalemia

Daniel B. Sims, MD; Laurence S. Sperling, MD

From the Department of Medicine, Emory University School of Medicine, Atlanta, Ga.

(*Circulation*. 2005;111:e295–e296.)

DOI: 10.1161/01.CIRCULATIONAHA.0000165127.41028.D1

A 20-year-old man with a history of type 1 diabetes mellitus presented to the emergency department with nausea, vomiting, and abdominal pain of 8 hours' duration. Diabetic ketoacidosis was diagnosed based on a glucose of 68.8 mmol/L (1240 mg/dL), bicarbonate of 5 mmol/L, pH of 6.92, and a positive urine dipstick for ketones. Serum potassium measured 9.4 mmol/L. An electrocardiogram (ECG) (Fig. 1) revealed ST-segment elevation (asterisks); a wide QRS complex tachycardia; absent P waves; and tall, peaked, and tented T waves (arrows). One hour after the patient received intravenous fluid, calcium gluconate, bicarbonate, and insulin, the electrocardiographic abnormalities had resolved (Fig. 2), leaving only sinus tachycardia secondary to volume depletion and minimal peaking of the T waves (arrows). Serum potassium now measured 5.7 mmol/L. Creatine kinase, creatine kinase-MB, and troponin I values were normal. At the time of discharge, the patient was in good condition, with a normal ECG.

Hyperkalemia can cause several characteristic ECG abnormalities that are often progressive. Initially, the T wave becomes tall, symmetrically peaked, and tented. Widening of the QRS complex with an intraventricular conduction delay then occurs. Additional elevation of serum potassium leads to a decrease in the amplitude of the P wave and its eventual disappearance from the ECG. Rarely, ST-segment elevation mimicking myocardial infarction, described as a "pseudoinfarction" pattern, is present. Further progression of hyperkalemia leads to a sine wave appearance of the ECG and eventual asystole.

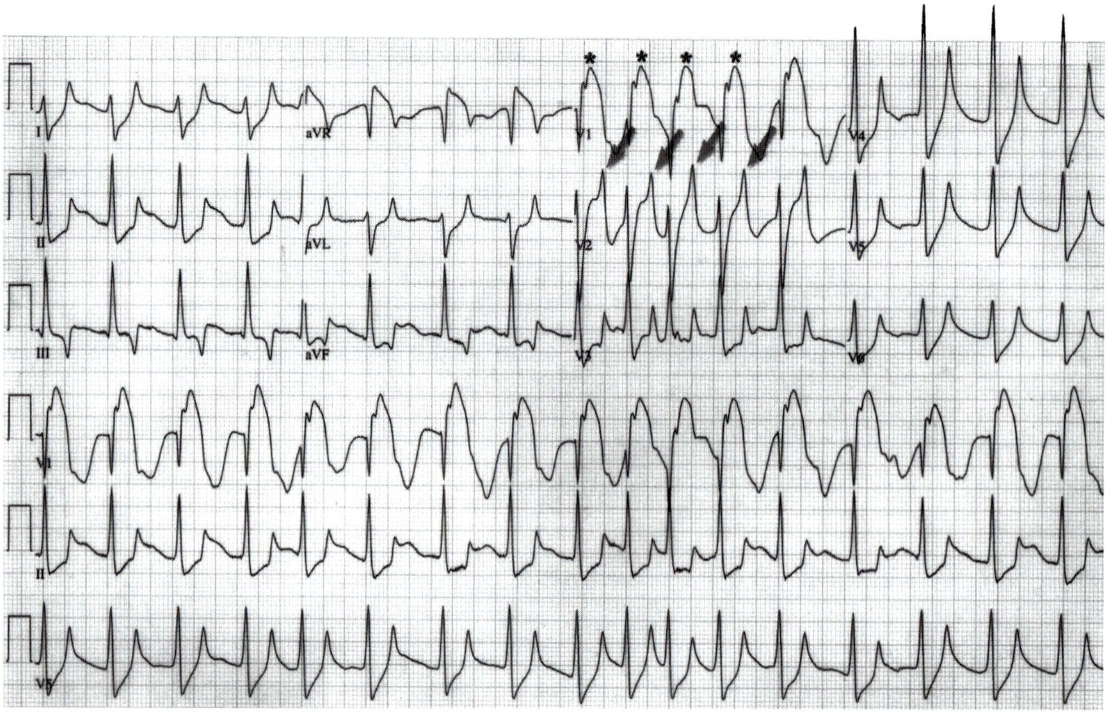

Figure 1. ECG obtained on presentation to the emergency department demonstrating a wide complex tachycardia, absent P waves, peaked T waves (arrows), and ST-segment elevation (asterisks) in leads V_1, V_2, and aVR. Serum potassium measured 9.4 mmol/L.

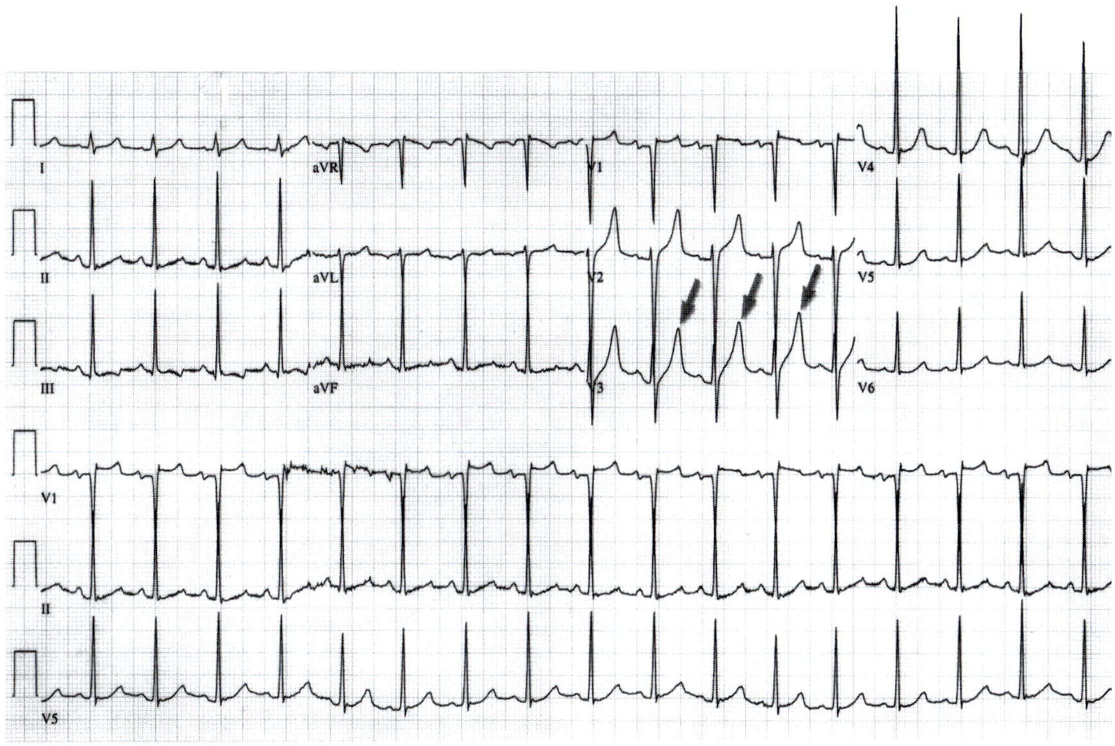

Figure 2. ECG 1 hour after initiation of treatment. Minimally peaked T waves (arrows) and sinus tachycardia remain. Serum potassium measured 5.7 mmol/L.

119 Left Ventricular Pseudoaneurysm: Echocardiographic and Intraoperative Images

Demetrio Tallarico, MD; Pier Andrea Chiavari, MD; Pasquale Mollo, MD; Giuseppe Campolongo

From the Institute of the Heart and Large Vessels "Attilio Reale," "La Sapienza" University of Rome, Italy.

(*Circulation*. 2005;111:e35–e36.)

DOI: 10.1161/01.CIR.0000153815.87329.ID

A 44-year-old hypertensive woman with fever for 1 week and a history of apical myocardial infarction (1 month before) was transferred to our institution with chest pain and dyspnea. On physical examination, her heart rate was 115 bpm, her arterial blood pressure was 85/50 mm Hg, and peripheral cyanosis was present. The electrocardiogram (ECG) showed sinus tachycardia and Q waves in the V_1 to V_2 leads. The serum concentrations of creatine phosphokinase-MB, troponin I, and myoglobin were within normal limits. A chest x-ray revealed an enlarged heart and a mild left pleural effusion. Two-dimensional (2-D) transthoracic echocardiography (TTE) showed a large apical ventricular discontinuity (widest diameter 2.82 cm; Fig. 1A in communication with an echo-free space, suggestive of a huge pseudoaneurysm with a partially stratified thrombus (Fig. 1B). A minimal pericardial effusion was present. The maximum internal end-systolic pseudoaneurysmal diameters were 11.27 × 10.45 cm (Fig. 2A) with a ratio of orifice to cavity diameter of 0.25. Color Doppler showed flow passage from the left ventricle into the pseudoaneurysm (Fig. 2B) and pulsed Doppler demonstrated systodiastolic flow through the false aneurysmal mouth (Fig. 3A). Coronary angiography revealed a midportion occlusion of the left anterior descending artery; ventricular angiography was not performed because of the high risk of pseudoaneurysmal rupture. Surgery confirmed the diagnosis (Fig. 3B), and the myocardial hole was repaired via endoventricular circular patch plasty. The postoperative course was uneventful.

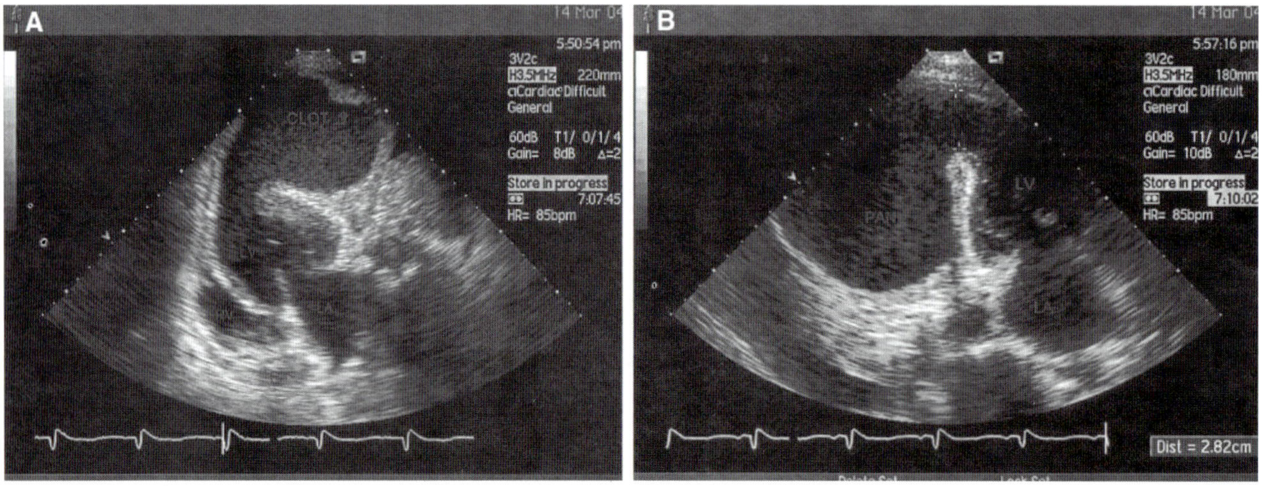

Figure 1. 2-D TTE, apical four-chamber modified view. **A,** Site of rupture with thin wall of large pseudoaneurysmal cavity (PAN) arising from left ventricular apex (A) and a protruding thrombotic mass **(B)**. LA indicates left atrium; LV, left ventricle; and RV, right ventricle.

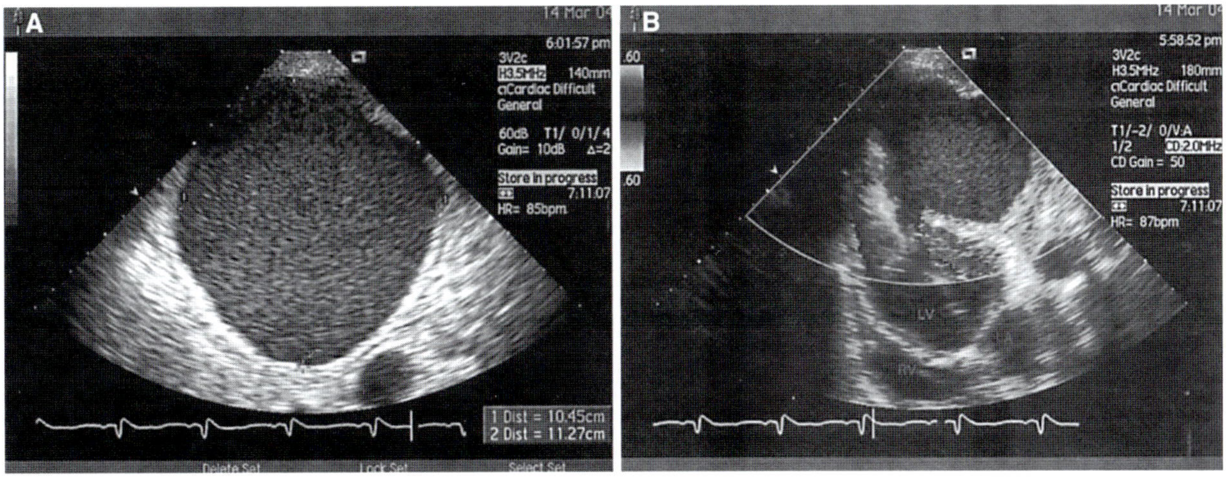

Figure 2. 2-D TTE images. **A,** Evident spontaneous echo-contrast inside pseudoaneurysm and maximum sac diameters. **B,** Color Doppler reveals communication between left ventricle and false aneurysm. Abbreviations as in Figure 1 legend.

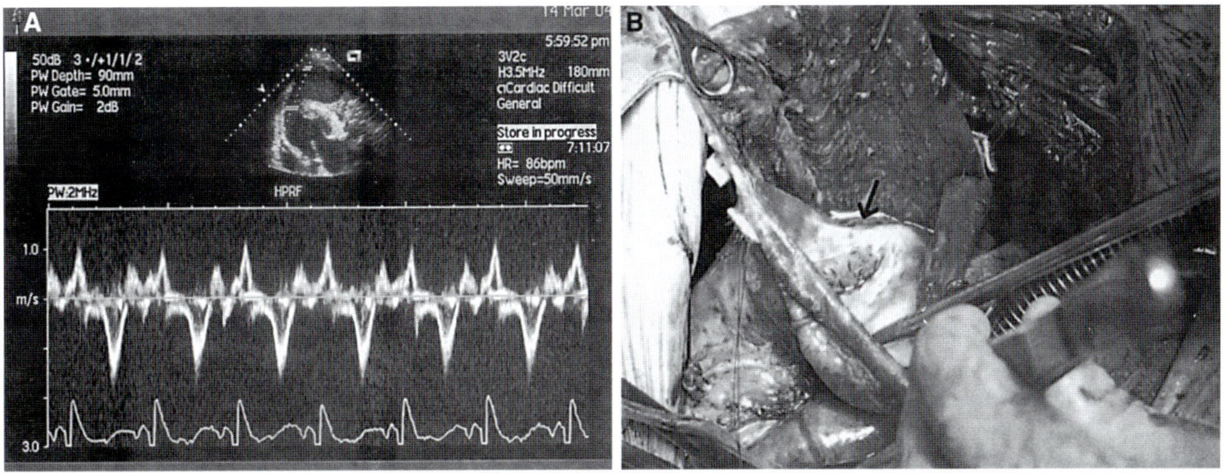

Figure 3. **A,** Pulsed Doppler across pseudoaneurysmal mouth shows bidirectional flow. **B,** Intraoperative finding; surgical probes indicate open cavity and pseudoaneurysmal neck (arrow).

120 Spontaneous Left Atrial Dissection Presenting as Pulmonary Edema

Jung-Hyun Choi, MD; Jun-Kyu Kang, MD; Kyung-Joo Park, MD; Jo-Won Jung, MD; So-Yeon Choi, MD; Myeong-Ho Yoon, MD; Gyo-Seung Hwang, MD; Seung-Jea Tahk, MD; Joon-Han Shin, MD

From the Departments of Cardiology (J.-H.C., J.-W.J., S.-Y.C., M.-H.Y., G.-S.H., S.-J.T., J.-H.S.), Cardiac Surgery (J.-K.K.), and Radiology (K.-J.P.), Ajou University Hospital, Suwon, Republic of Korea.

(*Circulation.* 2005;111:e372–e373.)

DOI: 10.1161/CIRCULATIONAHA.104.477463

A healthy 30-year-old man who had not had any prior medical or surgical history presented to the emergency department with substernal pain for 2 days that was sharp and exacerbated by inspiration and recumbency. Chest radiograph (Fig. 1A) showed mild left atrial enlargement. The electrocardiogram (ECG) showed normal findings. The next day, the patient complained of sudden onset of class 3 dyspnea and frothy blood-tinged sputum. Follow-up chest radiography showed increased interstitial pulmonary vascular markings with consolidation in the right lower lung field, suggestive of pulmonary edema (Fig. 1B). Transthoracic echocardiogram showed minimal pericardial effusion and a cyst-like, thin-walled, space-occupying lesion in the left atrium, which was not connected with the true lumen of the left atrium by color Doppler interrogation and contrast agent injection (Fig. 2). Contrast cardiac computed tomography revealed a large homogenous mass in the posterior wall of the left atrium with a severely compressed left atrial chamber, which extended along the pulmonary veins, with tight luminal narrowing of the low pulmonary veins (Fig. 3). The patient underwent emergency surgery, and the condition was diagnosed as spontaneous left atrial dissection with minimal hemopericardium.

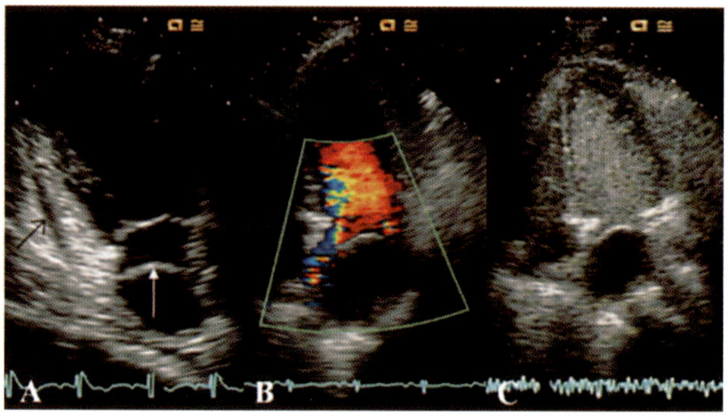

Figure 2. Transthoracic echocardiography showed abnormal membrane in left atrium (**A,** white arrowheads) with minimal pericardial effusion (black arrow). Background echo contrast of both sides in left atrium were nearly same. Color Doppler **(B)** and contrast echocardiography **(C)** revealed no communication of blood flow across membrane.

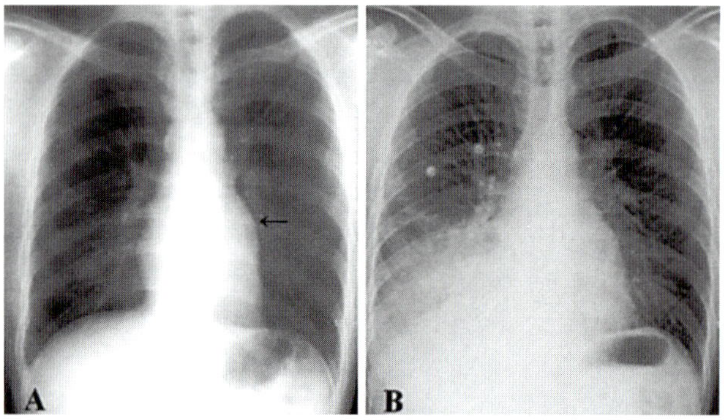

Figure 1. A, Initial chest radiograph showed bulging contour of left mid heart border (arrow), suggestive of left atrial enlargement with normal pattern of pulmonary vascularity. **B,** Chest radiograph taken 1 day later shows diffusely increased interstitial densities with septal lines and air-space consolidation predominantly in right lower lung zone.

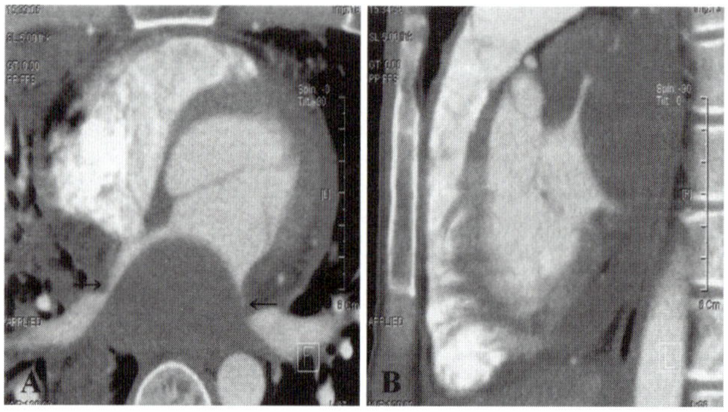

Figure 3. Axial **(A)** and sagittal reformatted **(B)** CT images show large mass in posterior part of left atrial wall with smooth surface and homogenous density without enhancement by contrast media. Note tight narrowing of both inferior pulmonary veins (arrows) and compressed left atrial chamber.

121 Reversible Right Ventricular Hypertrophy due to Cardiac Sarcoidosis

Hideo Okamura, MD; Yoichi Goto, MD, PhD; Masahiro Terashima, MD, PhD; Shuichi Takagi, MD, PhD; H. Ishibashi-Ueda, MD, PhD; Hiroshi Nonogi, MD, PhD

From the Division of Cardiology, National Cardiovascular Center, Osaka, Japan.

(*Circulation*. 2005;111:e383–e384.)

DOI: 101161/CIRCULATIONAHA.104.489294

A 42-year-old man was admitted to our hospital with shortness of breath on light effort. An electrocardiogram (ECG) revealed advanced arteriovenous (AV) block (Fig. 1A), and a chest computed tomography (CT) scan showed markedly increased thickness (12 mm) of the right ventricular wall (Fig. 2A). The endomyocardial biopsy showed a noncaseous epithelioid cell granuloma with giant cells, which supported the diagnosis of cardiac sarcoidosis (Fig. 3). There was no evidence of systemic inflammation, such as fever, elevated C-reactive protein, leukocytosis, or eosinophilia. Treatment with oral prednisolone

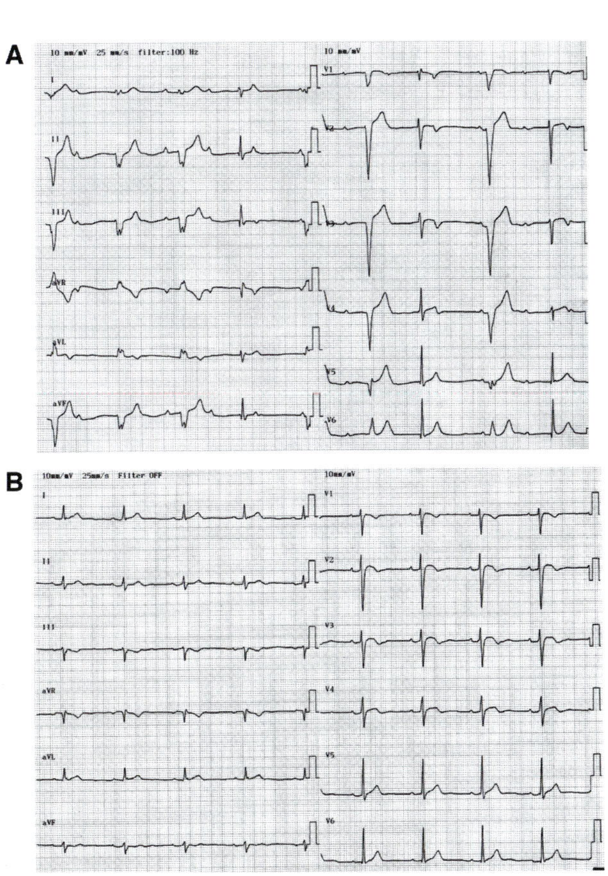

Figure 1. A, (Feb. 15, 2002) ECG on admission showed advanced AV block with ventricular escape complexes. **B,** (Apr. 22, 2002) After treatment with oral prednisolone for 1 month, AV conduction dramatically improved to normal PQ interval.

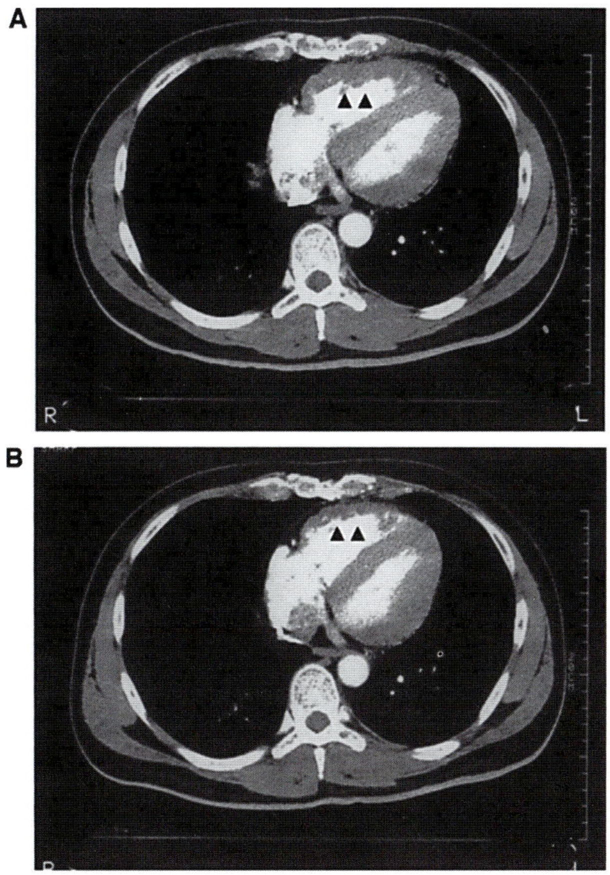

Figure 2. A, (Feb. 8, 2002) Chest CT scan showed markedly increased thickness (12 mm) of right ventricular wall (arrowheads). **B,** (Apr. 12, 2002) Hypertrophy of right ventricle disappeared (wall thickness 6 mm) within 2 months after steroid therapy (arrowheads).

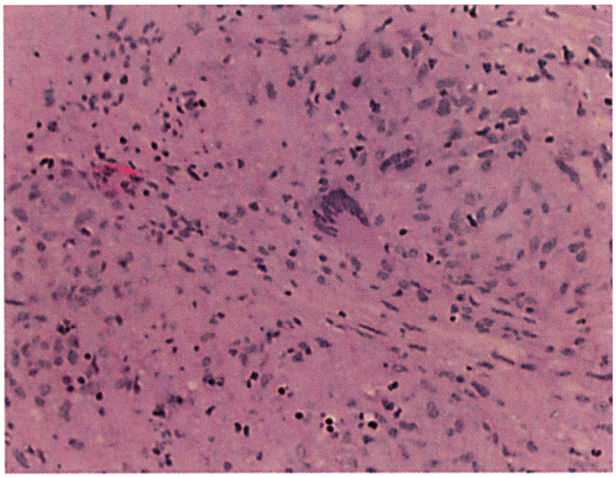

Figure 3. Photomicrograph of endomyocardial biopsy: Noncaseous epithelioid granuloma with giant cells is seen. (Hematoxylin and eosin stain [HE], ×200.)

(40 mg daily) was started, and the hypertrophy of the right ventricular wall disappeared (wall thickness 6 mm) and AV conduction normalized within 2 months (Figs. 1B and 2B). This reversible right ventricular hypertrophy was also confirmed by serial echocardiography. Because of the reversible nature, the right ventricular hypertrophy was considered to reflect myocardial cell infiltration or edema. No recurrence has been detected in the subsequent 2 years with a reduced dose of prednisolone (10 mg/d).

122 Three-Dimensional Imaging in Rupture of Papillary Muscle after Acute Myocardial Infarction

Vito Marangelli, MD, PhD; Luisa Cacciavillani, MD; Sara Pontarollo, MD; Francesca di Marco, MD; Gino Gerosa, MD; Sabino Iliceto, MD

From the Cardiology Division, Department of Cardiologic, Thoracic, and Vascular Sciences (L.C., S.P., S.I.) and Cardiac Surgery Unit (F.d.M., G.G.) of the University of Padova, Padova, Italy, and Azienda Ospedaliera Policlinico (V.M.), Bari, Italy.

(*Circulation*. 2005;e385–e387.)

DOI: 10.1161/CIRCULATIONAHA.104.489807

A 62-year-old male was referred to our hospital for cardiogenic shock. Two weeks before, he complained of transient epigastric pain; 1 hour before admission, he underwent advanced life-support maneuvers because of the onset of severe dyspnea and a syncopal attack with two episodes of asystole that occurred during transportation to our coronary care unit. A 12-lead electrocardiogram (ECG) tracing and cardiac enzyme levels were consistent with a diagnosis of myocardial infarction.

At admission, he underwent a routine two-dimensional (2-D) echocardiographic examination (Fig. 1A), which showed akinetic inferior and inferolateral left ventricular walls, complete rupture of the inferomedial papillary muscle of the left ventricle, and mitral regurgitation of a severe degree. Although a severe prolapse of the mitral leaflets was found, no images of the systolic eversion of the papillary muscle in the left atrium were recorded because of the presence of residual chordae binding the ruptured muscle to the ventricular free wall (Fig. 1B). A three-dimensional (3-D) echocardiographic examination was performed with a Sonos 7500 (Phillips) with the 3-D live mode (Figs. 2A and 2B). Thus, the exact

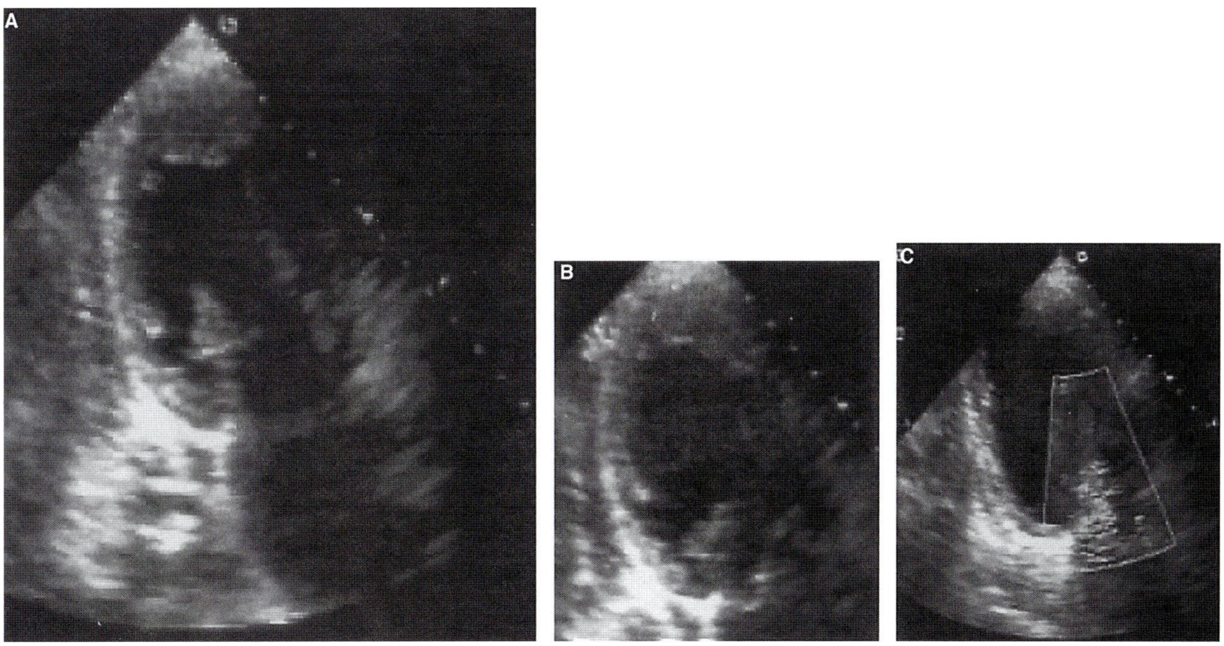

Figure 1. Ruptured papillary muscle and its base as seen in 2-D **(A** and **B)** color Doppler echocardiographic images **(C)** obtained at admission.

shape and movement of the ruptured papillary muscle and its ruptured base were imaged. The volume data-set analysis showed binding of the papillary muscle to the left ventricular wall as the cause of the absence of its systolic eversion in the left atrium. Eventually, the patient underwent successful prosthetic mitral valve implantation and single coronary artery bypass graft (CABG) implantation with complete restoration of neurological integrity and no extension of the left ventricular asynergic area. The ruptured papillary muscle and excised mitral valve are shown in Figure 3.

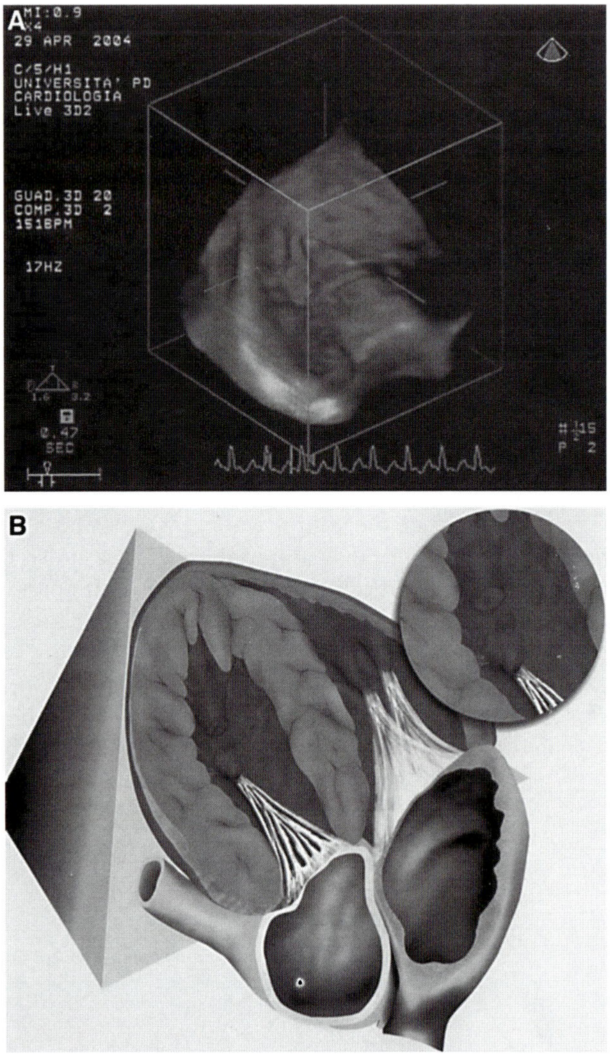

Figure 2. Ruptured papillary muscle and its base as seen in 3-D live mode **(A)** and artist graph representing imaged anatomic structures **(B)**.

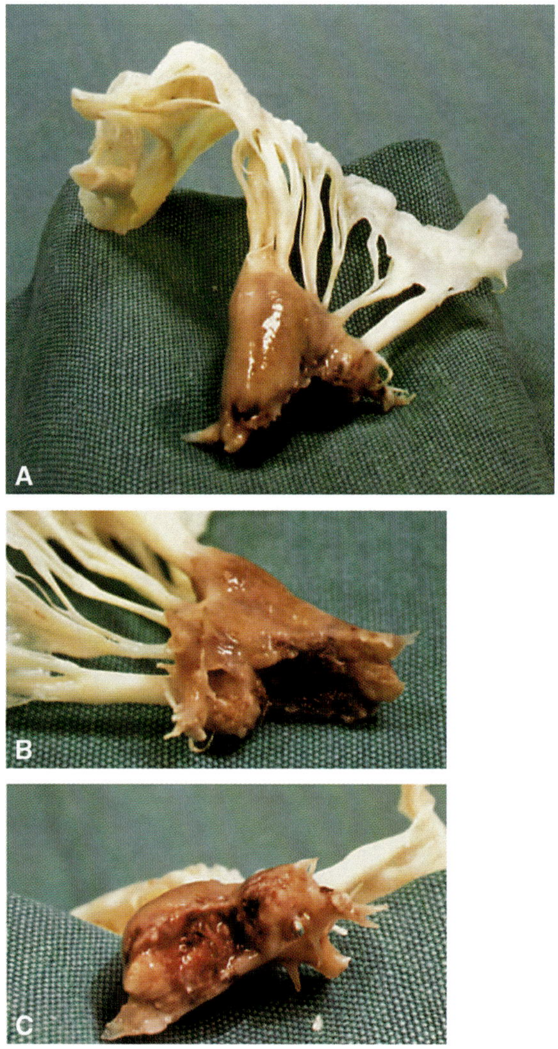

Figure 3. Ruptured papillary muscle as seen after heart surgery in multiple views (**A** through **C**). **C,** Details of its ruptured surface.

123 Angiosarcoma of the Pericardium: A Fatal Disease

Stijn L. Brinckman, MD; Poll van der Wouw, MD

From the Department of Cardiology, Onze Lieve Vrouwe Gasthuis, Amsterdam, the Netherlands.

(*Circulation*. 2005;111:e388–e389.)

DOI: 10.1161/CIRCULATIONAHA.104.492371

A 31-year-old male presented with increasing exertional breathlessness. He had been healthy previously, with no recent chest pain or fever. The only notable abnormalities on blood testing were a microcytic anemia and an elevated lactate dehydrogenase level. The chest radiograph showed an increased cardiothoracic ratio and mild pulmonary congestion. Transthoracic echocardiography showed reasonable left ventricular systolic function and chamber sizes within normal limits. Doppler study disclosed marked respiratory variations in transmitral flow without significant regurgitation. In the pericardium, a homogenous mass was seen surrounding the heart, but mainly posterolaterally, and there was minimal pericardial effusion (Fig. 1). His clinical situation deteriorated quickly, and he was sent for emergency thoracotomy. A large mass, which surrounded the entire heart but did not invade the myocardium, was discovered and partially removed (Fig. 2). One week after an initial clinical improvement, the patient developed signs of tamponade again. Cardiac magnetic resonance imaging (MRI) showed a mass surrounding both ventricles, atria, the ascending aorta, and the pulmonary trunk (Fig. 3). Unfortunately, the patient died a few days later owing to respiratory insufficiency. The final histological diagnosis was high-grade sarcoma that corresponded to an angiosarcoma.

Angiosarcomas are the most common primary cardiac malignant tumor. In autopsy series, the cumulative prevalence of cardiac angiosarcoma is 0.03–0.0002%. They tend to be found in patients aged 20 to 50 years. Angiosarcomas respond poorly to chemotherapy. Most patients do not survive beyond 6 months of diagnosis.

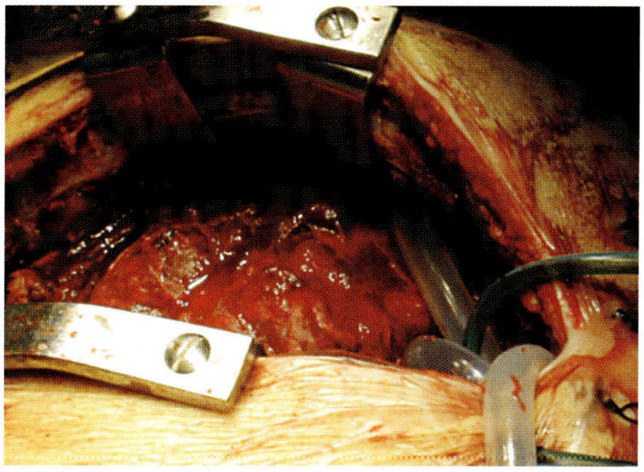

Figure 2. Intraoperative demonstration of heart showing inhomogeneous mass covering it.

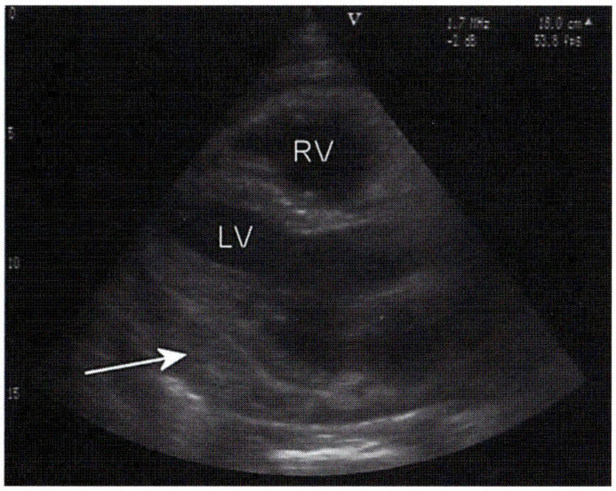

Figure 1. Parasternal long-axis transthoracic echocardiogram showing right (RV) and left (LV) ventricle and tumor (arrow).

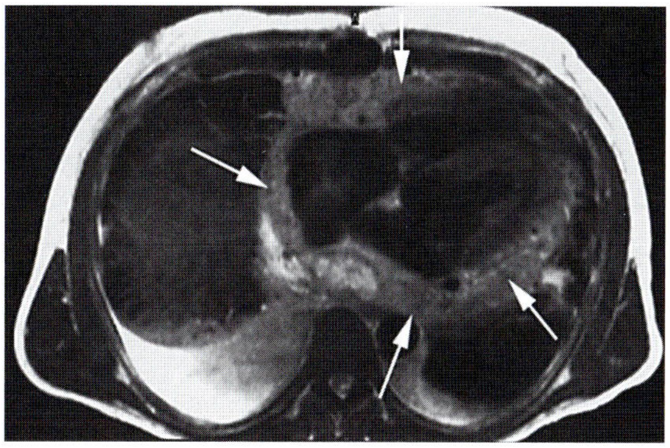

Figure 3. Magnetic resonance image showing tumor mass around heart (arrows).

124 Ventricular Septum Rupture after Myocardial Infarction Demonstrated by Multislice Computed Tomography

Halil Doğan, MD; Jeroen J. Bax, MD; Albert de Roos, MD; Lucia J.M. Kroft, MD

From the Departments of Radiology (H.D., A.R., L.J.M.K.) and Cardiology (J.J.B.), Leiden University Medical Center, Leiden, the Netherlands.

(*Circulation*. 2005; 111: e449–e450.)

DOI: 10.1161/CIRCULATIONAHA.104.478537

A 71-year-old man was referred to the emergency department of our hospital for chest pain associated with intense interscapular pain. At presentation, a significant difference in systolic/diastolic blood pressure between the left and right arm was measured, and shortly thereafter, the patient developed severe hypotension. Accordingly, multislice computed tomography (MSCT) of the chest was performed because dissection of the thoracic aorta was suspected. There was no dissection, but severe backflow of contrast agent in the inferior vena cava and hepatic veins was observed (suggesting right ventricular dysfunction), together with an enlarged heart and extensive coronary artery calcifications. A defect in the inferior part of the interventricular septum was observed at the midventricular level (Fig. 1). The electrocardiogram (ECG) revealed a ventricular rhythm (60 bpm), with QRS duration of 140 ms and right bundle-branch block configuration; however, ST-T-segment elevation was present in the inferior leads (II, III, AvF), suggesting acute inferior wall infarction. Severe hemodynamic and respiratory instability followed, and the patient was hospitalized in the intensive care unit. Transthoracic echocardiography with color Doppler imaging confirmed acute ventricular septal rupture (Fig. 2), with extensive akinesia of the inferior, posterior, and lateral walls, indicating acute inferior wall infarction. Secondary to the ventricular septal rupture, severe right ventricular dilatation had occurred. Shock persisted despite treatment with high doses of intravenous inotropics and noradrenaline.

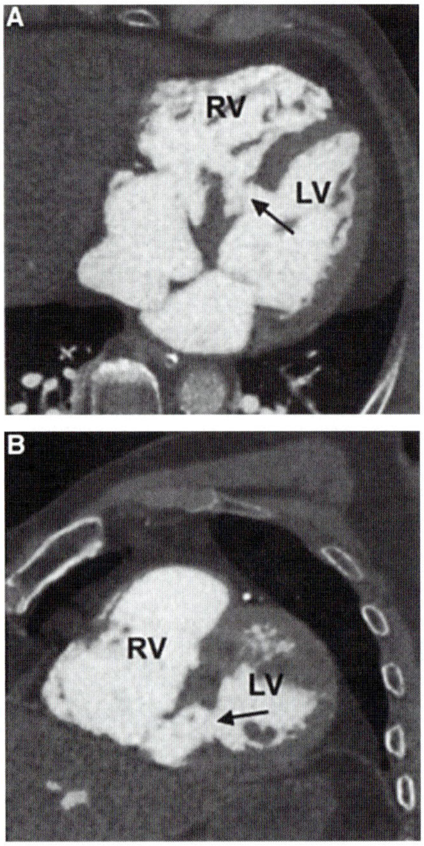

Figure 1. MSCT Images reconstructed in four-chamber view **(A)** and short-axis view **(B)** showing the ventricular septal rupture (arrow) and dilatated right ventricle. RV indicates right ventricle; LV, left ventricle.

The patient died before an intra-aortic balloon pump could be inserted. Autopsy confirmed the MSCT and echocardiographic findings of an acute inferior wall infarction with ventricular septal rupture and right ventricular dilatation. The right coronary artery reveled plaque rupture and occlusion.

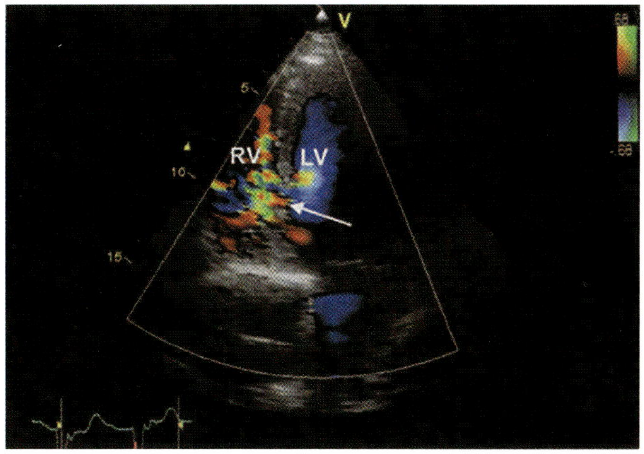

Figure 2. Ventricular septal rupture on two-dimensional (2-D) echocardiography (four-chamber view) with color Doppler flow. Abbreviations as in Figure 1.

Section VI

Congenital Heart Disease

125 Arteriovenous Fistula

Richard W. Lowry, MD; Mark J. Hausknecht, MD
From Baylor College of Medicine, The Methodist Hospital, Houston, Tex.
(*Circulation*. 1994;90:1077.)

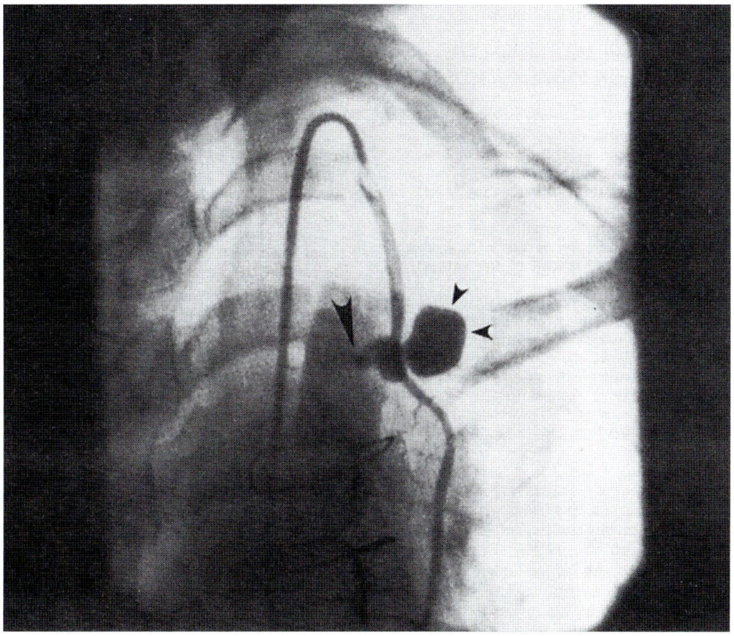

Figure 1. This patient presented with exertional angina and diffuse precordial T-wave inversions on electrocardiogram (ECG) 4 weeks after internal mammary artery to left anterior descending coronary artery bypass. Coronary angiography revealed a pseudoaneurysm (small arrows) of the proximal internal mammary artery with fistulous communication to the brachiocephalic vein (large arrow) and a significant left-to-right shunt. This unusual complication may have resulted from attempts to place a left subclavian central line postoperatively.

126 Vascular Ring

Zia Q. Farooki, MD

From the Children's Hospital of Michigan–Wayne State University, Detroit, Mich.

(*Circulation*. 1995;91:549–551.)

The accompanying figures illustrate a case of a vascular ring formed by the right aortic arch, aberrant left subclavian artery, and left ductus ligamentum.

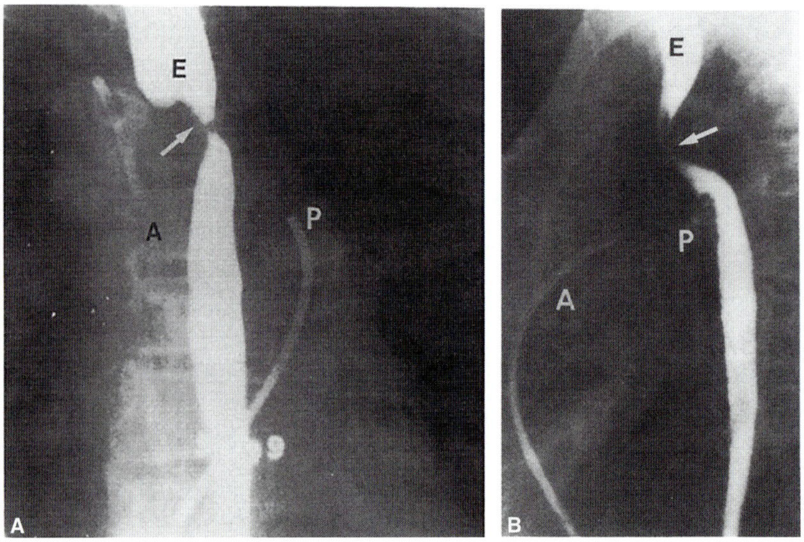

Figure 1. **A,** Frontal projection: A large right-sided filling defect is seen on the barium esophagogram (E) performed during cardiac catheterization (arrow). The positions of the transvenous catheter tip in the main pulmonary artery (P) and of the retrograde catheter in the ascending aorta (A) are shown. **B,** Lateral projection: A large posterior filling defect is seen on the barium esophagogram (arrow).

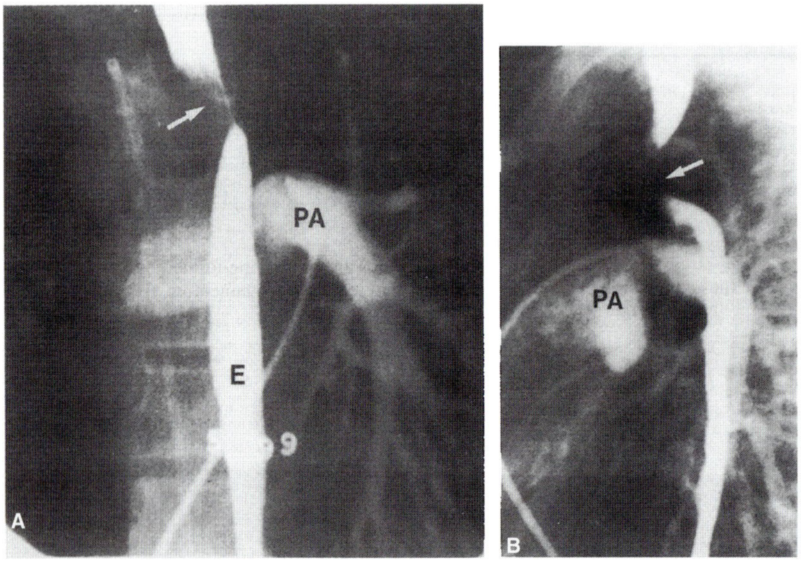

Figure 2. Pulmonary angiogram demonstrates the relation of the pulmonary artery (PA) to the filling defects in the frontal **(A)** and lateral **(B)** projections.

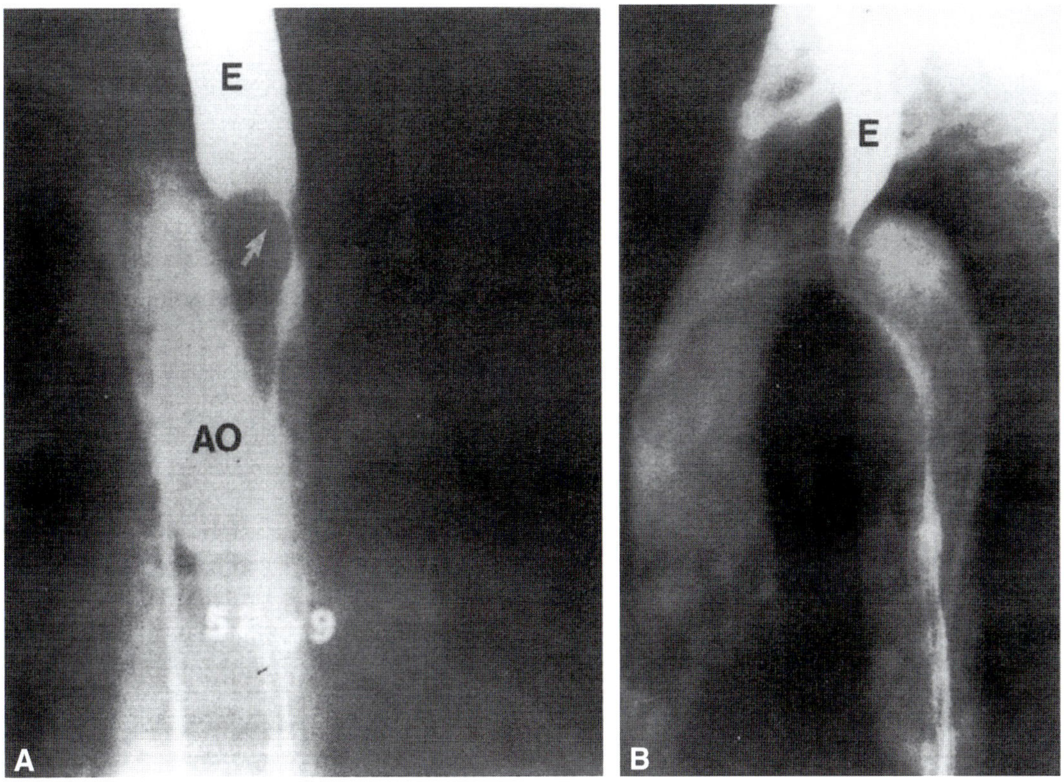

Figure 3. **A,** Frontal ascending aortogram demonstrates the right aortic arch, which is not related to the filling defect. **B,** Lateral view of the arch and descending aorta clearly demonstrates the spatial relation between the aorta and the filling defect. AO indicates aorta; E, barium esophagogram.

127 Mirror-Image Dextrocardia with Situs Inversus

Ayman S. Al-Khadra, MD

From the Department of Medicine, New England Deaconess Hospital, Harvard Medical School, Boston, Mass.

(*Circulation.* 1995;91:1602–1603.)

A 57-year-old white male was found to have an abnormal electrocardiogram (ECG) (Fig. 1) on admission for evaluation of rectal bleeding and anemia. The patient had no history of cardiac or sinopulmonary disease. Figure 1 shows the ECG with right-axis deviation of the P wave (negative in aVL and lead I and positive in aVR) and of the QRS complex indicating left to right activation, and low voltage in the left precordial leads. The chest x-ray (Fig. 2) shows dextrocardia and right-sided gastric air bubble. A barium enema was performed to evaluate his rectal bleeding; that showed a right-sided sigmoid colon (Fig. 3). Abdominal computed tomography (Fig. 4) was done to look for metastasis from a possible cancer, and that demonstrates the left-sided liver and right-sided stomach, spleen, and descending aorta.

Mirror-image dextrocardia is the most common form of cardiac malposition encountered and is almost always associated with situs inversus of the abdominal organs. The anatomic right ventricle is anterior to the left ventricle and the aortic arch curves to the right and posteriorly. The anatomic right lung with its three lobes is on the left side. Generally, there is no increased risk of an infracardiac malformation. Twenty-five percent of these patients will have associated sinusitis and bronchiactasis (Kartagener syndrome). The risk in these patients lies in the atypical presentation of diseases such as angina pectoris, myocardial infarction, acute cholecystitis, acute appendicitis, and diverticulitis where pain is referred to the "wrong" side. Recognizing the presence of dextrocardia will also help avoid unnecessary workup for abnormal ECG.

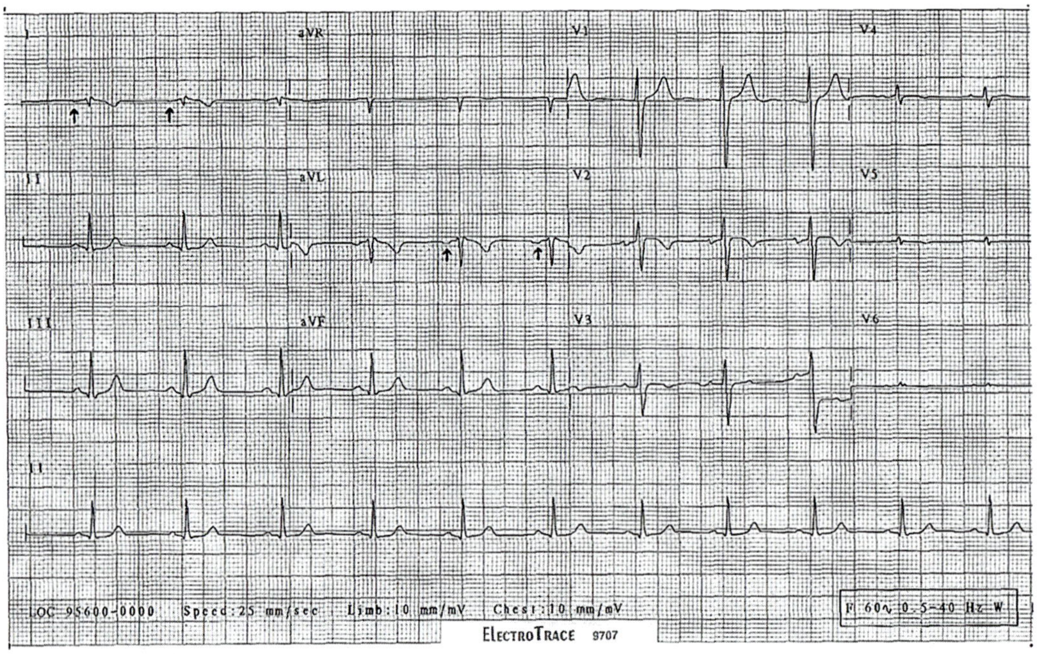

Figure 1. ECG showing marked right-axis deviation of the P wave (negative in aVL and lead I) and of the QRS complex, and low voltage in the precordial leads, V_4 through V_6. Lead aVR is similar to the normal aVL in the normal ECG.

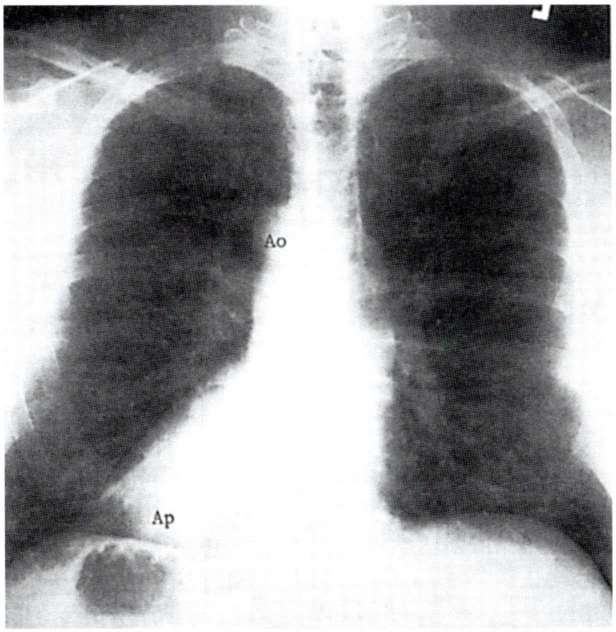

Figure 2. Chest x-ray showing dextrocardia and right-sided gastric air bubble indicating the presence of both dextrocardia and situs inversus (the most common combination) and showing the reason behind missing this diagnosis on the "routine" chest film.

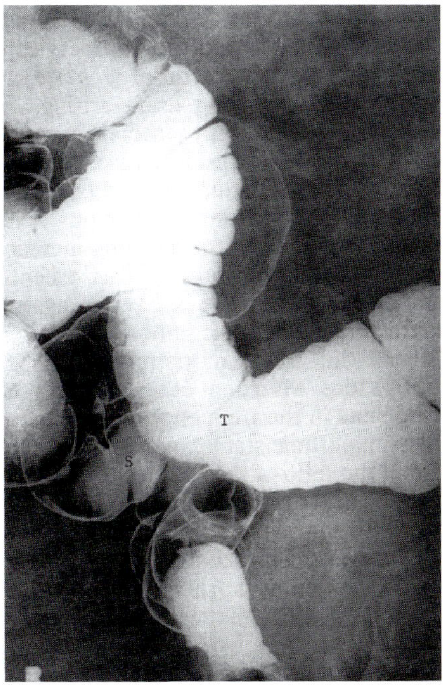

Figure 3. Barium enema showing right-sided sigmoid colon.

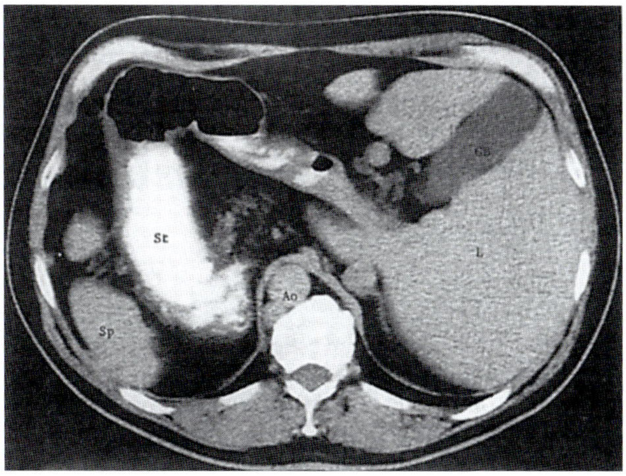

Figure 4. Abdominal computed tomography scan showing left-sided liver, gallbladder, and inferior vena cava and right-sided stomach, spleen, and abdominal aorta.

128

Muscle Bridging of the Left Anterior Descending Coronary Artery

P.R. Vogt, MD; P. Dubach, MD; M.I. Turina, MD

From the Clinic for Cardiovascular Surgery, University Hospital Zurich (P.R.V., M.I.T.), and the Department of Internal Medicine, Cantonal Hospital Chur (P.D.), Switzerland.

(*Circulation*. 1996;93:614.)

In a 62-year-old woman with a history of angina pectoris (New York Heart Association functional class 3) for 15 years, the stress exercise test revealed a significant ST-segment depression in leads V_5 and V_6. Coronary angiography showed the coronary arteries to be normal in diastole (Fig. 1A). In systole, however, a muscle bridge occluding the left anterior descending artery was observed (Fig. 1B). At operation, the muscle bridge over the middle third of the left anterior descending artery was transected (Fig. 1C). Postoperatively, the patient is free of angina pectoris, and the stress exercise test is normal.

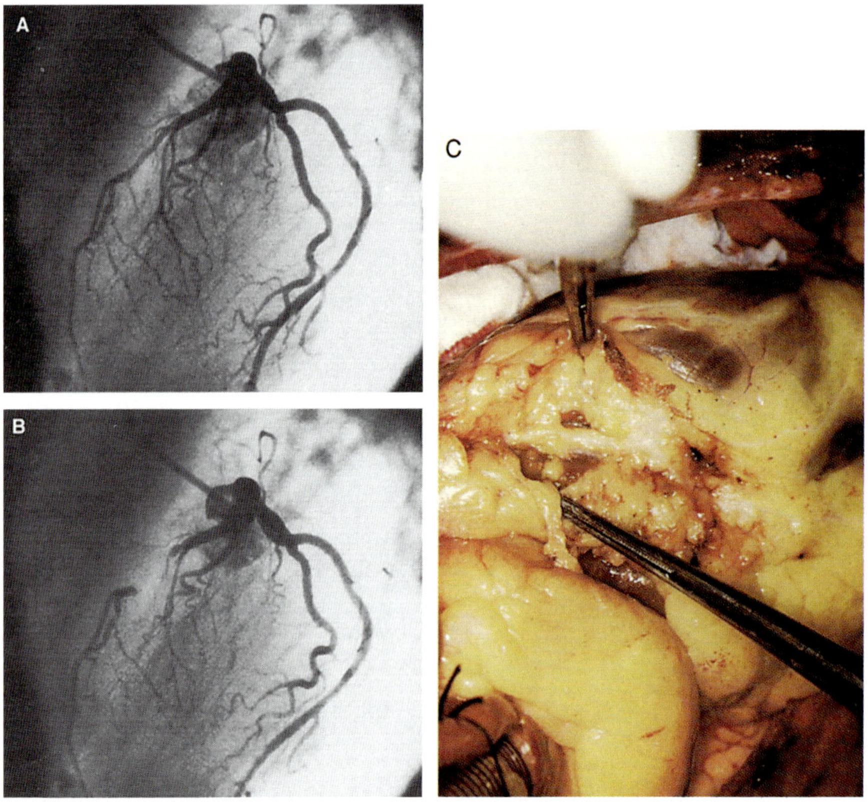

Figure 1.

129 Myocardial Bridges

Manfred Zehender, MD

From Abteilung Innere Medizin III, Klinikum der Albert-Ludwigs Universitat, Freiburg, Germany.

(*Circulation.* 1997;95:2455.)

In a 36-year-old long-distance runner with a history of palpitations and presyncope, an episode of sudden cardiac death occurred during competitive mountain racing. Endless-loop Holter monitoring (Fig. 1A) demonstrated rare episodes of nonsustained ventricular tachycardia, an episode of acceleration, and finally spontaneously terminating ventricular tachycardia followed by marked ST-segment alteration. Coronary angiography (Figs. 1B and 1C) excluded coronary artery disease but demonstrated a tunneled epicardial coronary artery (myocardial bridges) (Fig. 1C, arrows).

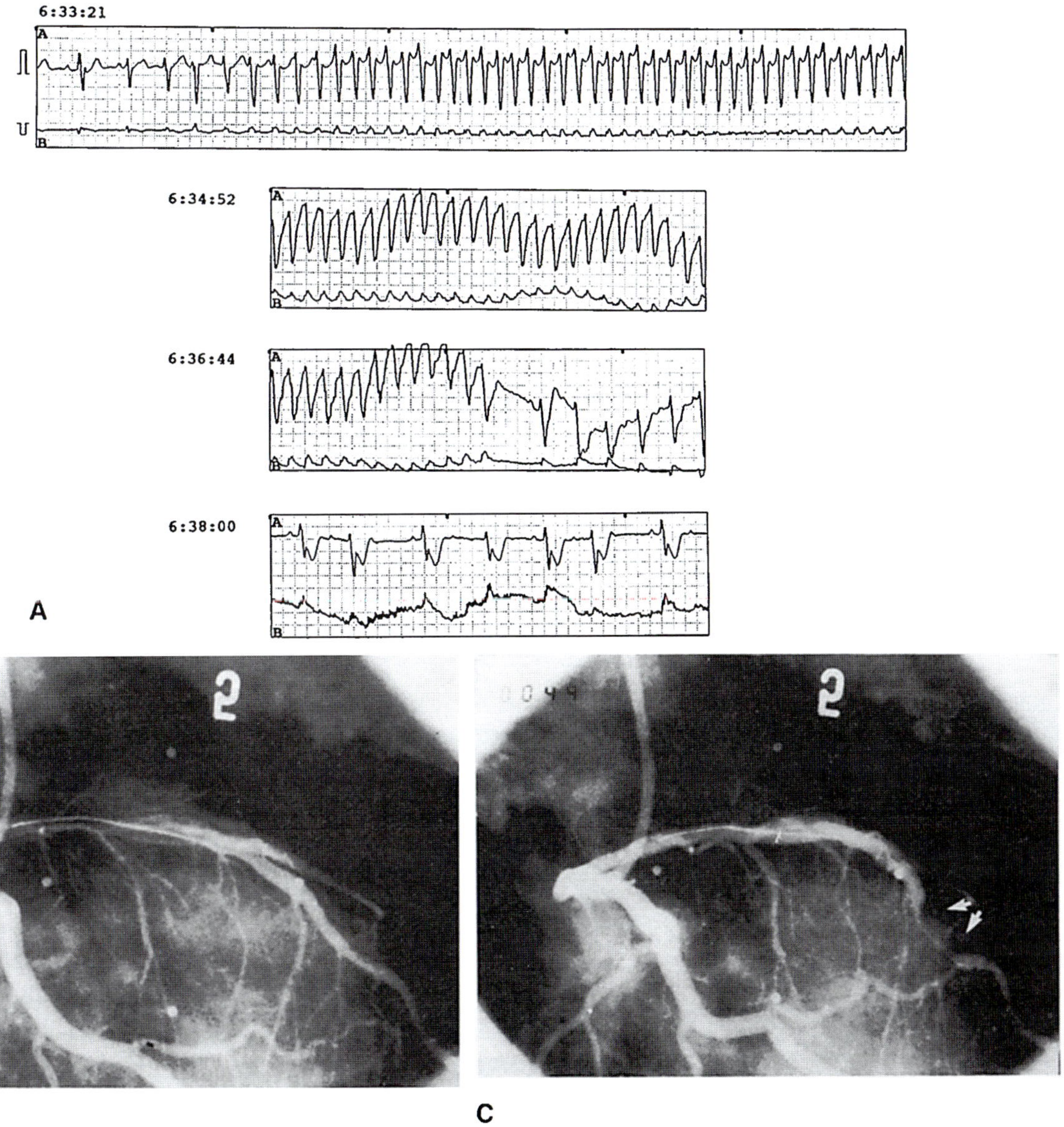

Figure 1.

130 Noninvasive Imaging of Anomalous Origin of the Left Coronary Artery from the Pulmonary Artery

Seiki Hamada, MD; Norihiko Yoshimura, MD; Makoto Takamiya, MD

From the Department of Radiology, National Cardiovascular Center, Osaka, Japan.

(*Circulation*. 1998;97:219.)

A 28-year-old woman presented with chest pain caused by progressive myocardial ischemia. In this case, a right coronary arteriogram confirmed an enlarged right coronary artery, and both the left anterior descending branch and the circumflex artery were supplied by collateral circulation. The left main artery was connected with the pulmonary trunk during the late phase of the right coronary arteriogram. Electron beam computerized tomography (EBCT) during intravenous administration of contrast medium showed an anomalous origin of the left coronary artery from the pulmonary artery, sometimes known as the Bland-White-Garland syndrome. These axial EBCT images (Fig 1) were performed with 3 mm thickness and 100 ms acquisition time. Cardiac motionless images allow clear visualization of both the anomalous origin of the left main coronary trunk and enlarged right coronary artery. We can see that the left main trunk supplied the left anterior descending branch and circumflex artery.

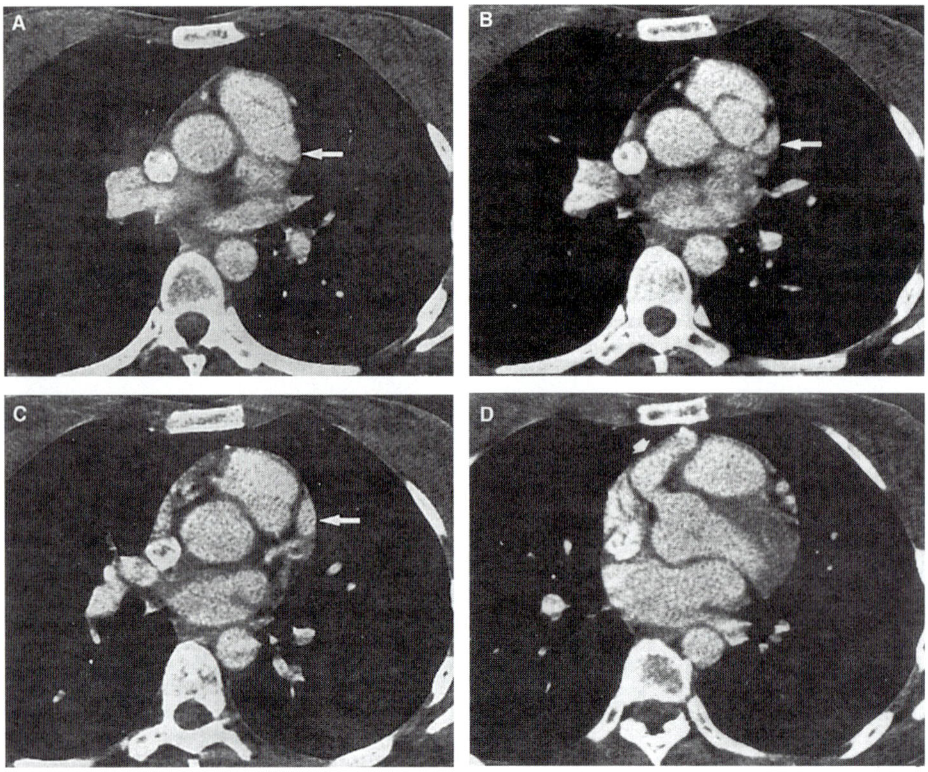

Figure 1. Serial EBCT axial view of anomalous origin of left coronary artery from pulmonary trunk. **A** through **C,** Left coronary artery (arrows) with its origin at pulmonary trunk. **D,** Dilated right coronary artery (arrow) with its origin at aortic root.

131 Noninvasive Diagnosis of Anomalous Origin of the Left Main Coronary Artery from the Pulmonary Artery

Guy Vaksmann, MD; Pierre Mauran, MD; Charles Francart, MD; Christian Rey, MD

From the Department of Pediatric Cardiology, Cardiologic Hospital, Lille, France.

(*Circulation*. 1998;97:1869.)

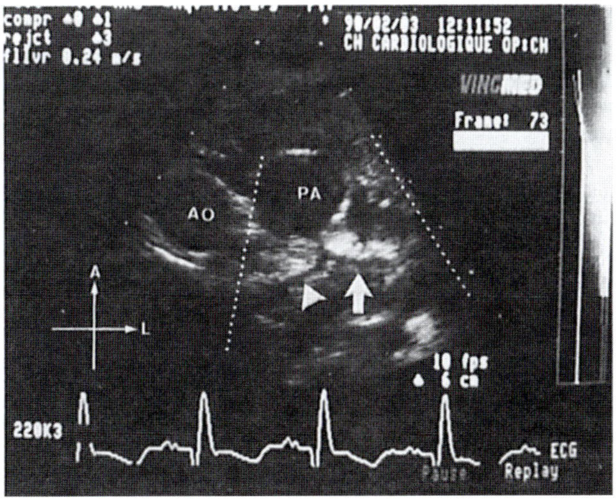

Figure 1. Two-dimensional echocardiography. High parasternal short-axis view demonstrating left coronary artery originating from pulmonary trunk posteriorly. Arrow shows left anterior descending coronary artery; arrowhead, left circumflex artery. A Indicates anterior; AO, aorta; L, left; and PA, pulmonary artery.

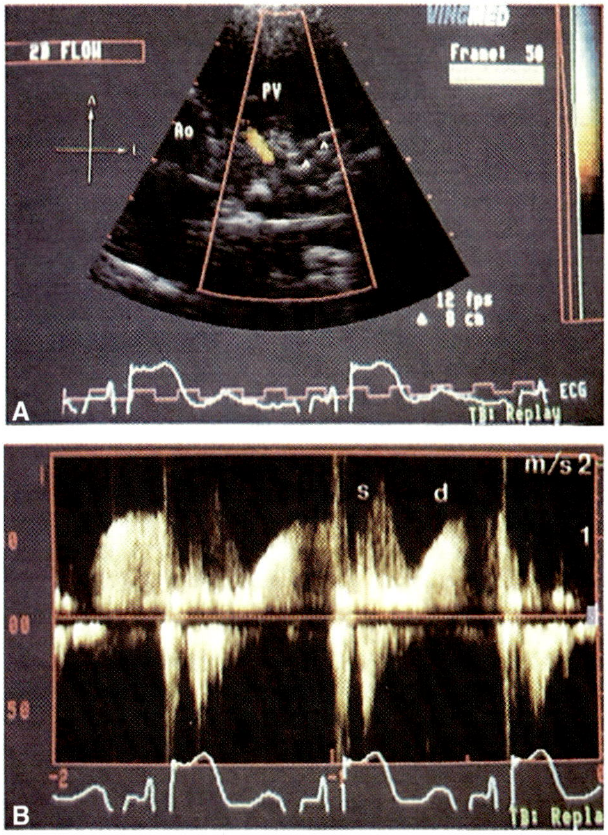

Figure 2. Echocardiographic images in a second patient. **A,** Color Doppler high parasternal short-axis view showing streaming of blood flow from left coronary artery to pulmonary artery. Arrowheads indicate left anterior descending coronary artery. **B,** Pulsed Doppler with interrogation of left coronary artery ostium showing biphasic signal with two velocity peaks in systole (s) and diastole (d).

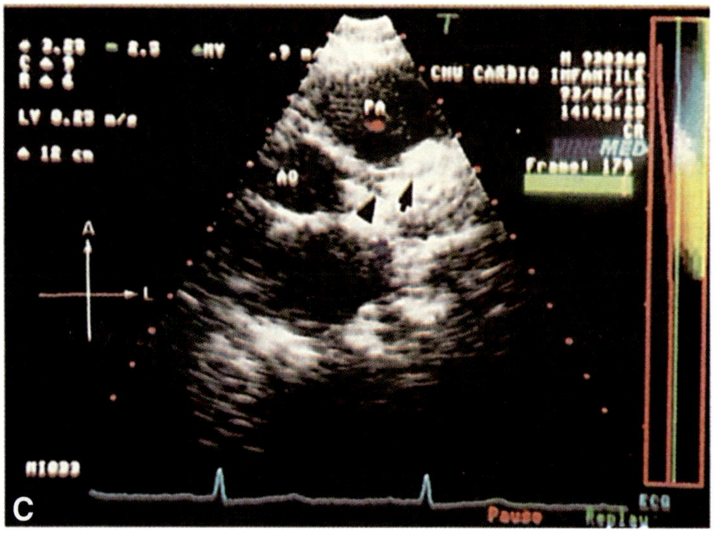

Figure 2. (*continued*) **C,** High parasternal short-axis view after direct reimplantation of left coronary artery on aorta. Arrow shows left anterior descending artery; arrowhead, left circumflex artery. A indicates anterior; Ao, aorta; PA, pulmonary artery; PV, pulmonary valves; and L, left.

132 Giant Coronary Fistula

Nicole Sekarski, MD; Maurice Payot, MD; Jean-Jacques Goy, MD
From the Division of Cardiology, CHUV, Lausanne, Switzerland.

(*Circulation,* 1998;97:1868.)

This African 3-year-old boy had had a systolic and diastolic murmur of 3/6 maximal at the left midsternal border in the neonatal period. He was diagnosed with a patent ductus arteriosus. At time of surgery, no ductus was found. Because the murmur was still present after the operation, the patient was sent to our institution for further investigation. He was asymptomatic, and his blood pressure was 135/90. The chest radiograph was normal. Mild right ventricular hypertrophy was noted on the electrocardiogram (ECG). The echocardiogram showed no ductus, but the ostium of the left coronary artery was dilated (6 mm in diameter) (Fig. 1A), and this artery ended in the apex of the right ventricle. A continuous flow between this artery and the right ventricle was documented. Aortic angiography confirmed the suspected coronary artery-to-right ventricle fistula (Fig. 1B). The fistula was ligated distally. The postoperative course was uncomplicated, and the child was discharged on day 7. Cardiac auscultation was normal, and a postoperative echocardiogram did not show any abnormal flow.

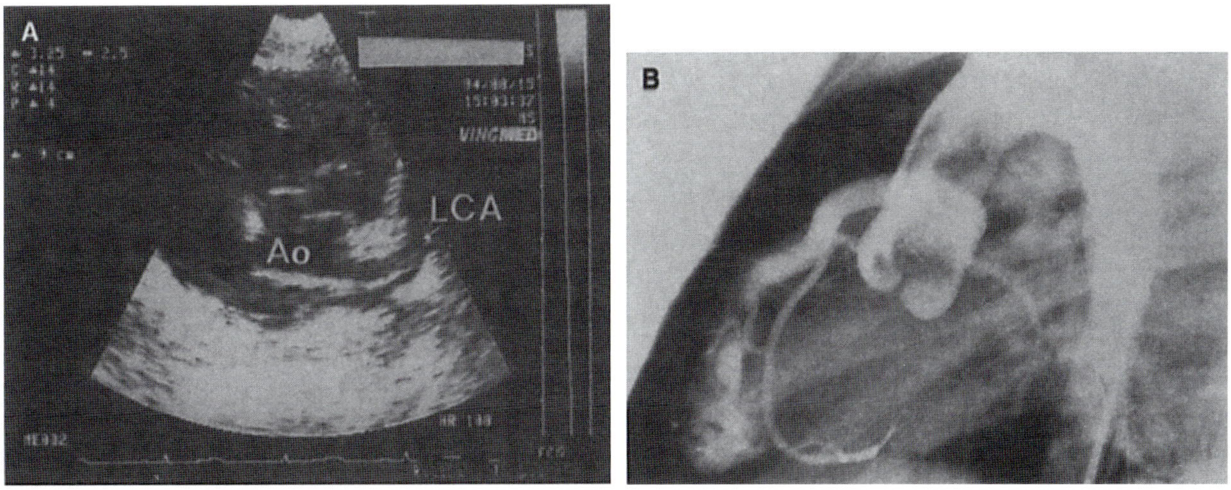

Figure 1. A, Transverse echocardiographic view of aorta (Ao) and ostium of dilated left coronary artery (LCA). **B,** Aortography (lateral view) showing normal right coronary artery and the left anterior descending coronary artery ending in the right ventricle.

133 "The Thrill is Gone": Visualization and Treatment of an Arteriovenous Fistula

James N. Topper, MD, PhD; Joshua A. Beckman, MD; Reza Malek, MD; Michael Meyerovitz, MD; Mark A. Creager, MD

From the Cardiovascular Division, Department of Medicine (J.N.T., J.A.B., M.A.C.), and the Department of Radiology (R.M., M.M.), Brigham and Women's Hospital, Boston, Mass.

(*Circulation*. 1998;98:375.)

An 87-year-old woman underwent placement of a permanent pacemaker for recurrent near-syncope and sick sinus syndrome. Left subclavian vein access was difficult to obtain despite multiple attempts, and the pacemaker was ultimately placed on the right side. After surgery, the patient developed a mediastinal hematoma necessitating transfusion. No other acute interventions were required. Over the next 8 weeks, the patient developed progressive fatigue, weakness, exertional dyspnea, and lower-extremity edema. The pacemaker was functioning normally. Diuretic and angiotensin converting enzyme (ACE) inhibitor therapies were instituted, which improved but did not resolve the patient's symptoms. The patient was referred to our institution for further evaluation.

The blood pressure was 105/80 mm Hg, and the heart rate was 72 bpm and regular. The lungs were clear to auscultation. A prominent thrill was appreciated adjacent to her left clavicle. A loud to-and-fro bruit was audible across her precordium.

The patient underwent angiography, which revealed an arteriovenous fistula. The arteriogram on the left is a visualization of the left subclavian artery and its branches, demonstrating a fistula between the left internal mammary artery (Fig. 1A, large arrow) and the left subclavian/brachiocephalic vein (Fig. 1A, small arrow). The left internal jugular vein is seen to be filling in a retrograde fashion. After coil embolization, the left internal mammary artery is occluded (Fig. 1B, arrow), and no venous structures are seen during arterial injection. The thrill was not palpable after the procedure. The patient was discharged the next day, and all of her symptoms resolved over the next week.

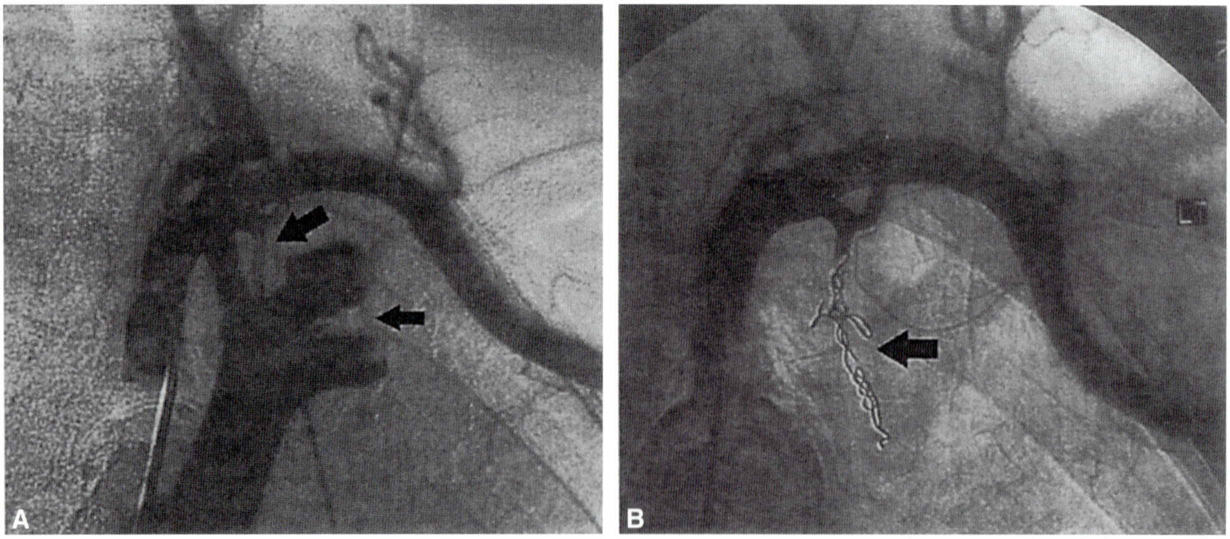

Figure 1. A, Pre embolization. **B,** Post embolization

134 Scimitar Syndrome

Victor A. Ferrari, MD; Muredach P. Reilly, MB; Leon Axel, PhD, MD; Martin G. St. John Sutton, MBBS, FRCP

From the Cardiac Noninvasive Imaging Laboratory and the Adult Congenital Heart Clinic, Cardiovascular Division, Department of Medicine (V.A.F., M.P.R., M.G.S.S.), and the Department of Radiology (L.A.), University of Pennsylvania Medical Center, Philadelphia, Pa.

(*Circulation*. 1998;98:1583–1584.)

A 27-year-old male truck driver presented with recurrent rapid palpitations associated with near-syncope for 6 months. He was noted to have had "isolated" dextrocardia soon after birth. There was no family history of congenital heart disease. Before a herniorrhaphy at age 4 years, a chest radiograph demonstrated anomalous venous drainage of the right lung. He was otherwise asymptomatic, with a normal exercise tolerance.

On examination, he was acyanotic, in sinus rhythm, with a blood pressure of 120/80 mm Hg. His apical impulse was not palpable, and heart sounds were best heard to the right of the sternum. The first heart sound was normal, and the second sound was widely split, with a holosystolic murmur of tricuspid regurgitation.

A chest radiograph showed dextrocardia and a small right lung with a prominent anomalous right pulmonary vein. Two-dimensional echocardiography demonstrated an enlarged right heart but an intact atrial septum by contrast injection. Cardiac-gated magnetic resonance imaging (MRI) showed dextrocardia, a dilated and hypertrophied right ventricle, and a large pulmonary vein that joined the inferior vena cava (IVC) below the level of the diaphragm (Fig. 1). Three-dimensional (3-D) MR angiography with gadolinium contrast enhancement unequivocally demonstrated that the venous drainage of the whole of the diminutive right lung was by an anomalous vein whose entire course to the suprahepatic IVC was visualized. The arterial supply of the right lung was seen to originate from a normal right pulmonary artery (Figs. 2 and 3). A 24-hour electrocardiogram (ECG) monitor revealed recurrent long R-P narrow complex tachycardia, with rates of up to 230 bpm. Cardiac catheterization showed a pulmonary artery systolic pressure of 38 mm Hg and a left-to-right shunt ratio of 1.8:1.

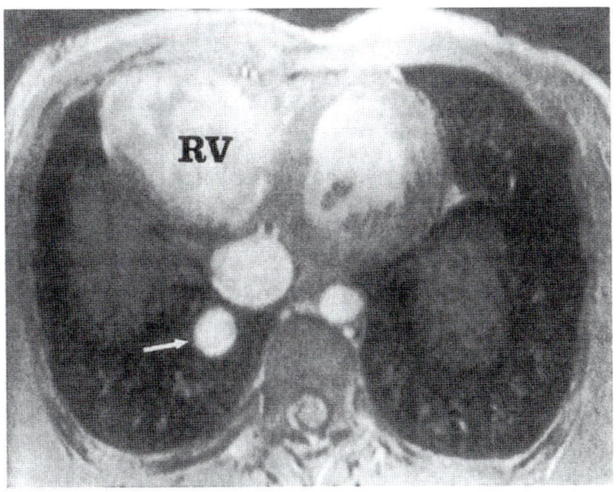

Figure 1. Two-dimensional cardiac-gated MRI at level of top of diaphragm in transverse plane using a fast segmented k-space gradient recalled echo technique demonstrates dextrocardia and a dilated right ventricle (RV). Anomalous draining pulmonary vein (arrow) is seen adjacent to dilated inferior vena cava just superior to diaphragmatic hiatus.

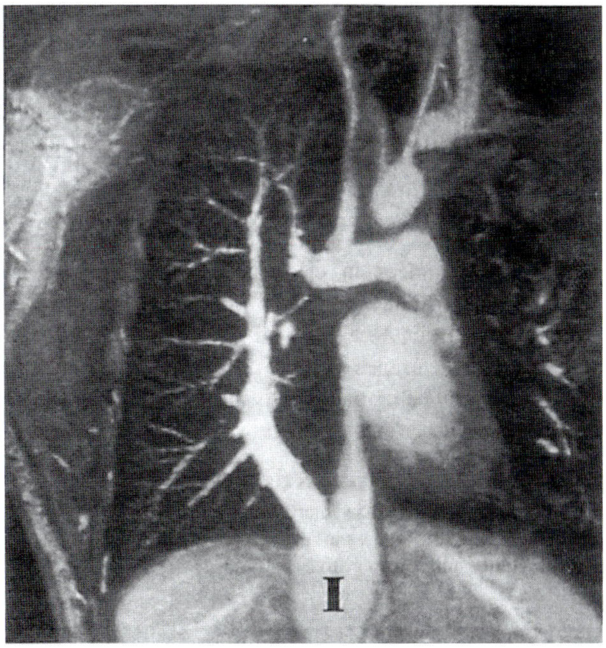

Figure 2. Reformatted oblique section through 3-D data set using gadolinium-DTPA contrast enhancement. In this coronal oblique view, superior and inferior pulmonary venous radicals are seen draining to anomalous (or scimitar) vein and into IVC (I) at diaphragmatic level. Proximal portion of right pulmonary artery is also seen adjacent to upper segment of anomalous vein. This 3-D magnetic resonance (MR) angiogram was acquired during a single breath-hold of 34 seconds.

The patient underwent electrophysiological testing and atrioventricular nodal modification to control his supraventricular tachycardia. He is off all medications and feeling well, without recurrence of arrhythmia, 8 months after the procedure and is being conservatively managed with respect to his anomalous venous drainage.

Acknowledgments

The authors acknowledge the contributions of Jeffrey Goldman, MD, and Janice Dawson, RN, and the expert technical assistance of Norman Butler and Tanya Kurtz.

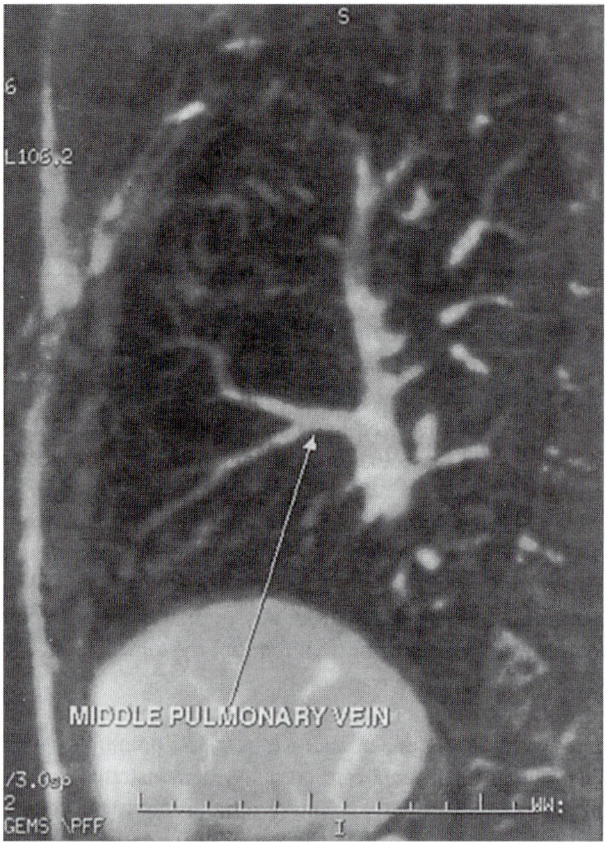

Figure 3. A reformatted sagittal oblique view through contrast-enhanced 3-D data set (spine to right of image) demonstrating course of right middle pulmonary vein, which drains into main body of anomalous vein. All lobes of right lung were thus seen to drain via the anomalous vein.

135 Holt-Oram Syndrome

Michael Böhm, MD

From the Klinik III für Innere Medizin der Universitat zu Köln, Köln, Germany.

(*Circulation*. 1998;98:2636–2637.)

A 29-year-old woman presented with dizziness. Physical and radiographic examinations showed skeletal hand malformations, i.e., digitalized triphalangeal thumbs and dystrophy of the carpal bones. When she was 15 years old, an atrial septal defect had been repaired. Electrocardiogram (ECG) recordings showed abnormalities of atrial excitation such as a wandering pacemaker, atrial ectopic activity, AV-nodal block, and sinus bradycardia of <60 bpm.

A clinical diagnosis of Holt-Oram syndrome was made. Holt-Oram syndrome is the prototype of heart-hand syndromes and has recently been mapped to the long arm of chromosome 12 (12q2). It must be differentiated from heart-hand syndrome type II (Tobatznik's syndrome) and heart-hand syndrome type III (MIM No. 140450), which are phenotypically similar. The latter do not map to 12q2, and atrial septal defects do not occur in these conditions. Approximately 350 cases have been published. The autosomal dominant syndrome has a strong variance in phenotype expression. Approximately 50% of the patients have cardiac malformations. The limb malformations can vary from mild thumb abnormalities to complete absence of the arm. The presence of upper-limb abnormalities in a patient with cardiac disease can be the clue to the diagnosis of a complex congenital syndrome.

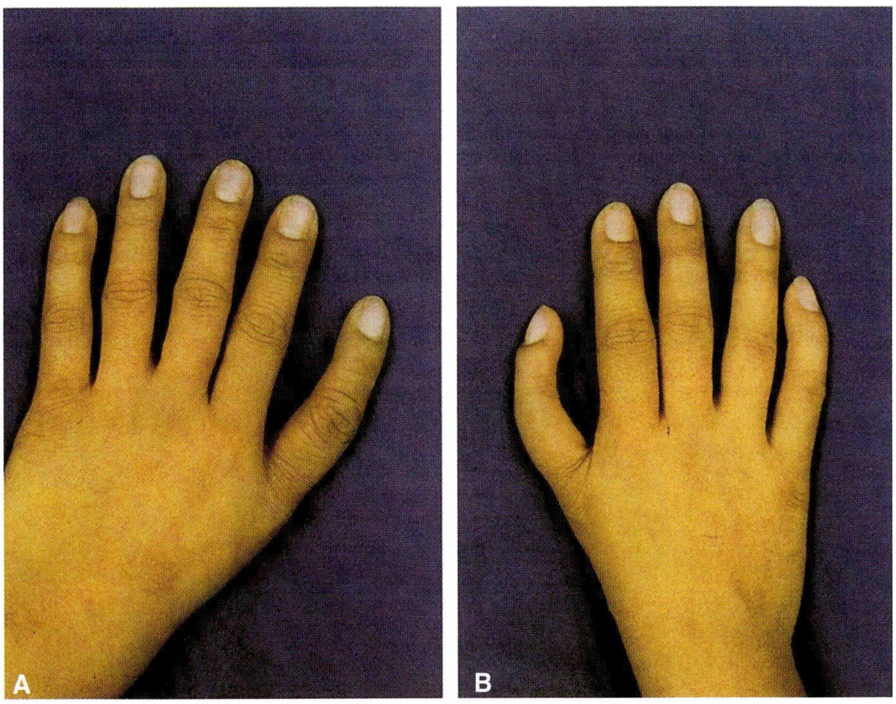

Figure 1. Photograph of patient's hands.

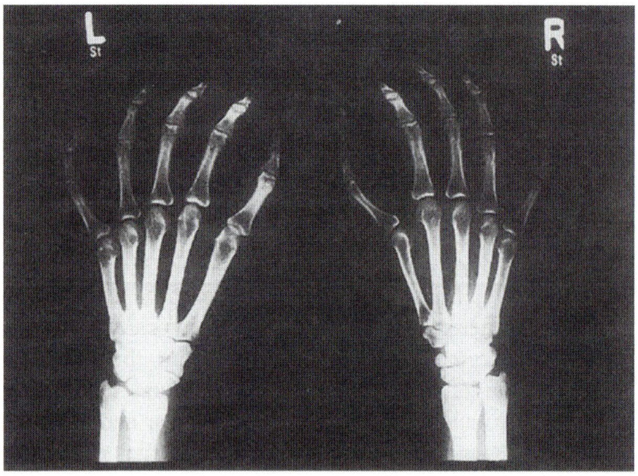

Figure 2. Radiograph of both hands. Note triphalangeal thumbs, slightly hypoplastic thumb of right hand, and asymmetrical dysplastic carpal bones.

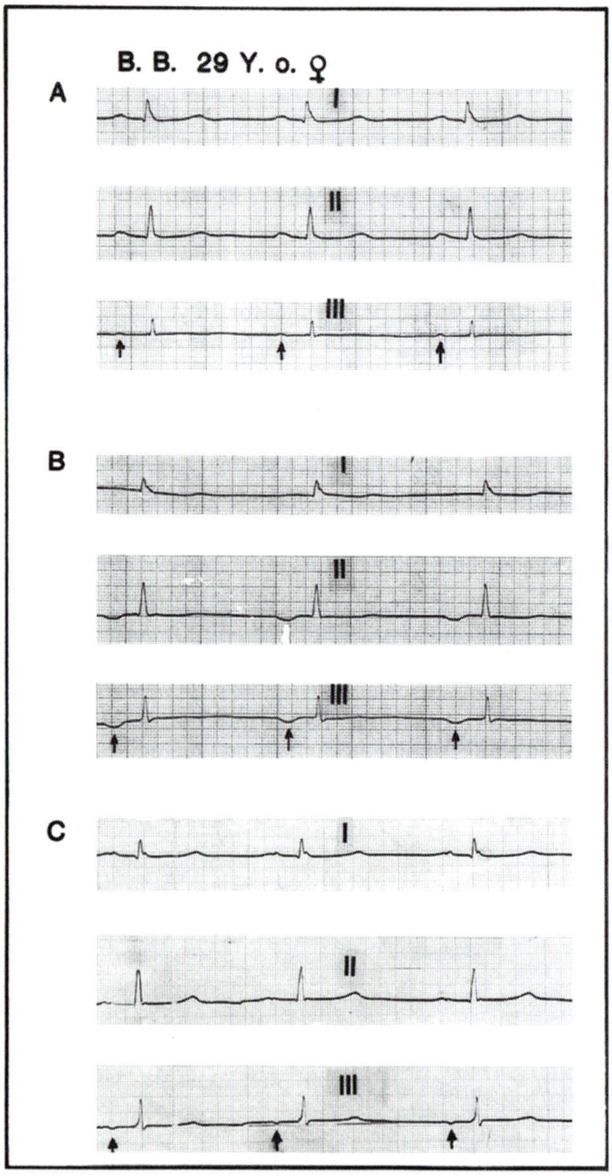

Figure 3. ECGs recorded on admission **(A)** and 6 **(B)** and 24 **(C)** hours after admission. Note differently shaped P wave marked with arrows at III in all recordings.

136 Cor Triatriatum

Ivan Godoy, MD; Wiwun Tantibhedhyangkul, MD; Robert Karp, MD; Roberto Lang, MD

From the Noninvasive Cardiac Imaging Laboratories, Section of Cardiology, Department of Medicine (LG., W.T., R.L.), and Section of Cardiac Surgery, Department of Surgery (R.K.), The University of Chicago Medical Center, Chicago, Ill.

(*Circulation*. 1998;98:2781.)

A 70-year-old woman was evaluated for worsening angina. Physical examination disclosed a harsh diastolic murmur. Transesophageal echocardiography (TEE) showed a membrane (Fig. 1A, arrow) attached laterally to the junction of the left upper pulmonic vein and left atrial appendage. This membrane divided the left atrium into 2 chambers: (1) a posterosuperior chamber that received blood from the pulmonic veins (PS-LA) and (2) an anteroinferior (AI-LA) chamber that contained the left atrial appendage and mitral valve. The presence of a large communicating orifice together with multiple fenestrations of the membrane was clearly visualized from the 3-dimensional reconstruction of the TEE-acquired images (Fig. 1B, reconstructed left atrium and Fig. 1C, view from the roof of the posterosuperior chamber). The atrial membrane was excised during surgery, which was recommended because of the presence of associated significant coronary artery disease. Fig. 1D corresponds to the surgical view from the roof of the posterosuperior chamber showing the identical membrane perforations previously diagnosed by 3-dimensional echocardiography (Fig. 1C). LV indicates left ventricle; AML, anterior mitral leaflet; and PML, posterior mitral leaflet.

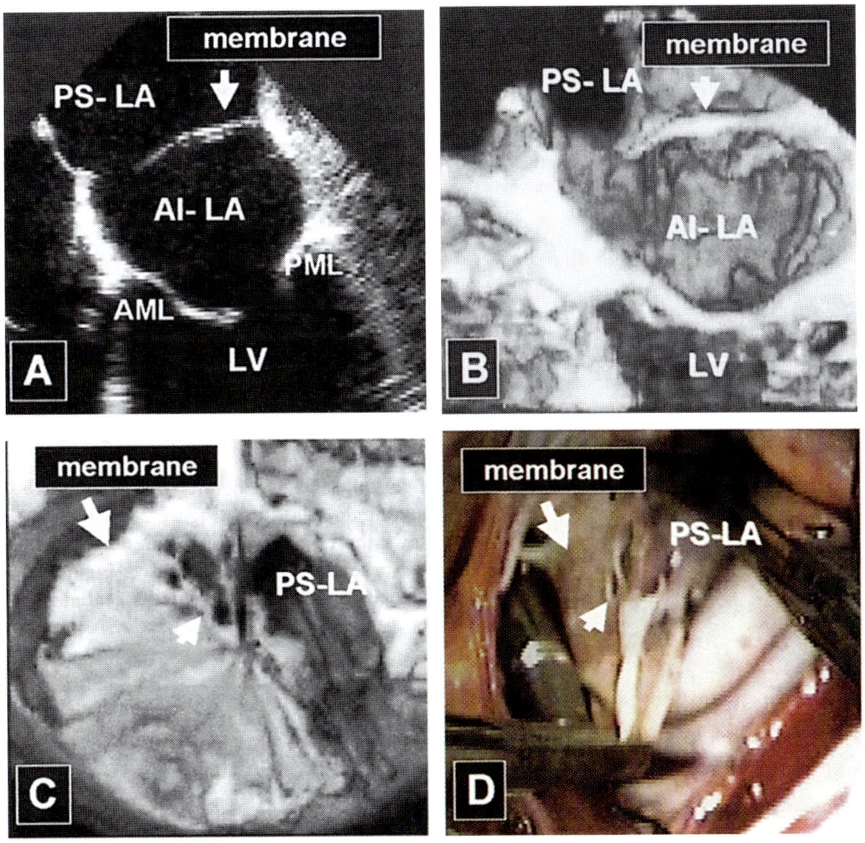

Figure 1.

137 Combined Angiography and Three-Dimensional Computed Tomography for Assessing Systemic-to-Pulmonary Collaterals in Pulmonary Atresia with Ventricular Septal Defect

Emmanuel Le Bret, MD; Loïc Mace, MD; Patrice Dervanian, MD; Thierry Folliguet, MD; Armand Bourriez, MD; Joy Zoghby, MD; Virginie Lambert, MD; Jean Losay, MD; Yves Martin-Bouyer, MD; Jean Yves Neveux, MD

From the Department of Cardiovascular and Cardiopediatric Surgery, Centre Chirurgical Marie Lannelongue, Le Plessis Robinson, France.

(*Circulation*. 1998;98:2930–2931.)

A 12-month-old child was evaluated for pulmonary atresia with ventricular septal defect. Assessment of the whole arterial pulmonary arborization was first done by angiography. This examination revealed that the left lung received vascularization by the native pulmonary artery via a central shunt performed during the neonatal period and by 2 aortopulmonary collateral arteries. The positions of these two arteries and their spatial relationship with the left bronchus were clearly visualized before unifocalization by three-dimensional computed tomography (CT).

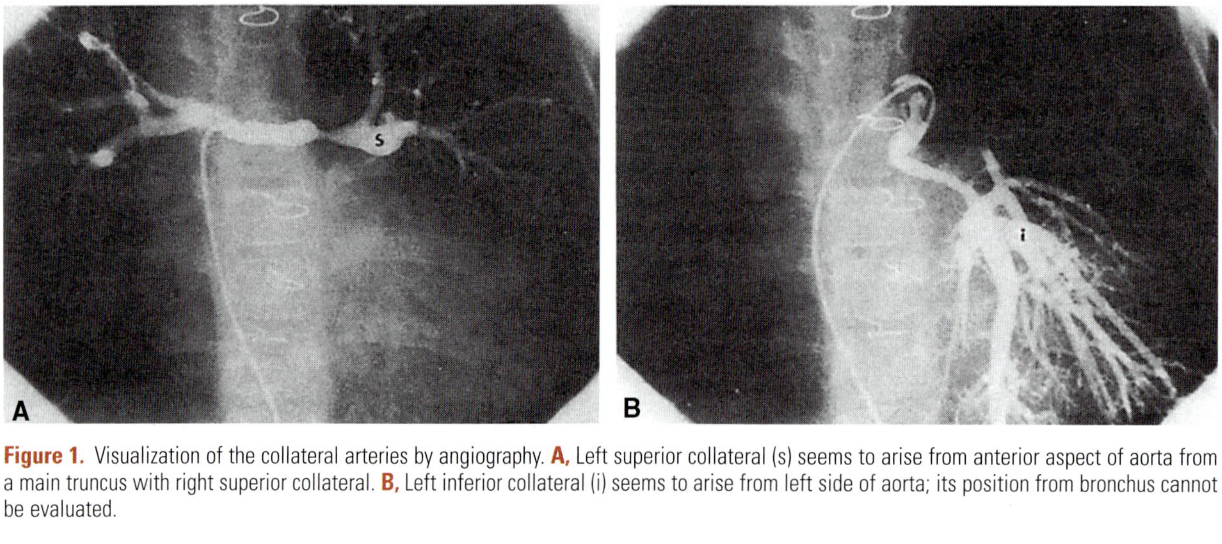

Figure 1. Visualization of the collateral arteries by angiography. **A,** Left superior collateral (s) seems to arise from anterior aspect of aorta from a main truncus with right superior collateral. **B,** Left inferior collateral (i) seems to arise from left side of aorta; its position from bronchus cannot be evaluated.

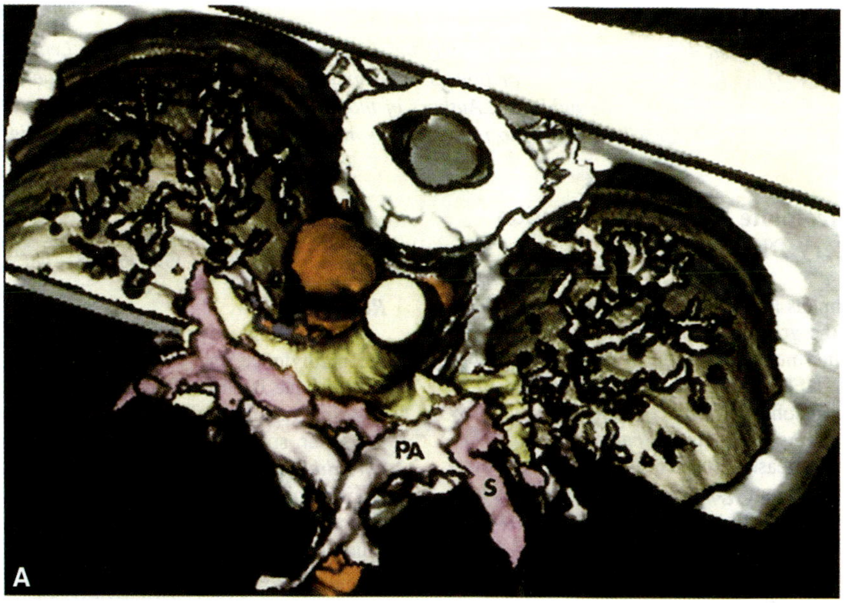

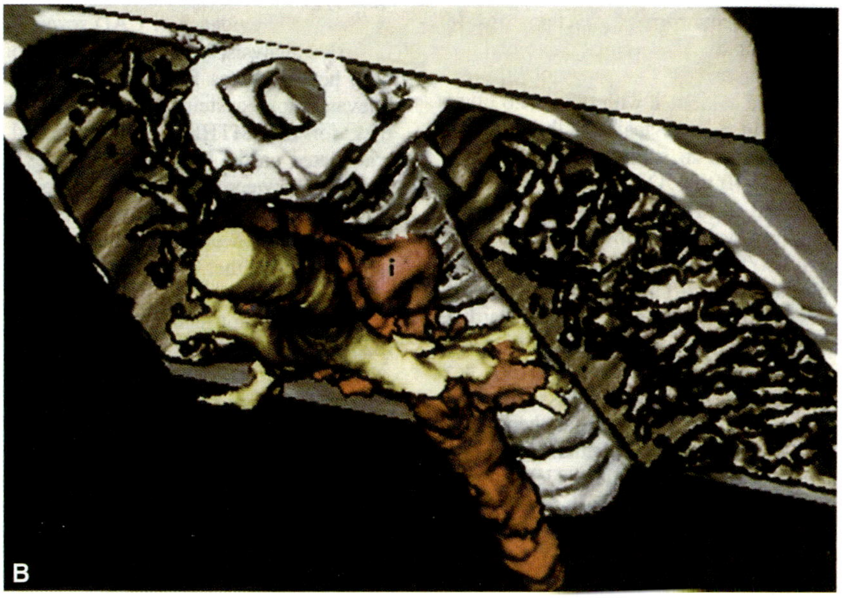

Figure 2. Visualization of collateral arteries by three-dimensional CT. **A,** Left superior collateral (s) arises from anterior aspect of aorta by a main truncus that passes under carena and then appears in front of left bronchus under native pulmonary artery (PA). **B,** Left inferior collateral (i) arises from left side of aorta, making a loop behind left main truncus, and then crosses inferior aspect of bronchus.

138 Isolated Congenital Absence of the Pulmonary Valve

Fause Attie, MD; Maria Rijlaarsdam, MD; Eduardo Chuquiure, MD

From the Instituto Nacional de Cardiologia Ignacio Chavez, Mexico DF, Mexico.

(*Circulation*. 1999;99:455–456.)

A 66-year-old man was admitted for evaluation of a heart murmur, atypical thoracic pain, and exertional dyspnea. Physical examination disclosed a harsh systolic ejection murmur and a single second heart sound followed by an early diastolic murmur best heard at the left second and third intercostal space. A chest radiograph showed moderate cardiomegaly and massively dilated main pulmonary trunk (Fig. 1). The electrocardiogram (ECG) showed atrial fibrillation and right bundle-branch block.

A transthoracic echocardiogram revealed dilated right chambers with aneurysmal dilation of the pulmonary trunk and branches. Pulmonary valve leaflets were not visualized. Doppler examination at the pulmonary annulus demonstrated back-and-forth flow, with a mild systolic gradient of 15 mm Hg (Fig. 2). Color Doppler showed moderate pulmonary regurgitation. MRI depicted an enlarged main pulmonary artery and the absence of pulmonary valve leaflets (Fig. 3). Cardiac catheterization ruled out the presence of intracardiac shunts. The right ventricular systolic pressure was 42 mm Hg, and pulmonary arterial systolic pressure was 28 mm Hg. Coronary arteriography was normal. Considering the echocardiographic and MRI findings, a right ventriculogram was not performed. Cardiac surgery was not considered because the patient improved with digitalis and diuretic therapy and is in New York Heart Association (NYHA) functional class I.

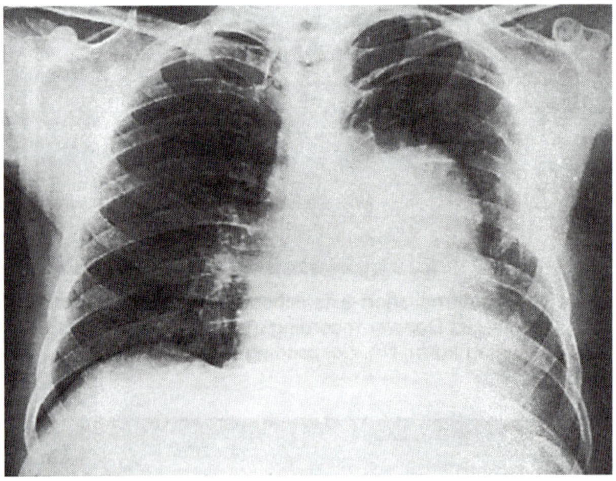

Figure 1. Posteroanterior chest x-ray. Heart is enlarged. Observe bulging of main pulmonary artery.

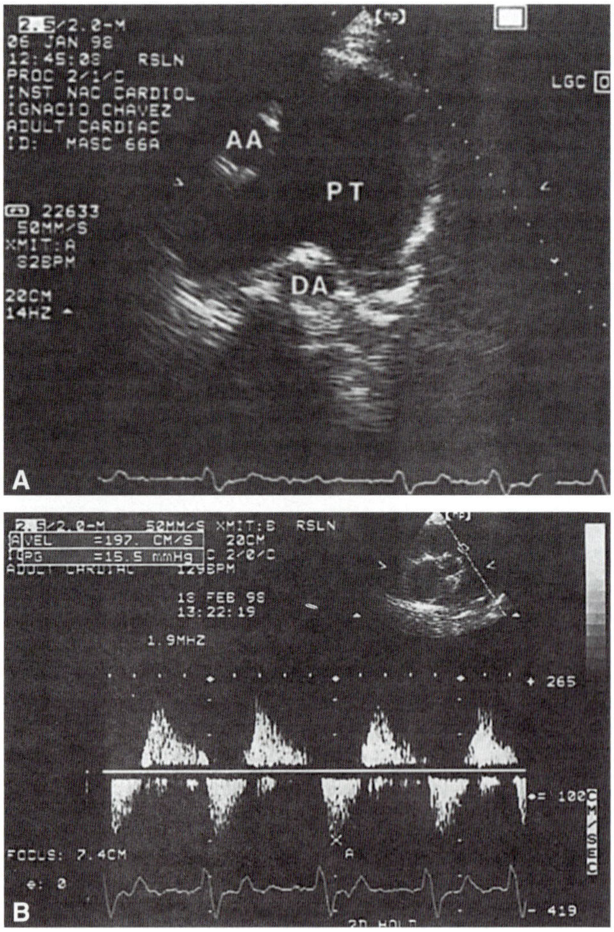

Figure 2. Parasternal short-axis echocardiogram of pulmonary artery. A, Observe grossly dilated pulmonary trunk (PT) and branches. B, Continuous Doppler recording at pulmonary annulus demonstrates a small systolic gradient and diastolic regurgitation. AA indicates ascending aorta; DA, descending aorta.

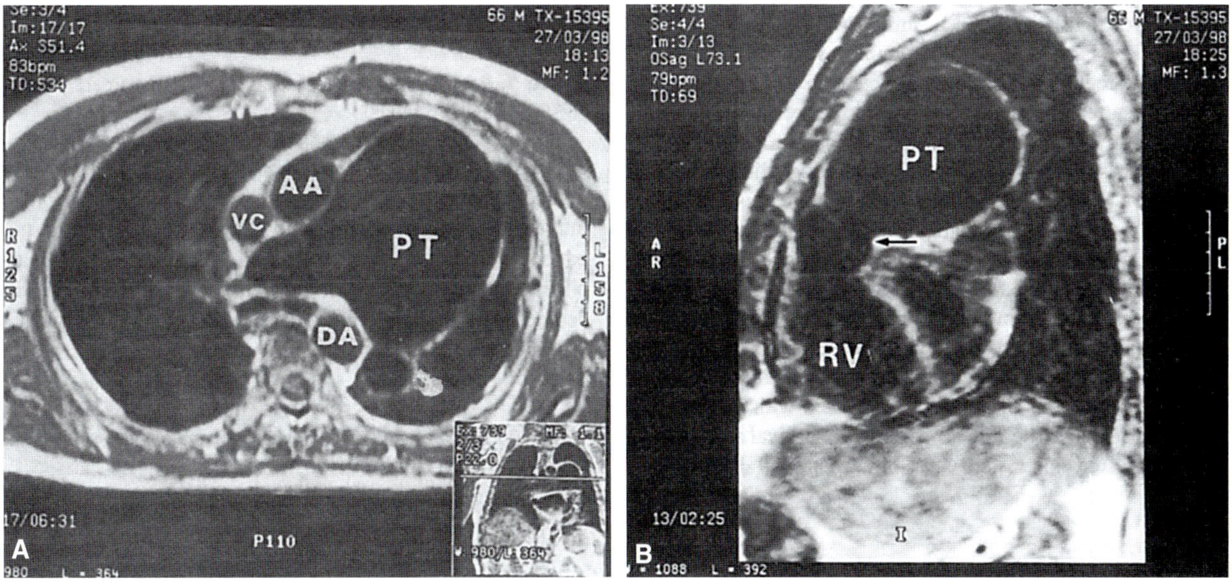

Figure 3. MRI of pulmonary artery. **A,** Transverse image of enlarged pulmonary trunk (PT). **B,** Sagittal image showing absence of pulmonary valve leaflets (arrow). VC indicates superior vena cava; AA, ascending aorta; DA, descending aorta; and RV, right ventricle.

Congenital absence of the pulmonary valve is rarely found as an isolated lesion. Usually it is associated with a ventricular septal defect. The critical period for survival is during infancy. Most symptoms are caused by respiratory distress or infection secondary to airway obstruction produced by the dilated pulmonary artery compressing the bronchus or by intractable cardiac failure. The long-term survival of this patient can be explained by the absence of significant obstruction at the level of the pulmonary ring due to the degree of pulmonary regurgitation and by the absence of associated defects.

139 Evolutionary Persistence of Spongy Myocardium in Humans

Annalisa Angelini, MD; Paola Melacini, MD; Fabio Barbero, MD; Gaetano Thiene, MD

From the Departments of Pathology (A.A., G.T.) and Cardiology (P.M., F.B.), University of Padua Medical School, Padua, Italy.

(*Circulation*. 1999;99:2475.)

A 15-year-old boy underwent successful cardiac transplantation for severe congestive heart failure. His sister had died at the age of 9 years of undefined congenital heart disease. At the age of 10 years, during a school medical screening, the patient was diagnosed with a cardiomyopathy. At cardiac catheterization, the right ventricle disclosed an increased trabecular pattern, mainly in the region of the apex, and the left ventricle showed an increased wall thickness, with mild hypokinesia. Subsequently, the patient complained of dyspnea on effort and presented signs of congestive heart failure. Five years later, the boy was admitted to an intensive care unit requiring a continuous inotropic drug infusion. Two-dimensional echocardiography disclosed biventricular dilatation with diffuse hypokinesia and a hyperechogenic coarse endocardial shape (Figs. 1A and 1B) interpreted as apical mural thrombi (arrow). The heart removed at transplantation was markedly dilated (weight, 720 g) and revealed the gross morphological features of noncompaction (spongy myocardium) with numerous, excessively prominent trabeculations and deep intertrabecular recesses penetrating into the endocardium (Fig. 1C). Histological examination confirmed that the spongy appearance was due to the deep intertrabecular recesses, lined by endothelium, which spread close to the epicardial surface (Fig. 1D). This feature strongly resembles the spongy myocardium pattern of nonmammalian vertebrates such as fish, amphibians, and reptiles.

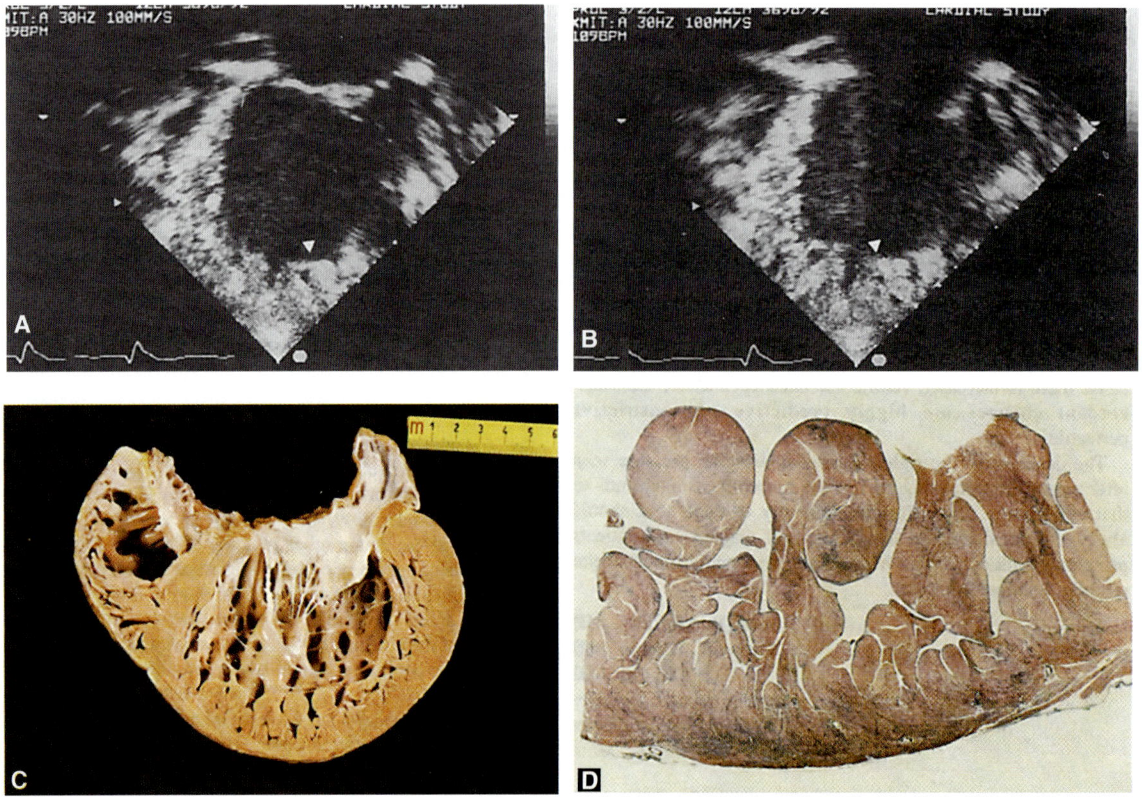

Figure 1.

140 Three-Dimensional Visualization of Recurrent Coarctation of the Aorta by Electron-Beam Tomography and MRI

Paul T. Pitlick, MD; Courtney L. Anthony, MD; Phillip Moore, MD; Roger Y. Shifrin, MD; Geoffrey D. Rubin, MD

From the Departments of Pediatrics (P.T.P.) and Diagnostic Radiology (R.Y.S., G.D.R.), Stanford University School of Medicine; the Department of Pediatrics, California-Pacific Medical Center (C.L.A.); the Department of Pediatrics, University of California, San Francisco (P.M.); and The Lucile Salter Packard Children's Hospital, Stanford.

(*Circulation*. 1999;99:3086–3087.)

The patient was a 12-year-old boy who was born with a coarctation of the thoracic aorta. He underwent a Gore-Tex patch angioplasty of the coarctation at 13 days of age. Subsequent restenosis led to subclavian flap angioplasty at age 7 months. He presented now with upper extremity hypertension and decreased femoral pulses.

Attempted visualization of the aortic isthmus by cross-sectional echocardiography was inadequate. The family was initially reluctant to consent to a cardiac

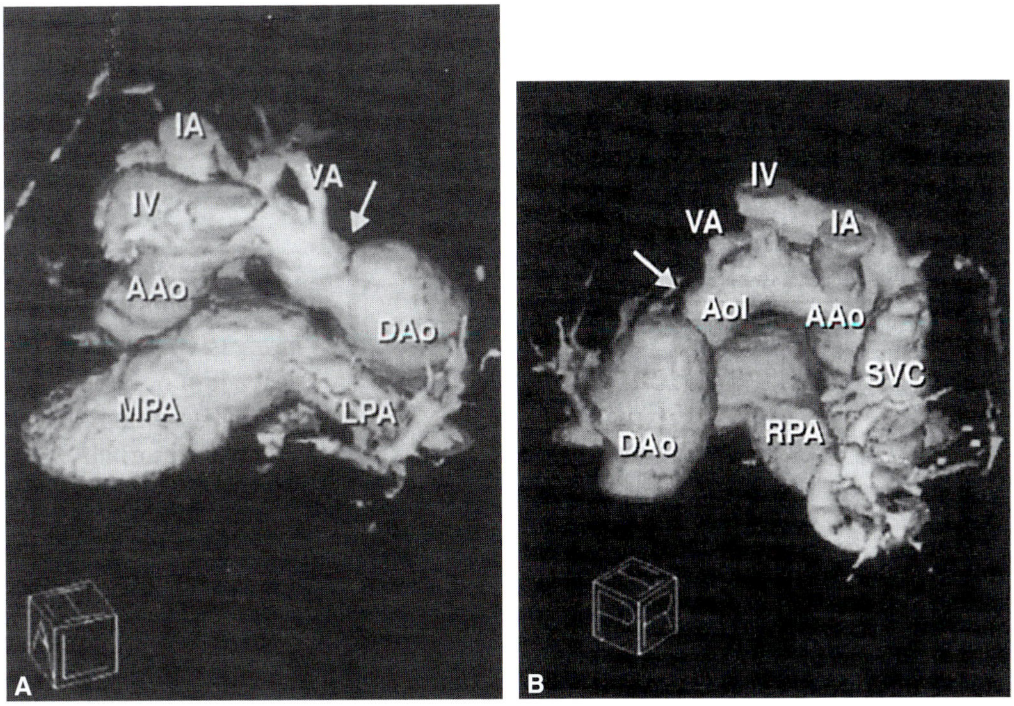

Figure 1. Shaded-surface reconstruction of aortic arch, innominate vein, and pulmonary arteries from EBT. Blocks in lower left-hand corners show orientation. A indicates anterior; H, head; L, left; R, right; P, posterior; AAo, ascending aorta; AoI, aortic isthmus; DAo, descending aorta; IA, innominate artery; IV, innominate vein; LCC, left common carotid; LPA, left pulmonary artery; LSA, left subclavian artery; LV, left ventricle; MPA, main pulmonary artery; RPA, right pulmonary artery; RV, right ventricle; SVC, superior vena cava; and VA, vertebral artery. **A,** View from left, front, and slightly cephalad. A web is suggested along upper surface of aortic isthmus (arrow), possibly because previous operations were from left thoracotomies, and this would be region of operation. Aorta below coarctation site is aneurysmal. **B,** View from right, posterior, slightly cephalad. A web is well-defined here (arrow). Please see the Online version of Figure 1 for 3D rotation.

catheterization. After three-dimensional (3-D) reconstruction of electron-beam tomography (EBT) and magnetic resonance imaging (MRI) (Figs. 1 and 2), the pathological condition was more fully appreciated. The patient then underwent cardiac catheterization, angiography (Fig. 3), and balloon angioplasty of the recurrent coarctation.

Parameters for the EBT images were image thickness 1.5 mm, spacing 1.5 mm, scan duration 0.1 second, 40 slices, and 3 mL/kg of contrast delivered by injection into the right antecubital vein. The scan was performed with breath-holding, and the scans were triggered to late diastole (80% of the R-R interval) for every heartbeat. The EBT shaded-surface displays were created with MagicView software (Siemens Medical Systems) on a Sun workstation; the chest wall was subtracted from the source images before the display. The MRI shaded-surface displays were created from a 3-D fast spoiled-gradient-recalled acquisition in steady state data set obtained during a bolus infusion of gadolinium.

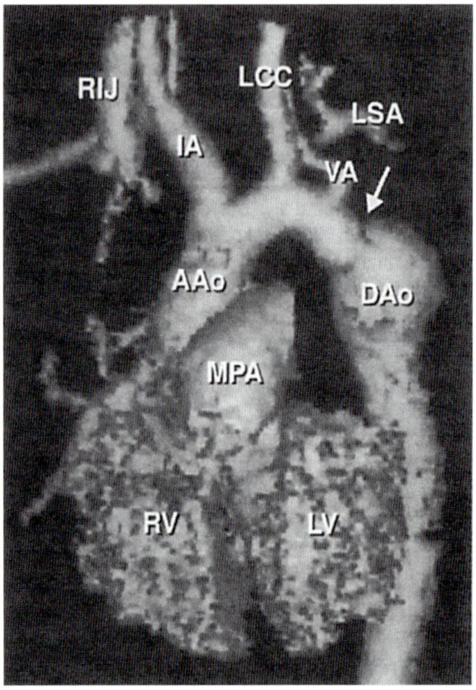

Figure 2. 3D reconstruction of MRI data set. Left anterior oblique projection shows to good advantage the web in region of aortic isthmus, as well as poststenotic dilation. Left pulmonary artery has been edited out of image to facilitate visualization of aorta. RIJ indicates right internal jugular vein; other abbreviations as in Figure 1.

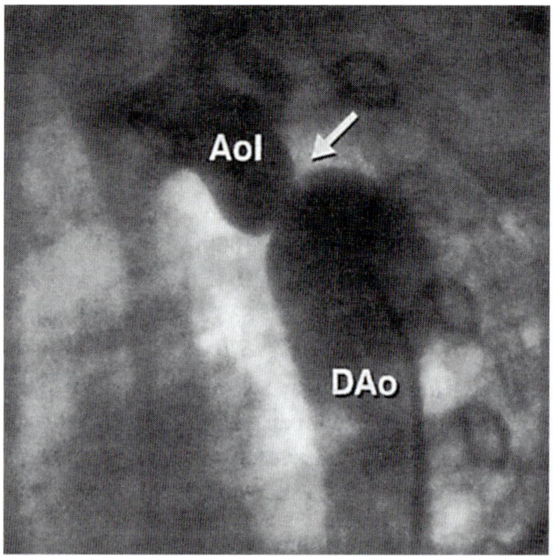

Figure 3. Aortogram, 70° left anterior oblique view. A discrete web is present, with an aneurysm of descending aorta. Abbreviations as in Figure 1.

141 Cardiovascular Evaluation in Thoracopagus Twins

Alfonso Casta, MD

From Harvard Medical School, Children's Hospital, Boston, Mass.

(*Circulation*. 1999;100:103.)

Thoracopagus is the most common form of conjoined twins. Cardiovascular evaluation is necessary to establish the existence of two separate hearts before planning surgical separation of the twins. This is usually done by cardiac ultrasound, cardiac catheterization, documenting two separate pulse rates on physical examination, and the presence of two independent QRS complexes on simultaneously recorded electrocardiograms (ECGs). A set of thoracopagus twins underwent cardiac catheterization to confirm the presence of severe congenital heart defect in one of the twins before surgical separation. The other twin had no congenital heart defect. ECG electrodes were placed in the chest of the twins, and the recording is shown in the figure. Two independent QRS complexes were recorded in ECG lead III. One QRS complex (small arrow) appears to be marching through the other complex (larger arrow). Heart rates are similar.

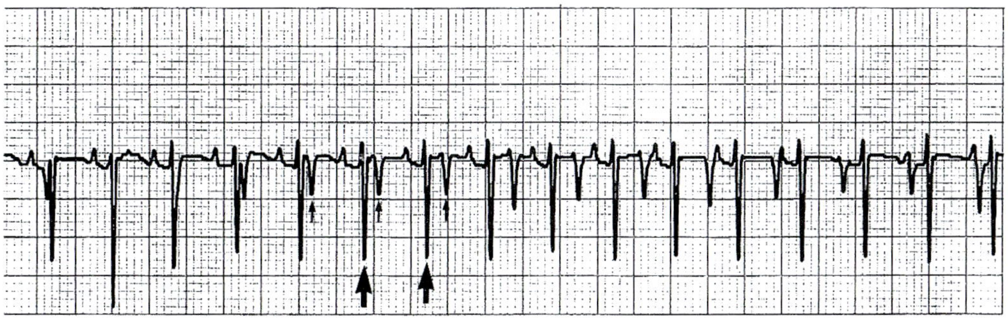

Figure 1.

142 Is This Right? (. . . or Is It Left?)

Peter G. Danias, MD, PhD; Warren J. Manning, MD

From the Charles A. Dana Research Institute and the Harvard-Thorndike Laboratory of the Department of Medicine, Cardiovascular Division (P.G.D., W.J.M.), and the Department of Radiology (W.J.M.), Beth Israel Deaconess Medical Center and Harvard Medical School, Boston, Mass.

(*Circulation*. 1999;100:209–210.)

An asymptomatic 57-year-old woman presented with dextrocardia and situs inversus. The surface electrocardiogram (ECG) (Fig. lA) reveals a rightward QRS axis. Poor R-wave progression is present in the standard precordial leads, whereas the right chest leads (rV_1 through rV_6), conversely, demonstrate progression of the R wave. The repolarization abnormality seen in leads rV_4 through rV_6 is secondary to left ventricular hypertrophy related to long-standing systemic hypertension.

The posteroanterior chest radiograph (Fig. 1B) is a mirror image of the normal radiograph, with the heart located at the right hemithorax, the ascending aorta (arrows) and aortic knuckle forming the left heart border, and the left hemidiaphragm positioned higher than the right hemidiaphragm. The letters L and R indicate the patient's left and right side, respectively.

The coronal magnetic resonance imaging (MRI) (Fig. 1C) of the chest and upper abdomen demonstrates the relationship of the thoracic and abdominal organs. AAo indicates ascending aorta; LV, left ventricle; PA, pulmonary artery; and RA, right atrium.

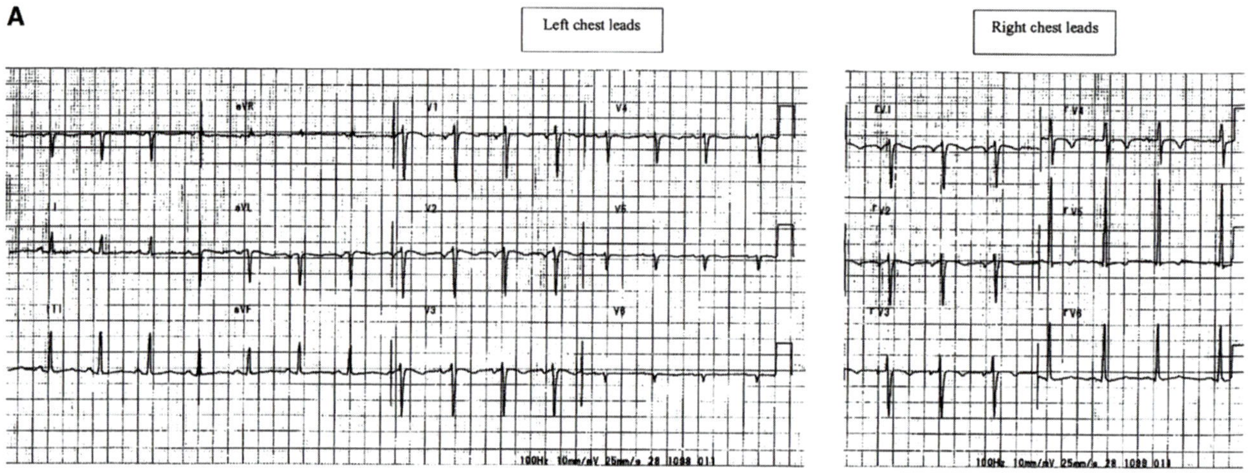

Figure 1.

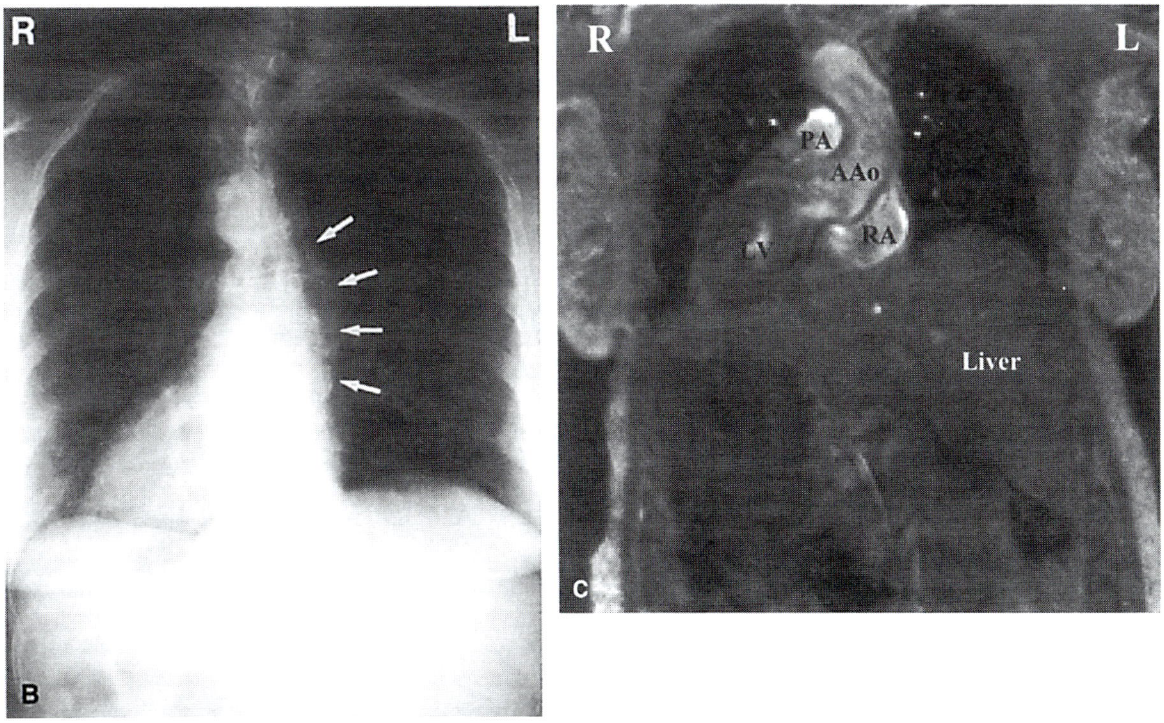

Figure 1. (*continued*)

143 Corrected Transposition of the Great Vessels and Situs Inversus Viscerum in a 65-Year-Old Oligosymptomatic Woman

Sabino Scardi, MD; Peter Knoll, MD; Claudio Pandullo, MD

From the Centro Cardiovascolare, Azienda per i Servizi Sanitari No. 1 Triestina, Trieste (S.S., C.P.), and the Divisione di Cardiologia, Ospedale Regionale Bolzano, Bolzan (P.K.), Italy.

(*Circulation*. 1999;100;777.)

Corrected transposition of the great vessels (atrioventricular discordance and ventricular discordance) is a rare congenital heart disease and is very singular if it is associated with situs inversus viscerum. This is the case in a 65-year-old woman in New York Heart Association (NYHA) functional class II.

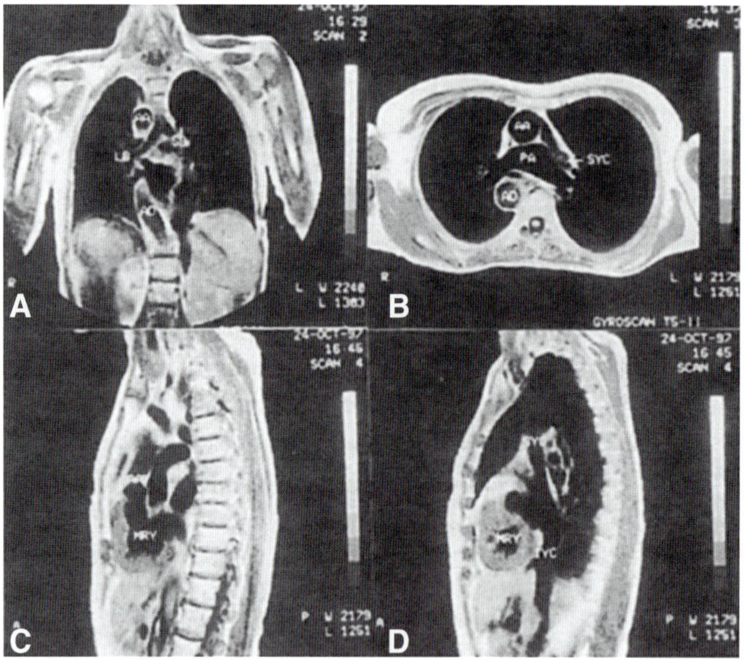

Figure 1. The nuclear magnetic resonance (NMR) image shows the liver (L) on the left side and the spleen (S) on the right side of the abdomen **(A)**. The pulmonary artery (PA) is posterior to the aorta (AA) **(B)** and is connected to the posterior ventricle, morphologically the left one. Conversely, the aorta (AA) is anterior to the pulmonary artery (PA) and is connected to the anterior ventricle, morphologically the right one (MRV) **(C)**. The superior and inferior venae cavae are on the left side and are connected to the right atrium **(D)**. The aortic arch and the thoracic aorta are located on the right side. AA indicates aorta ascendens/aortic arch; AD, aorta descendens; LB, long bronchus; SB, short bronchus; MRV, morphologically right ventricle; SVC, superior vena cava; and IVC, inferior vena cava.

144 Recognition of Left Atrial Aneurysm by Fetal Echocardiography

Robin R. Fountain-Dommer, MD; Henry B. Wiles, MD; C. Osborne Shuler, MD; Scott M. Bradley, MD; Girish S. Shirali, MD

From Children's Heart Center of South Carolina, Charleston (R.R.F.-D., H.B.W., C.O.S., S.M.B., G.S.S.), and the University of South Carolina School of Medicine, Columbia (C.O.S.).

(*Circulation*. 2000;102:2282–2283.)

A fetus was noted to have a mediastinal mass on prenatal ultrasound. Fetal echocardiography at 26 weeks of gestation demonstrated a large cystic structure adjacent to the left atrium and left ventricle (Fig. 1). The baby was born full-term. Echocardiography revealed a large, thin-walled aneurysm (3 × 3 cm) lateral to the left atrium and communicating with it through an orifice posterior to the base of the left atrial appendage. As determined by magnetic resonance imaging (MRI), this aneurysm extended from the transverse aortic arch to the cardiac apex (Fig. 2). Angiograms were obtained with the catheter tip positioned within the aneurysm (Fig. 3). None of these imaging modalities revealed thrombus within the aneurysm.

At 29 days of age, the aneurysm was approached surgically through a median sternotomy under cardiopulmonary bypass; it appeared thin-walled and

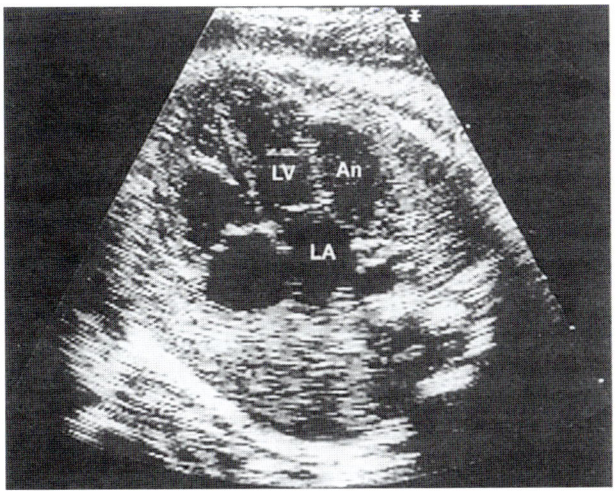

Figure 1. Four-chamber fetal echocardiogram at 26 weeks of gestation reveals a large cystic structure lateral to the left atrium (LA) and left ventricle (LV). This structure appears to communicate with the left atrium. An indicates aneurysm.

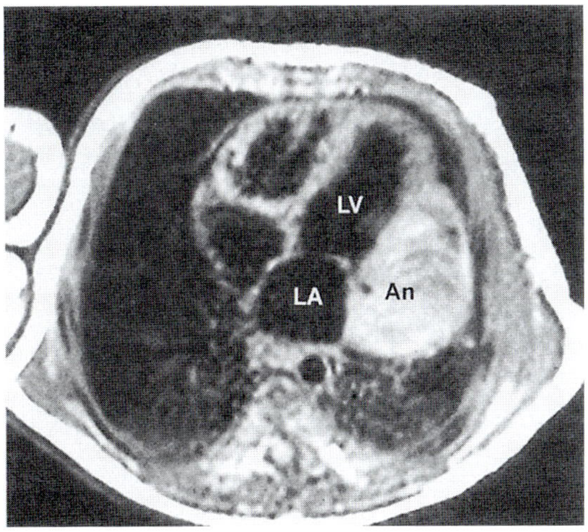

Figure 2. Coronal T1-weighted magnetic resonance (MR) spin echo image shows the aneurysm (An) on the lateral surface of the left ventricle (LV) and left atrium (LA). Significant signal is present within the aneurysm, indicating nonflowing fluid.

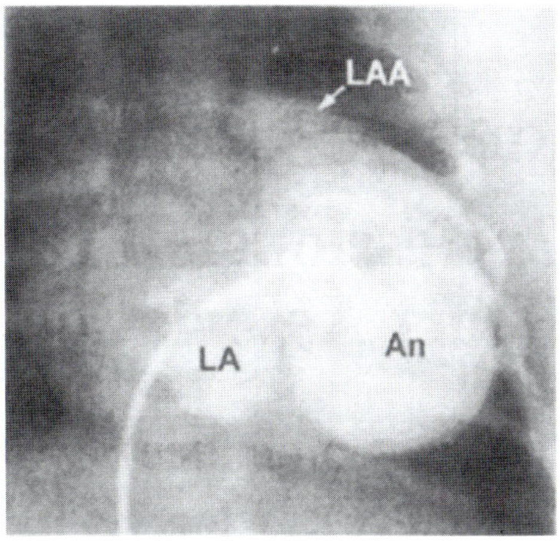

Figure 3. Angiogram with catheter tip in left atrial aneurysm (An). Communication between left atrium (LA) and aneurysm is evident. Left atrial appendage (LAA) is visible superior to and separate from the aneurysm.

translucent and extended along the lateral aspect of the left ventricle (Fig. 4). When the aneurysm was opened, it was evident that a portion of its medial wall consisted of left ventricular epicardium (Fig. 5). The aneurysm was resected, and its left atrial orifice was closed using autologous pericardium. Follow-up echocardiography revealed no recurrent aneurysm.

Most patients with left atrial aneurysms present with arrhythmia or abnormal cardiac silhouette on chest radiography. This is the first case to be recognized by fetal echocardiography.

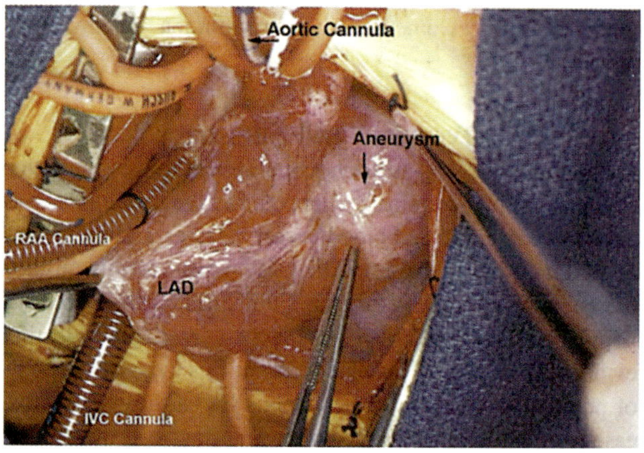

Figure 4. Intraoperative photograph taken before opening aneurysm. Lower forceps is located at margin between left ventricle and aneurysm. RAA indicates right atrial appendage; IVC, inferior vena cava; LAD, left anterior descending coronary artery.

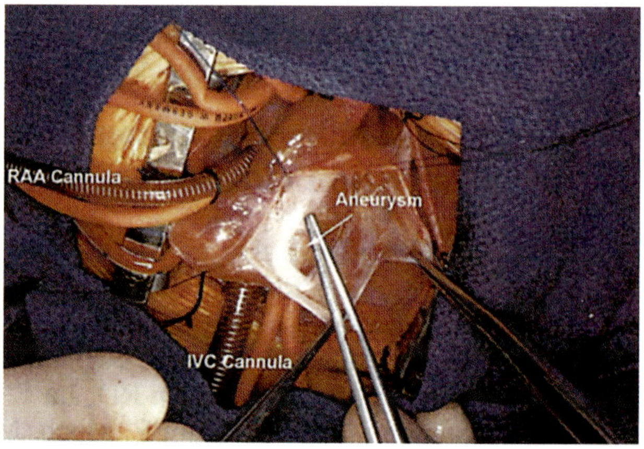

Figure 5. Intraoperative photograph showing inside of aneurysmal sac draped over left ventricle, revealing left ventricular epicardium. RAA indicates right atrial appendage; IVC, inferior vena cava.

145 Congenital Complete Absence of the Pericardium

Osman Ratib, MD; Joseph K. Perloff, MD; William G. Williams, MD

From the Department of Radiological Sciences (O.M.) and the Ahmanson/UCLA Adult Congenital Heart Disease Center (J.K.P.), University of California, Los Angeles, and the Department of Surgery (W.G.W.), the Toronto Hospital, Toronto, Ontario, Canada.

(*Circulation*. 2001;103:3154–3155.)

A 38-year-old woman with ill-defined chest pain had an abnormal x-ray 8 years before her only pregnancy. She had been unable to bear down during delivery, but gestation was otherwise uncomplicated, yielding a normal female offspring. She subsequently experienced left-sided chest pain that awakened her from sleep when turning into either a right or left lateral decubitus position. The pain was pulsating, stabbing, heavy, moderate in severity, and sometimes lasted for hours. Thoracic MRI in the supine and left lateral recumbent positions diagnosed congenital complete absence of the pericardium (Fig. 1A). The pain was ascribed to torsion at the thoracic inlet because of striking positional changes (mobility) of the heart (Fig. 1A). Congenital complete absence of the pericardium was confirmed during an operation designed to stabilize the cardiac position (Figs. 1B and 2). The heart was encapsulated in a Gore-Tex sack. The postoperative magnetic resonance images are shown in Figures 1 and 2. Figure 3 shows hypoplasia of the left lung and left pulmonary artery, which sometimes coexist with congenital complete absence of the pericardium.

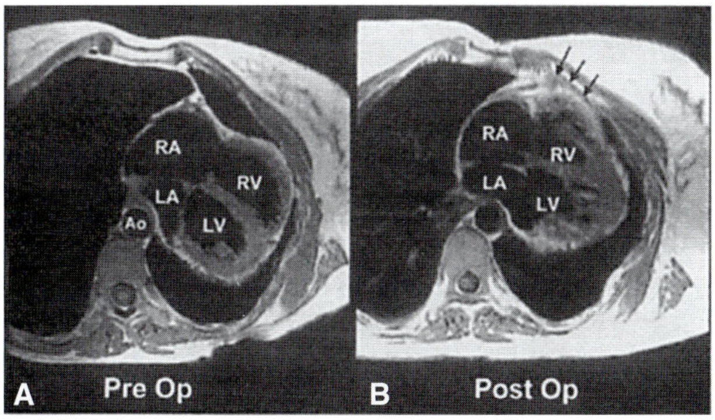

Figure 1. Axial views. The preoperative (Preop) image shows the mobile, unfixed heart. The postoperative (Postop) image shows adhesion (fixation) of the lateral wall of the right ventricle to the chest wall (arrows) after surgical anchoring. RA indicates right atrium; RV, right ventricle; LA, left atrium; LV, left ventricle; and Ao, aorta.

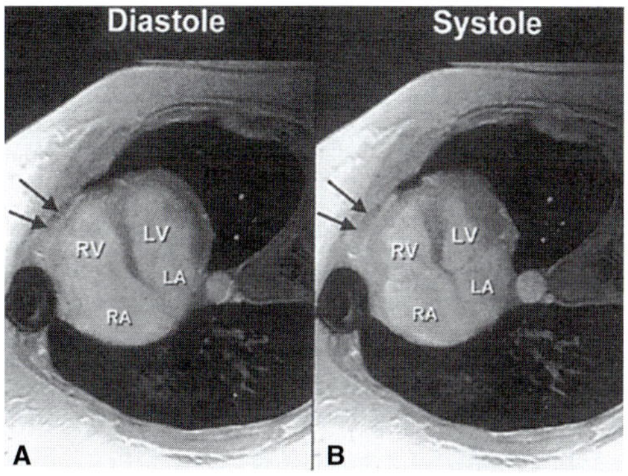

Figure 2. Dynamic images obtained in a horizontal long axis (four-chamber) view in diastole and systole with the patient positioned on her right side. These images illustrate the absence of significant cardiac motion after surgical fixation of the heart to the chest wall (arrows). Abbreviations as in Figure 1.

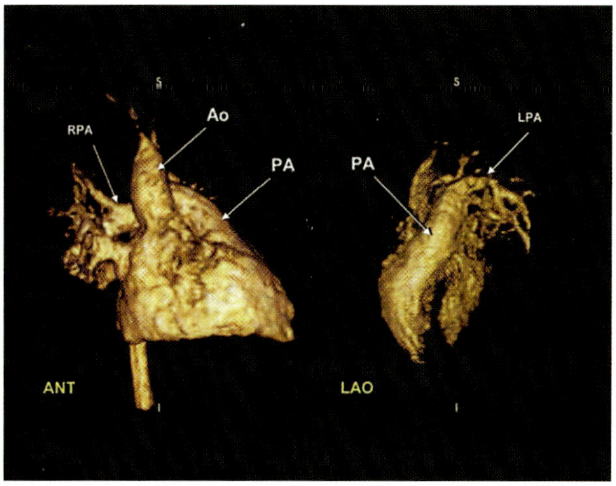

Figure 3. Three-dimensional reconstruction of gadolinium-enhanced MR angiography of the heart and great arteries in the anterior (ANT) and left anterior oblique (LAO) views. The left anterior oblique view shows the hypoplastic left pulmonary artery (LPA). RPA indicates right pulmonary artery; Ao, aorta; PA, pulmonary artery; S, superior; I, inferior.

146 Identification of Fetal Atrial Flutter by Doppler Tissue Imaging

John L. Cotton, MD

From the Division of Pediatric Cardiology, University of North Carolina at Chapel Hill.

(*Circulation*. 2001;104:1206–1207.)

A 26-year-old woman presented at 33 weeks of gestation with a singleton fetus with tachycardia. A complete fetal echocardiogram revealed a structurally normal fetal heart without signs of hydrops. The fetal heart rate was between 200 and 220 bpm. Evaluation of the rhythm with pulsed Doppler and M-mode scanning was not definitive. Fetal Doppler tissue imaging color M-mode scanning was performed by placing the cursor across the atrium and ventricle and increasing the color tissue scale while decreasing the overall gain to optimize visualization of the tissue motion. A diagnosis of atrial flutter with 2:1 block was made (Fig. 1). The mother was treated with digoxin and flecainide to control the flutter, without success. After documentation of fetal lung maturity, the mother underwent delivery. The newborn was noted to be in atrial flutter with 2:1 block (Fig. 2) and was eventually cardioverted to normal sinus rhythm after failure of further medical treatment.

Fetal arrhythmias occur in 1% to 2% of all pregnancies. Current methods used to evaluate these rhythm disturbances during fetal echocardiography include M-mode and pulsed Doppler scanning. Because color facilitates visual interpretation in difficult cases, color M-mode Doppler tissue imaging can be an important adjunct to the usual imaging techniques in the differentiation of arrhythmias in the fetus.

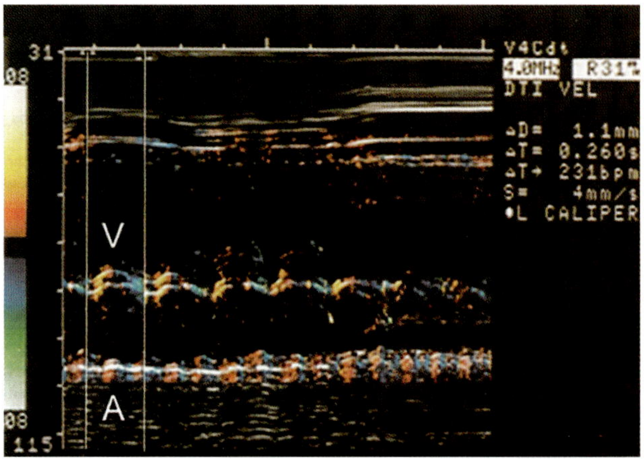

Figure 1. Fetal color Doppler M-mode tracing of atrial flutter. Atrial contractions (A) are seen at bottom of tracing and ventricular contractions (V) in middle of tracing. One contraction-relaxation cycle is represented by blue and red signal. Two atrial contractions (at a rate of 440 bpm) are seen for every ventricular contraction (at a rate of 220 bpm), suggesting fetal atrial flutter with 2:1 block.

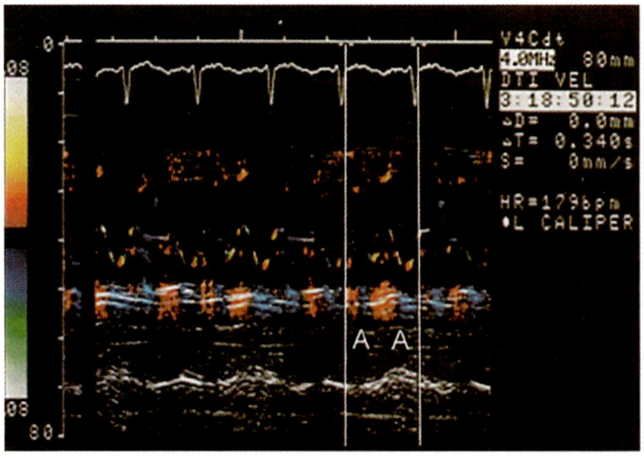

Figure 2. Postnatal color Doppler M-mode tracing of atrial flutter. Two atrial contractions (A) are seen for each ventricular contraction, as noted on electrocardiogram (ECG) at top of screen.

147 Magnetic Resonance Angiography of Criss-Cross Heart

Philip A. Araoz, MD; Gautham P. Reddy, MD; Pate D. Thomson, MD; Charles B. Higgins; MD

From the Department of Radiology, University of California, San Francisco (P.A.A., G.P.R., C.B.H.); and the Berkeley Cardiovascular Group (P.D.T.), Berkeley, Calif.

(*Circulation*. 2002;105:537–538.)

A 29-year-old man presented with a history of cyanotic congenital heart disease. During childhood, cardiac catheterization and angiography had demonstrated atrial situs solitus, L-ventricular loop, L-transposition of the great arteries, and crisscross atrioventricular connections. The patient had a Mustard procedure at age 13 that improved the cyanosis. He was now reporting decreasing exercise tolerance.

The patient underwent cardiac magnetic resonance imaging (MRI) with magnetic resonance angiography (MRA) as the first step in his evaluation. MRI showed L-transposition of the great arteries and an L-ventricular loop (inversion of the ventricles). The ventricles also had a superior/inferior relationship, in which the morphological right ventricle was to the left of and superior to the morphological left ventricle (Fig. 1). The atria were normally positioned (atrial situs solitus), and the atrioventricular connections were concordant. The concordant atrioventricular connections occurred because the pulmonic and systemic blood streams crossed in the midheart, so that the normally positioned atria supplied the appropriate but abnormally positioned ventricles. This type of atrioventricular relationship has been called the "crisscross heart" or "twisted atrioventricular connection."

Many patients with crisscross atrioventricular connections have discordant ventriculoarterial connections, as did this patient. This patient was cyanotic at birth, despite the presence of an L-ventricular loop and L-transposition, which usually cause a physiological correction and an acyanotic state. With the crisscross atrioventricular relationship, the right atrium remained connected to the right ventricle, causing systemic venous (desaturated) blood to flow to the right ventricle and into the aorta (Fig. 2). Thus, systemic venous blood flow was rerouted by the Mustard procedure across the mitral valve, into the left ventricle, and out the pulmonary artery.

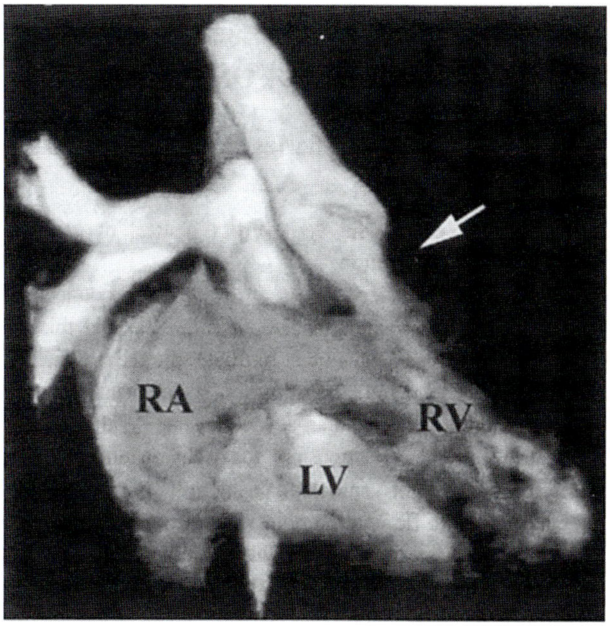

Figure 1. Volume-rendered, 3-D reconstruction of gadolinium-enhanced MRA. The projection is equivalent to a right anterior oblique view in conventional angiography. The morphological right ventricle (RV) is superior and to the left of the morphological left ventricle (LV). Note the infundibulum (arrow) and trabeculations that define the morphological right ventricle. The right atrium (RA) attaches to the right ventricle via a long, superior connection that crosses over the left atrium-to-left ventricle connection. Ventriculoarterial connections are discordant, with the aorta arising from the morphological right ventricle and the pulmonary artery arising from the morphological left ventricle. The patient's previous Mustard procedure was best visualized from posterior views and is not shown.

In cases of complex congenital heart disease such as the current case, MRI has the advantage of a large field-of-view and the ability to image in multiple planes. This capability has been increased with the advent of gadolinium-enhanced, breath-hold MRA (Fig. 3). Gadolinium-enhanced MRA images have a higher spatial resolution than most conventional MR sequences and lend themselves to three-dimensional (3-D) reconstructions.

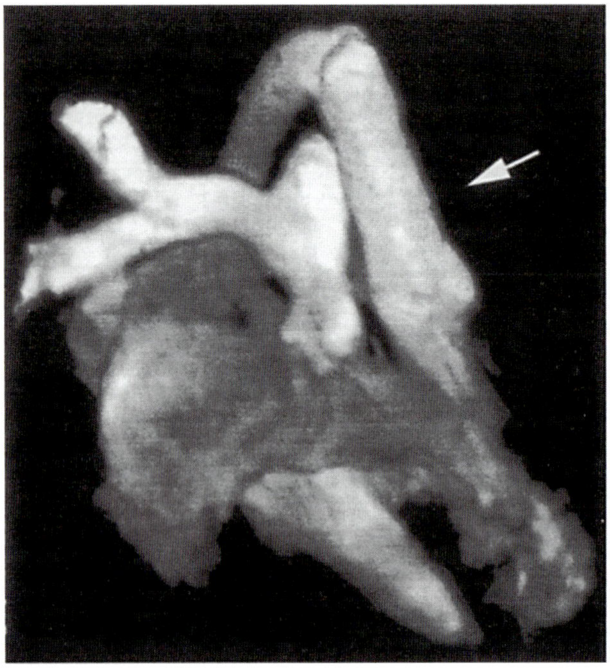

Figure 2. The same volume-rendered reconstruction is shown in a projection equivalent to a cranially angled right anterior oblique view to profile the great vessels better. This patient had concordant atrioventricular connections with discordant ventriculoarterial connections (complete transposition). However, note that the aorta (arrow) is anterior and to the left of the pulmonary artery. In crisscross heart, the relative position of the great vessels does not predict the atrioventricular connection or ventricular looping.

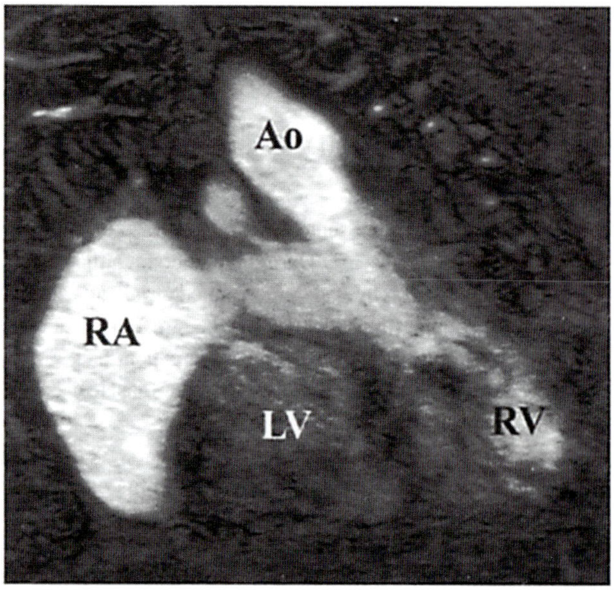

Figure 3. Single source image from gadolinium-enhanced MRA. The MRA was obtained by acquiring multiple coronal images in a single breath-hold during bolus intravenous injection of gadolinium. This single image shows the right atrium (RA)-to-right ventricle (RV) connection passing superior to the left ventricle (LV). These volume-rendered, 3-D images were made during postprocessing. Ao indicates aorta.

148 Three-Dimensional Computed Tomography Showing Partial Anomalous Pulmonary Venous Connection Complicated by the Scimitar Syndrome

Teruo Inoue, MD; Michiko Ichihara, MD; Toshihiko Uchida, MD; Yoshihiko Sakai, MD; Terumi Hayashi, MD; Shigenori Morooka, MD

From the Department of Cardiology, Koshigaya Hospital Dokkyo University School of Medicine, Saitama, Japan.

(*Circulation*. 2002;105:663.)

The patient is a 41-year-old woman who was referred to our hospital because of an abnormal chest radiograph. On admission, she was asymptomatic, but her cardiac silhouette was shifted to the right on chest radiograph. From contrast-enhanced chest computed tomography (CT), we suspected that the right upper pulmonary vein connected to the inferior vena cava. The CT also revealed hypoplasia of the right lung. The three-dimensional (3-D) imaging reconstructed from the CT clearly showed the right upper pulmonary vein connected to the inferior vena cava (Fig. 1). During cardiac catheterization, oxymetry sampling showed a step up of the blood oxygen content at the inferior vena cava level just below the border of the right atrium, which indicated left-to-right shunting at this level. In addition, the upper pulmonary venous drainage into the inferior vena cava was also shown by pulmonary arteriography. This partial anomalous pulmonary venous connection associated with hypoplasia of the right lung and dextroposition of the heart is designated Scimitar syndrome. Left-to-right shunt was slight and pulmonary hypertension was not present. Consequently, no surgical treatment was required.

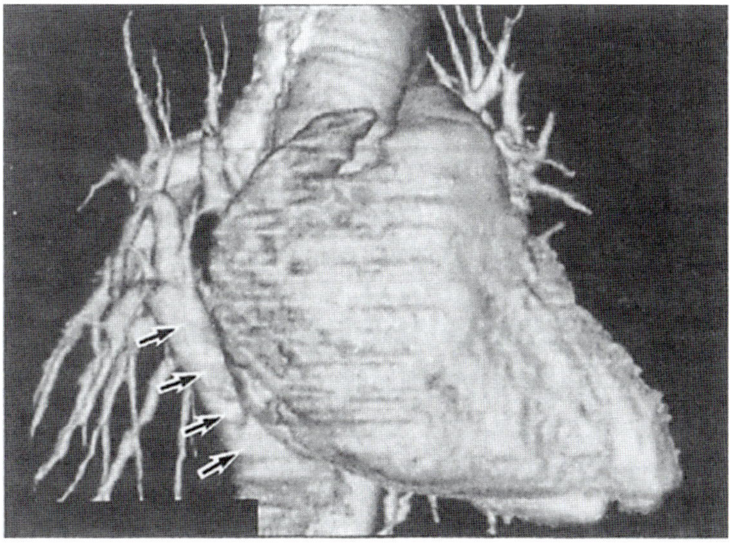

Figure 1. 3-D imaging in the right anterior oblique view, reconstructed from contrast-enhanced CT. The image clearly shows that the right upper pulmonary vein was connected to the inferior vena cava (arrow).